EPIDEMIOLOGY

An Introductory Text

JUDITH S. MAUSNER, M.D., M.P.H.

*Associate Professor, Department of
Community and Preventive Medicine,
Medical College of Pennsylvania*

ANITA K. BAHN, Sc.D., M.D.

*Associate Professor, Department of
Community and Preventive Medicine,
Medical College of Pennsylvania;
Associate, Department of Epidemiology,
Johns Hopkins University School of Hygiene
and Public Health; State Epidemiologist;
Chief, Division of Communicable Diseases,
Maryland State Department of Health and
Mental Hygiene; Consulting Epidemiologist,
Institute for Cancer Research,
Fox Chase Cancer Center, Philadelphia;
Professor of Epidemiology,
University of Pennsylvania School of Medicine*

W. B. SAUNDERS COMPANY
Philadelphia • London • Toronto

W. B. Saunders Company: West Washington Square
Philadelphia, PA 19105

1 St. Anne's Road
Eastbourne, East Sussex BN21 3UN, England

1 Goldthorne Avenue
Toronto, Ontario M8Z 5T9, Canada

Listed here is the latest translated edition of this book together with the language of the translation and the publisher.

Spanish—Nueva Editorial Interamericana S.A. de C.V.,
     Mexico 4 D.F., Mexico

Epidemiology   ISBN 0-7216-6180-7

Last digit is the print number: 9   8

To

F.K.S., B.M., and R.B.

PREFACE

This text is designed to provide a background in epidemiology for an introductory course in community medicine, health administration, or public health. It is also intended as a review for students preparing for examinations in preventive medicine.

We consider it important that all physicians, not just those who serve as health officers or do research in epidemiology, be familiar with epidemiologic principles and methods. Epidemiology and biostatistics, no less than physiology and pathology, are basic disciplines essential to both clinical and community medicine. They provide a way of thinking about health and disease.

Further, in reading the medical literature, all physicians should be able to follow critically a chain of evidence and to avoid the major pitfalls of epidemiologic inference. Epidemiologic sophistication fosters a questioning attitude toward medical practices which may be introduced and accepted without adequate support from well-controlled studies.

Finally, physicians and other health workers have an increasing role in providing preventive services and in maintaining the health of a community. This makes it desirable for them to know the common indices of community health, the analytic methods of demography, and the theory behind screening programs, as well as the methods appropriate to the epidemiologic study of acute and chronic diseases.

The text is intended to be a general introduction to epidemiology. Certain diseases are cited for purposes of illustration, but no attempt is made to present a comprehensive survey. However, the basic principles presented should provide the background for understanding the epidemiology of specific diseases.

Several technical subjects are explained in appendices to the appropriate chapters; they may be omitted without loss of continuity. To aid in self-teaching, at the end of each chapter there are study questions, including key concepts to be defined. Detailed answers to most of these questions are provided at the end of the book. For those readers unfamiliar with medical terminology, definitions have been provided when they seemed necessary.

We hope that our text will serve, at least for some, as a stepping stone to more advanced studies in epidemiology and preventive medicine. There is a great need for epidemiologists and other specialists in preventive medicine to participate actively in the prevention of disease and maintenance of health in population groups.

Many persons have helped, directly and indirectly, in the writing of this book. An early version of the entire manuscript was read by Drs. Frederic Bass, Jean D. Galkin, Nicholas Petrakis, Raymond Seltser, and Charlotte Silverman. Portions of the text were reviewed by Mr. Nathan Mantel; Drs. William H. Barker, Thomas C. Chalmers, Helen C. Chase, Ira W. Gabrielson, Frederick Hoesly, and Anders S. Lunde; and other colleagues at The Medical College of Pennsylvania, the Maryland State Department of Health and Mental Hygiene, the Washington (D.C.) Hospital Center, the Center for Disease Control, and the National Center for Health Statistics. Special thanks are due to Dr. Richard Morton, who reviewed a large portion of the manuscript. We benefited greatly from his keen pedagogic insights and judgment. We also profited from the comments and suggestions of several classes of medical students at The Medical College of Pennsylvania and of graduate students in public health nursing and health administration at the University of Pennsylvania. Of course, any errors in fact or interpretation in the book are entirely the responsibility of the authors.

This book was developed and used in teaching in the Department of Community and Preventive Medicine at The Medical College of Pennsylvania as part of activities supported from 1966 to 1973 by training grant PHT 6–76 and 5 DO4 AH 00676 "Expansion of Training Program in Epidemiology and Biostatistics" from the Bureau of Health Manpower Education of the National Institutes of Health. Drs. Katharine Boucot Sturgis, Glen A. Leymaster, and Ira W. Gabrielson, former and current chairpersons of the department, contributed to our enterprise in many ways. The secretarial staff, especially Miss Carolyn Pratt, uncomplainingly typed innumerable drafts and duplicated earlier versions for our students.

Lastly, we want to thank the staff of W. B. Saunders Company for their skilled and friendly assistance in helping us bring this project to completion.

The debt we owe our husbands for unfailing support and encouragement is beyond measure.

JUDITH S. MAUSNER   ANITA K. BAHN

CONTENTS

4

5

6

7

8

9

13

EPIDEMIOLOGIC ORIENTATION TO HEALTH AND DISEASE

1

POPULATION MEDICINE AND EPIDEMIOLOGY

Knowledge about human health and disease is the sum of the contributions of a large number of disciplines — anatomy, microbiology, pathology, immunology, clinical medicine, pediatrics, radiology — the list is potentially very long. However, the various disciplines can be grouped according to their methods and underlying concepts. When this is done three major categories emerge: one consists of the basic sciences (e.g., biochemistry, physiology, pathology), another the clinical sciences (e.g., adult medicine, neonatology, obstetrics and gynecology, urology, and so on), and the third population medicine. In different settings, population medicine is also referred to as community medicine, preventive medicine, or social medicine. This is the field concerned with the study of health and disease in human populations. Its goal is to identify the totality of health problems and needs of defined populations and to consider mechanisms by which these needs are, or should be, met.

The concerns of population medicine are quite different from those of the clinical disciplines. **Clinical medicine** focuses largely on the medical care of individuals. Typically, these have been **sick** people who have presented themselves for help; in recent years examination of apparently well people has been encouraged in order

1

to detect disease in early stages. In **population medicine** the community replaces the individual patient as the primary focus of concern. The problem here is to evaluate the health of a defined community, including those members who would benefit from, but do not seek, medical care. This approach requires specific techniques and skills in addition to those needed for clinical practice. The principles and methods underlying population medicine form the subject matter of this book.

It is readily apparent that clinical and population approaches to health and disease are highly interrelated and, together with the basic sciences, complement each other. A physician is guided toward a correct diagnosis in an individual patient by his knowledge of the distribution of diseases according to such factors as age, sex, and ethnicity. He is also aided by information about the illnesses prevalent in a given community. For a patient with fever and respiratory disease, for example, he will want to know if an influenza epidemic is in progress or if there has been a recent upsurge in streptococcal isolations. The answers to such questions will assist him in decisions about the avenues he should explore to reach a diagnosis.

Conversely, community diagnosis is dependent on the accuracy of the diagnoses made on individual patients and on the completeness with which reportable diseases are, in fact, made known to those responsible for the public's health. In addition, the accuracy of both individual diagnoses and epidemiologic assessments is dependent on adequate laboratory support.

Tuberculosis provides a good illustration of the three different approaches to a specific disease. The basic sciences are concerned with various aspects of the tubercle bacillus, its structure and antigenic composition, growth in different media, resistance to specified antibiotics, and with host responses, such as the extent to which tubercles become walled off by fibrous tissue. Clinical study of a case entails diagnosis, estimation of the extent and activity of disease, choice of therapy, appraisal of the patient's response, and adequate follow-up.

The questions pertinent to tuberculosis as a community problem concern the frequency of the disease, the relative contributions of different programs to identification of cases, and the environmental and cultural factors which serve to maintain or reduce its frequency of occurrence. How many new cases are diagnosed each year? What age groups and segments of the community are primarily affected and why? Who has been exposed to a newly discovered active case? What proportion of known active cases and their contacts are under adequate medical supervision? How many deaths a year are due to tuberculosis? What proportion of cases become known to health agencies only after the death certificate is filed? Other community problems concern medical care needs, such as the number of hospital beds and clinic visits required.

Each of the three approaches outlined here has its characteristic locus of activity. The basic sciences are primarily based in the laboratory; clinical activities are carried out in hospital wards, emergency rooms, ambulatory care clinics, and private physicians' offices; and the locus of population medicine is the community. For a comprehensive picture of disease in a community, information is needed about the health problems and needs of all its segments. In part this is derived from the records of clinical facilities. However, since the entire population generally does not utilize the available clinical services, diagnosis of community health problems may require surveys of samples of the population to gather information about people not under medical supervision. On the basis of such information, health services needed to supplement those already in existence may be developed in health departments and other neighborhood health centers and through associated outreach activities.

Thus we see that for population medicine we need a systematic way of studying both the diseases present in a community and the patterns of delivery of medical care, since these influence the amount and nature of disease. Epidemiology is the discipline which provides this systematic approach.

Epidemiologists have traditionally concerned themselves with the elucidation of disease entities and with the practical aspects of containment of disease. Epidemiology, often under the label of "disease control" or "communicable disease control," has been one of the traditional services of local and state health departments. Recently there has been a move to apply epidemiologic methods in hospitals, mainly for the control of infections, but also for monitoring adverse drug reactions. Epidemiologists are now also applying epidemiologic principles and methods to studies of medical care systems and of the anticipated effects of new approaches to health care.

EPIDEMIOLOGY DEFINED

Epidemiology may be defined as **the study of the distribution and determinants of diseases and injuries in human populations.**

That is, epidemiology is concerned with the *extent* and types of illnesses and injuries in *groups* of people and with the *factors* which influence their distribution. This implies that disease is not randomly distributed throughout a population, but rather that subgroups differ in the frequency of different diseases. Further, knowledge of this uneven distribution can be used to investigate etiologic factors and to lay the groundwork for programs of prevention and control. The contribution of epidemiology to the advance of medical science was expressed well by Frost (1936) some 40 years ago.

Epidemiology at any given time is something more than the total of its established facts. It includes their orderly arrangement into chains of inference which extend more or less beyond the bounds of direct observation. Such of these chains as are well and truly laid guide investigation to the facts of the future; those that are ill-made fetter progress.

Need for Rates

Inherent in the definition of epidemiology is the necessity for measuring the amount of disease in a population or community by relating cases to a population base. Epidemiologic statements often consist of fractions, or *rates*, in which the *numerator* is the number of people with the disease and the *denominator* is the population in the same area at the same time. Rates of disease are called *morbidity* rates, rates of death *mortality* rates.

$$Rate = \frac{number\ of\ cases\ or\ deaths}{population\ in\ same\ area}\ in\ a\ time\ period$$

Clinical and epidemiologic studies deal with the same phenomena, but from somewhat different vantage points. In contrast to epidemiologic investigations, clinically oriented studies usually focus on sick people who come for care (i.e., the numerator only) and are not concerned with identifying and enumerating the population from which the cases arise. An example of the difference in the two approaches follows. A *clinical* report on ulcer disease bore the title, "Problem of the gastric ulcer reviewed: Study of 1000 cases" (Smith et al., 1953). An *epidemiologic* study of ulcer (Pulvertaft, 1959) presented mean annual incidence rates of peptic ulcer for a defined population base (York, England) and showed, for instance, that the rate was only 0.17 per 1000 females under 25 years of age but 0.96 for males.

Low as well as high rates of disease have provided useful clues to etiology. For example, absence of pellagra in attendants in mental hospitals at a time when it was prevalent in patients led Goldberger (1914) to reject the then popular hypothesis that pellagra is of infectious origin in favor of an hypothesis of nutritional deficiency. The virtual absence of carcinoma of the cervix among nuns (Gagnon, 1950) in contrast to the high rate among prostitutes (Røjel, 1953) suggested that sexual activity was probably an important etiologic factor. To quote a contemporary British epidemiologist (Morris, 1955):

> The main function of epidemiology is to discover groups in the population with high rates of disease, and with low, so that causes of disease and of freedom from disease can be postulated. . . . The biggest promise of this method lies in relating diseases to the ways of living of different groups, and by doing so to unravel "causes" of disease about which it is possible to do something. . . .
>
> The great advantage of this kind of approach to prevention is that it may be applicable in the early stages of our knowledge of diseases, to disrupt the pattern of causation before the intimate nature of diseases is understood. Sufficient facts may be established for this by epidemiological methods alone, or in combination with others. The opportunity may thus offer to deal with one "cause," or with various combinations of causes. . . .

Health and Disease

The preceding paragraphs stress the importance of rates in epidemiology. However, even though epidemiologists are primarily interested in occurrence of disease, they are also concerned with distributions of physiologic variables, such as blood pressure, blood glucose, serum uric acid, and serum cholesterol, in healthy and diseased individuals. Studies of these variables permit evaluation of their contribution, singly and in combination, to the development of disease.

The fact that we have defined epidemiology operationally in terms of measurement of *disease* should not obscure the ultimate concerns of epidemiology, which are the *prevention* of disease and the *maintenance of health*. Unfortunately it is easier to define and measure disease, disability, and death than to produce an operational definition of health.

Health is a rather elastic concept; it may be defined merely as the absence of disease and disability or it may be given a much more positive meaning, as in the widely cited Constitution of the World Health Organization (1948):

> Health is a state of complete physical, mental and social well-being and not merely the absence of disease or infirmity.

Attempts by national and international committees to quantify health status have led to some promising suggestions for its measurement (Sullivan, 1966). Nevertheless, both physical and mental health are still measured mainly through their converse, disease and death. Thus, of necessity, this text too will focus primarily on measurement of disease and ill health even though our ultimate goal is a positive one.

NATURAL HISTORY OF DISEASE

When morbidity rates are constructed, each person in the group under study must be classified as having or not having a specific disease. This decision is often difficult to make. The development of disease is often an irregularly evolving process, and the point at which a person should be labelled "diseased" rather than "not diseased" may be arbitrary. Many diseases, especially chronic disease which may last years or decades, have a *natural life history*. Just as we think of the "seven ages of man," so chronic disease may be considered to extend over time through a sequence of stages. As knowledge accumulates, it has become apparent that factors favoring the development of chronic disease often are present early in life, antedating the appearance of clinical disease by many years.

Since each disease has its own life history, any general formulation is necessarily arbitrary. Nevertheless, it may be useful to develop a schematic picture of the natural history of disease as a framework within which to understand different approaches to prevention and control.

Stage of Susceptibility

In this stage disease has not developed, but the groundwork has been laid by the presence of factors which favor its occurrence. For example, fatigue and acute and chronic alcoholism heighten susceptibility to pneumonia; inadequate maternal nurturing predisposes to emotional illness; high serum cholesterol levels increase the likelihood that overt coronary heart disease will develop.

Factors whose presence is associated with an increased likelihood that disease will develop at a later time are called *risk factors*. The need to identify such factors is becoming more apparent as awareness grows that chronic diseases present our major health challenge. Some risk factors can be altered, as when smokers can be persuaded to give up smoking. Others are not now amenable to change, but their identification may still be useful for tagging persons who deserve close medical supervision. Still other unalterable attributes such as age and sex may be considered risk factors.

Stage of Presymptomatic Disease

There is no manifest disease, but usually through the interaction of factors, pathogenetic changes have started to occur. At this stage, the changes are essentially below the level of the "clinical horizon," the imaginary dividing line above which disease manifests itself through detectable signs or symptoms. Examples of presymptomatic disease are atherosclerotic changes in coronary vessels before any signs or symptoms of illness, and premalignant (and, unfortunately, sometimes malignant) alterations in tissue.

Stage of Clinical Disease

By this stage sufficient anatomic or functional changes have occurred so that there are recognizable signs or symptoms of disease. It is important to subdivide this stage whenever possible for better management of cases and for epidemiologic purposes. There are several possible bases for subdivision. For example, cancer is usually classified on morphologic grounds (i.e., location of tumor and histologic type). The disease is generally staged by categorization of cases as localized, with regional metastases, and with distant spread. Quite a different approach has been proposed by Feinstein (1967), a staging based on symptomatology rather than morphologic extent of disease.

Functional and therapeutic classification is exemplified by the widely used categorization of cardiac disease of the New York Heart Association (1964). The following is adapted from their schema:

Functional Classification
Class I   No limitation of physical activity because of discomfort
Class II   Slight limitation of physical activity; patient comfortable at rest but ordinary activity produces discomfort
Class III Marked limitation of physical activity; comfortable at rest, but less than ordinary activity causes discomfort
Class IV Unable to carry out any physical activity without discomfort
Therapeutic Classification
Class A   Physical activity need not be restricted in any way
Class B   Ordinary physical activity need not be restricted, but patient is advised against severe efforts
Class C   Ordinary physical activity should be moderately restricted
Class D   Ordinary physical activity should be markedly restricted
Class E   Complete bed rest advised; patient confined to bed or chair

Note that functional and therapeutic classifications do not always parallel each other. For example, a patient with a recent heart attack or active rheumatic carditis (inflammation of the heart) may not have symptoms upon physical exertion, but may be advised to remain at complete rest (Class I, E).

A functional (psychosocial) classification of psychiatric disorders has also been proposed (Bahn, 1971).

As suggested above, classification, or staging, of disease is of great importance for epidemiologic study. Effective grouping reduces variability, yielding relatively homogeneous subgroups. This is important for evaluation of the effect of prophylactic or therapeutic agents (see discussion of clinical trials in Chapter 6), as well as for comparative studies of disease in different groups, i.e., international, regional, occupational and so on (as discussed in Chapter 3).

At present we do not have a complete understanding of the natural history of many diseases. We do not know why an individual with a number of risk factors, for example, does not progress to clinical disease. Much research in recent years has been directed to the follow-up of large groups over time (longitudinal studies) to gain this understanding.

Stage of Disability

Some diseases run their course and then resolve completely, either spontaneously or under the influence of therapy. However, there are a number of conditions which give rise to a residual defect of short or long duration, leaving the person disabled to a greater or lesser extent. On occasion a disease which is usually self-limited may later give rise to chronic disability. For example, a small proportion of cases of measles are followed by development of subacute sclerosing panencephalitis, a progressive neurologic disorder (Brody et al., 1972).

Although disability can be defined in various ways, in community surveys it usually means any limitation of a person's activities, including his psychosocial role as parent, wage earner, and so on. The National Health Survey (see Chapter 8) defines disability as "any temporary or long-term reduction of a person's activity as a result of an acute or chronic condition" (1958). Note that the emphasis is on loss of function rather than on structural defect. Individuals vary widely in their reaction to physical impairment. Two persons with the same amount of residual loss from poliomyelitis, for example, may show marked differences in their resultant level of disability. While there is a substantial amount of disability associated with acute illness, the extent of protracted disability resulting from chronic illness is of greater significance for society.

LEVELS OF PREVENTION

Implicit in the scheme just presented is the notion that a disease evolves over time and that as this occurs pathologic changes may become fixed and irreversible. Therefore, the aim is to push back the level of detection and intervention to the precursors and risk factors of disease. This lays the emphasis squarely on preventive rather than curative medicine.

With *prevention* a dominant theme, it may be well to elaborate upon this word. In a narrow sense, prevention simply means inhibiting the development of a disease before it occurs. However, in current usage, the term has been extended to include measures which interrupt or slow the progression of disease. For this reason several levels of prevention are said to exist. *Primary* prevention (appropriate in the stage of susceptibility) is prevention of disease by altering susceptibility or reducing exposure for susceptible individuals; *secondary* prevention (applied in early disease, i.e., preclinical and clinical stages) is the early detection and treatment of disease; *tertiary* prevention (appropriate in the stage of advanced disease or disability) is the alleviation of disability resulting from disease and attempts to restore effective functioning.

Primary Prevention

Prevention of the occurrence of disease consists of measures which fall into two major categories: general health promotion and specific protective measures. *General health promotion* includes provision of conditions at home, work, and school which favor healthy living, e.g., good nutrition, adequate clothing, shelter, rest, and recreation. It also encompasses the broad area of health education, which includes not only instruction in hygiene, but also such diverse areas as sex education, anticipatory guidance for children and parents, and counselling in preparation for retirement. *Specific protective measures* include immunizations, environmental sanitation (e.g., purification of water supplies), and protection against accidents and occupational hazards.

The past successes of public health in developed countries

have been accomplished largely by primary prevention of infectious disease through environmental manipulation and immunization. The most pressing unsolved problems in these countries today are chronic diseases whose prevention requires modification of deeply-rooted individual behavior, such as dietary patterns, physical activity, and the use of alcohol, tobacco, and other drugs. Equally obdurate and important is the problem of deaths and injuries from accidents, especially motor vehicle crashes. Future efforts at primary prevention of these conditions will probably focus both on attempts to influence individual behavior and on environmental controls (e.g., air-bags in cars, altered composition of dietary fats) which will in part shift health-related decisions from the individual to social institutions.

Secondary Prevention

With early detection and prompt treatment of disease, it is sometimes possible to either cure disease at the earliest stage possible or slow its progression, prevent complications, limit disability, and reverse communicability of infectious diseases. On a community basis, early treatment of persons with infectious diseases (e.g., venereal infections) may protect others from acquiring infection and thus provides at once secondary prevention for the infected individuals and primary prevention for their potential contacts. Examples of diseases in which efforts at control center primarily around secondary prevention are diabetes, *in situ* carcinoma of the cervix, and glaucoma.

As is true of primary prevention, secondary prevention is a responsibility of both physicians in private practice and those in community posts. Health departments and other community agencies often conduct screening surveys in which asymptomatic persons are tested to uncover disease in its early stages.

Tertiary Prevention

This consists of *limitation of disability* and *rehabilitation* where disease has already occurred and left residual damage. Physiotherapy to an affected limb to restore motion and prevent contractures exemplifies measures for the limitation of disability.

Rehabilitation is the name given to attempts to restore an affected individual to a useful, satisfying, and, where possible, self-sufficient role in society. Its major theme is maximal utilization of

PSYCHOSOCIAL

Social Evaluation
Social Service
Psychologic Service
  Psychometrics
  Evaluation
  Counselling
Psychiatric Service
Spiritual Counselling
Recreation

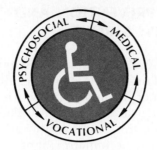

MEDICAL

Medical Diagnosis,
  Treatment and Super-
  vision of Medical
  Services

VOCATIONAL

Evaluation
  Vocational History
  Vocational Diagnostic Services
    Psychometrics and evaluation
    Prevocational interests
      and aptitude exploration
Counselling
Vocational Training
Placement
  Selective Industrial
  Transitional—Sheltered Workshop
Homebound

Figure 1–1 A schematic diagram of rehabilitation services. (Adapted from Rehabilitation Service, Hospital of the University of Pennsylvania.)

the individual's residual capacities, with emphasis on his remaining abilities rather than on his losses. Since modern rehabilitation includes psychosocial and vocational as well as medical components, it calls for good teamwork by people from a variety of professions, as shown in Figure 1–1. It may also require extensive physical facilities and sufficient funding to provide a variety of services over a prolonged period of time.

Until the occurrence of death, it may be possible at each stage of the evolution of a disease process to apply appropriate measures to prevent continued progression and deterioration of the patient's condition. The different levels of prevention can be fully understood only in relation to the natural progression or natural history of disease. The clearer our understanding of the natural history of a disease, the greater may be the opportunities for developing effective points of intervention. The interrelations between natural history and levels of prevention will be illustrated by a specific example, stroke.

APPLICATION OF PREVENTION AND NATURAL HISTORY: STROKE

Stroke, a term familiar to laymen as well as physicians, refers to a symptom complex of neurologic deficit resulting from damage to the brain by alteration of its blood supply. An equivalent term for stroke is cerebrovascular accident (CVA). The manifestations are variable and depend on the extent and location of the damage to nervous tissue; there may be impairment of speech or cerebration, or paralysis of one or more portions of the body.

Cerebrovascular disease is an important health problem. It is the third leading cause of death in the United States, resulting in some 200,000 deaths annually. It is also a major contributor to disability. The National Center for Health Statistics (1962) estimated that there are over 300,000 noninstitutionalized people in this country paralyzed as the result of a stroke.

There are several mechanisms of stroke: thrombosis, hemorrhage, and embolism.* Since cerebral thrombosis accounts for more than half of all strokes, the following section will focus primarily on cerebral thrombosis and its consequence, brain infarction.

The onset of stroke is often sudden. For many years stroke was regarded as a disease of older persons which comes on without warning and without any relation to the person's health status in earlier life. True, persons with markedly elevated blood pressure were known to be at high risk of hemorrhagic stroke, but infarction was regarded as an unpredictable occurrence. Since little was known about prevention, stroke was regarded fatalistically. At best there was a modest concern for rehabilitative measures.

In the past few decades advances in different disciplines have converged to bring new perspectives to the problem of stroke. Among them are increased awareness of the importance of the extracranial vessels (carotids and vertebral-basilar system) in the production of stroke, anticoagulant therapy and other pharmacologic advances, and technical achievements in vascular surgery and diagnostic radiology. Two specific *epidemiologic* advances, both relating to the natural history of stroke, also deserve notice. One is

---

*Robbins (1967) defines hemorrhage as "the escape of blood from vessels... (this) implies rupture of a vessel." Thrombosis consists of "the formation of a blood coagulum within a vessel or the heart." When a thrombus or other physical mass (e.g., clump of bacteria) is carried by the blood from its point of origin to a distant site this is referred to as embolism. The significance of both thrombosis and embolism "lies in their capacity to occlude vessels, impair the flow of blood and give rise to ischemic necrosis and infarction (death) of tissues."

the knowledge that stroke does not strike at random but that factors identifiable in early adult life influence the likelihood that stroke will develop years later. The other is the realization that fleeting episodes, called transient ischemic attacks (TIA), occur in a substantial portion of people who later suffer a definite stroke.*

Underlying Risk Factors. Much of our information about the life history of stroke is derived from populations placed under observation years ago, primarily for study of coronary heart disease (Kannel, 1966; Kannel et al., 1970; Chapman et al., 1966). The kind of information recorded at entry into these studies has made it possible subsequently to identify several factors related to occurrence of stroke. The information to be presented in this section will be

---

*The following terms are used to describe the syndromes associated with disturbance of cerebral blood flow:

Transient ischemic attack (TIA)—a focal neurologic deficit of abrupt onset and brief duration which is followed by complete recovery.

Progressive stroke (stroke in evolution)—a neurologic impairment which evolves over several hours or even days.

Completed stroke—a stable, focal neurologic deficit which persists for at least 24 hours. The extent of dysfunction with completed stroke is either stable or lessened. If progressive loss of function is observed, the patient is considered to have a stroke in evolution.

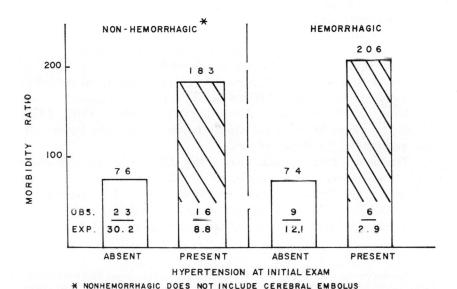

Figure 1-2 Risk of CVA according to blood pressure at initial examination. Men aged 30–62 years at entry. (From Kannel, W. B., Wolf, P. A., et al.: Epidemiologic assessment of the role of blood pressure in stroke. J.A.M.A., *214*:301, 1970.)

drawn mainly from a study carried out in Framingham, Massachu-setts, where a community sample of approximately 5000 people has been followed biennially over many years (Kannel et al., 1970). Several risk factors for stroke have been identified, but the major finding has been the overwhelming importance of hypertension as a precursor not only of intracerebral hemorrhage but also of throm-bosis. In terms of numbers affected, its role in thrombosis is of greater importance.

Figure 1–2 demonstrates the clear relation between blood pressure and subsequent stroke experience in the Framingham data. For both nonhemorrhagic stroke (i.e., brain infarction) and hemorrhagic stroke the morbidity ratio* is seen to be much higher for persons with hypertension than for those with normal blood pressure on initial examination.

The role of blood lipids as a possible risk factor in stroke is less clear (Greenhouse, 1971). The Framingham study (Kannel, 1966) did find that elevated blood lipid levels were associated with an increased risk of stroke, but only when lipids were measured in persons under the age of 50. This study also demonstrated that ciga-rette smoking and diabetes mellitus are risk factors. In a more recent analysis of the Framingham data (Wolf et al., 1973), cardiac abnormalities (left ventricular hypertrophy on electrocardiogram or cardiac enlargement on chest x-ray) were found to be associated with increased risk of cerebral infarction. This effect, which ap-pears to be independent of hypertension, suggests that inadequate cardiac function may adversely affect cerebral blood flow.

The potential value of knowing about these risk factors is that their reduction or elimination might provide a means of reducing the incidence of stroke. This has been achieved for hypertension, as shown by the Veterans Administration studies (1967, 1970, 1972). It remains to be tested whether changes in other factors can also reduce the incidence of stroke.

Transient Ischemic Attack. Since the 1950's it has become clear that strokes do not always occur unheralded. Estimates vary, but pehaps one-third to one-half of patients with stroke have had one or more transient ischemic attacks (Browne and Poskanzer, 1969). The prognostic import of TIA is not clearly understood, and there is lit-

---

*Morbidity ratio was defined in this study as "cases observed divided by cases expected multiplied by 100. The expected number of cases was calculated by apply-ing the age-specific incidence rates for CVA in the total study cohort to the age com-position of each blood pressure category in the population at risk." This is a method of age-adjustment (Chapter 7).

tle chance for further expansion of knowledge in this regard since it is now accepted that either of the two therapeutic approaches available, anticoagulation or surgery, yields better results than no therapy at all. Whether either form of treatment has a definitive advantage over the other is still being debated (Frank, 1971; Fields et al., 1970).

Implications for Prevention. Review of the considerations just outlined indicates that stroke may be viewed not as an isolated occurrence, but as the late or final manifestation in a long chain of events. Before facts about risk factors and TIA as precursors of stroke were available, the only intervention was through tertiary prevention, i.e., rehabilitation after a stroke had occurred. Following a period of relative fatalism, efforts at tertiary prevention became more active, with emphasis on early physical therapy to prevent contractures and muscle atrophy, early ambulation to prevent thromboembolic complications, and active occupational and psychologic rehabilitation. However, no attempt was made to intervene earlier in the life history of the disease.

With the aid of current knowledge, prevention of stroke is being implemented at the primary and secondary levels. Primary prevention attempts to alter the risk factors known to be related to stroke. Drug therapy to reduce blood pressure in hypertension is a major contribution to this stage of prevention, as are identification and treatment of correctable causes of hypertension. Secondary prevention is carried out through recognition and treatment of TIA to prevent the development of completed stroke. Thus a disease of the second half of life once considered an inevitable accompaniment of the process of aging is now being approached through preventive efforts applied to younger people earlier in the natural history of the disease.

SUMMARY

This chapter has set the stage for epidemiology within the framework of population medicine. Clinical and epidemiologic approaches to the study of disease were contrasted, as were the concepts of health and disease. Morbidity and mortality rates were presented as fundamental tools in epidemiology.

The chapter introduced a model of the natural history of disease over time, emphasizing precursors which antedate the appearance of clinically detectable disease and which increase the likelihood that disease will develop in future. The term "risk factor" was introduced to identify such predisposing conditions in the individual. The importance of subdividing the stage of clinical disease on anatomic or functional grounds was stressed, as was the personal and societal impact of the stage of disability.

The concept of levels of prevention—primary, secondary, and tertiary—was outlined and developed in relation to the natural history of disease. This was illustrated by reference to stroke. The modern approach to this disease extends beyond rehabilitation to include identification of risk factors and early detection and therapy.

In the next chapter we will expand the definition of epidemiology, delineate its scope, and present several epidemiologic models of the causation of disease.

STUDY QUESTIONS

1–1 Define the following terms and give an example when appropriate:

Population medicine (page 1)
Epidemiology (page 3)
Rate (page 4)
Health (page 5)
Natural history of disease (page 6)
Risk factor (page 6)
Disability (page 8)
Levels of prevention—primary, secondary, tertiary (page 9ff.)
Rehabilitation (page 10)

1–2 A serious problem for hospitals is that of accidents to patients. The following data come from an article entitled "The patients' accident pattern" (Williams, 1948):

Age Distribution of 82 Injured Patients

Age in Years	Number of Accidents
0–2	5
2–5	6
5–14	18
14–21	8
21–31	5
31–41	8
41–51	7
51–61	4
61 and over	21

The article stated:

Statistical analysis . . . by patient age group reveals that patients 61 years and older are most prone to accidents. The next greatest incidence occurs among the the 5 to 14 age group. We found an almost equal number of accidents among the 2 to 5, 14 to 21, 31 to 41, and 41 to 51 age groups. The fewest number occurred among those 51 to 61.

Comment on this interpretation. What further information would you need to evaluate the occurrence of accidents in relation to age?

Answer on page 341.

1–3 Clinical and epidemiologic approaches to the prevention, identification (diagnosis), and management of health problems differ. Following are examples of clinical and epidemiologic approaches to a commonly encountered problem, mental retardation. Add further examples to each category.

	Clinical Approach	Epidemiologic Approach
Prevention	Genetic counselling of parents	Studies to identify causes of mental retardation
Identification (Diagnosis)		Case-finding in schools
Management	Diet, e.g., for phenylketonuria (PKU)*	

Answer on page 341.

1–4 The following procedures might be undertaken in the diagnosis and management of mental retardation. For each indicate the level of prevention which is represented.

Example: Pap smears to detect *in situ* cancer of the cervix
Answer: Secondary
A. Nutritional counselling for pregnant women
B. Screening of newborn infants for PKU
C. Genetic counselling for parents with one retarded child
D. Immunization against rubella (German measles)
E. Developmental screening of infants
F. Placement of retarded children in institutions for special education

Answer on page 342.

---

*An inherited metabolic abnormality associated with mental retardation.

1-5 Chronic pulmonary emphysema is defined as a progressive disease of the lungs characterized by distention and destruction of lung tissue (terminal respiratory alveolar sacs). This results in trapping of air in the lung, with impairment of ventilation and circulation in the affected tissues. The predominant symptom is shortness of breath (dyspnea).

Population samples indicate that about 10 per cent of adult males in the United States are affected. Figure 1–3 shows the marked increase in deaths from this disease over the 15 year period from 1955 to 1970. Although females are susceptible, the typical emphysematous patient is a male, heavy smoker, aged 50 to 70, living in an urban industrialized area. List possible control measures which would provide primary, secondary, and tertiary prevention of this disease.

Answer on page 342.

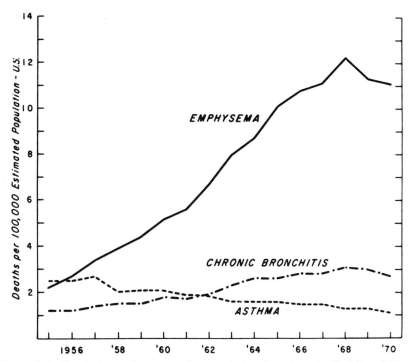

Figure 1–3 Trends in emphysema, asthma, and chronic and unspecified bronchitis as reported causes of death, United States, 1955–1970. Data for 1969–1970 are provisional. (From Chronic Obstructive Pulmonary Disease, A Manual for Physicians, 3rd ed. National Tuberculosis and Respiratory Disease Association, New York, 1972.)

1–6 Select a disease and develop its natural history using the discussion of stroke as a model.

List any identifiable risk factors (precursors).

List the stages of the disease.

List possible measures for primary, secondary, or tertiary prevention.

REFERENCES

Bahn, A.: A multidisciplinary psychosocial classification scheme. Am. J. Ortho-psychiatry, *41*:830, 1971.

Brody, J. A., Detels, R., et al.: Measles-antibody titres in sibships of patients with subacute sclerosing panencephalitis and controls. Lancet, *1*:177, 1972.

Browne, T. R., 3rd, and Poskanzer, D. C.: Treatment of strokes I. N. Eng. J. Med., *281*:594, 1969.

Chapman, J. M., Reeder, L. G., et al.: Epidemiology of vascular lesions affecting the central nervous system: The occurrence of strokes in a sample population under observation for cardiovascular disease. Am. J. Public Health, *56*:191, 1966.

Constitution of the World Health Organization, 1948. In Basic Documents, 15th ed. WHO, Geneva, 1964.

Feinstein, A. R.: Clinical Judgment. The Williams & Wilkins Company, Baltimore, 1967.

Fields, W. S., Maslenikov, V., et al.: Joint study of extracranial arterial occlusion. J.A.M.A., *211*:1993, 1970.

Frank, G.: Comparison of anticoagulation and surgical treatments of TIA. A review and consolidation of recent natural history and treatment studies. Stroke, *2*:369, 1971.

Frost, W. H.: Introduction to Snow on Cholera. Commonwealth Fund, New York, 1936. Reprinted by Hafner Publishing Company, New York, 1965.

Gagnon, F.: Contribution to study of etiology and prevention of cancer of cervix of uterus. Am. J. Obstet. Gynecol., *60*:516, 1950.

Goldberger, J.: The cause and prevention of pellagra. Public Health Rep., 29: 2354, 1914. Reprinted in Terris, M. (ed.), Goldberger on Pellagra. Louisiana State University Press, Baton Rouge, 1964.

Greenhouse, A. H.: Blood lipids and strokes; Are they related? J. Chronic Dis., 23:823, 1971.

Kannel, W. B.: An epidemiologic study of cerebrovascular disease. In Siekert, R. G., and Whisnant, J. P. (eds.), Fifth Conference on Cerebral Vascular Diseases, Millikan, C. H., Chairman, Grune and Stratton, New York and London, 1966, pp. 53–66.

Kannel, W. B., Wolf, P. A., et al.: Epidemiologic assessment of the role of blood pressure in stroke. The Framingham study. J.A.M.A., *214*:301, 1970.

Morris, J. N.: Uses of epidemiology. Br. Med. J., 2:395, 1955.

National Center for Health Statistics: Selected impairments by etiology and activity limitation. United States, July 1959–June 1961. USPHS Pub. No. 584–B35, U.S. Govt. Printing Office, Washington, D.C., 1962.

National Health Survey: Concepts and definitions in the Health Household—Interview Survey. USPHS Pub. No. 584–A3, U.S. Govt. Printing Office, Washington, D.C., 1958.

New York Heart Association, Inc.: Diseases of the Heart and Blood Vessels—Nomenclature and Criteria for Diagnosis, 6th ed. Little, Brown and Company, Boston, 1964.

Pulvertaft, C. N.: Peptic ulcer in town and country. Br. J. Prev. Soc. Med., *13*:131, 1959.

Robbins, S. L.: Pathology, 2nd ed. W. B. Saunders Company, Philadelphia, 1967.

Røjel, J.: The interrelation between uterine cancer and syphilis. Acta. Pathol. Microbiol. Scand. supp. 97:3, 1953.

Smith, F. H., Boles, R. S., Jr., et al.: Problems of the gastric ulcer reviewed: Study of 1000 cases. J.A.M.A., 153:1505, 1953.

Sullivan, D. F.: Conceptual problems in developing an index of health. U.S. Dept. of Health, Education, and Welfare, USPHS Pub. No. 1000, Series 2, No. 17, U.S. Govt. Printing Office, Washington, D.C., 1966.

Veterans Administration Cooperative Study Group on Antihypertensive Agents: Effects of treatment on morbidity in hypertension: I. Results in patients with diastolic blood pressures averaging 115 through 129 mm Hg. J.A.M.A., 202:116, 1967.

Veterans Administration Cooperative Study Group on Antihypertensive Agents: Effects of treatment on morbidity in hypertension: II. Results in patients with diastolic blood pressure averaging 90 through 114 mm Hg. J.A.M.A., 213:1143, 1970.

Veterans Administration Cooperative Study Group on Antihypertensive Agents: Effects of treatment on morbidity in hypertension: III. Influence of age, diastolic pressure, and prior cardiovascular disease; further analysis of side effects. Circulation, 45:991, 1972.

Williams, W. R.: The patients' accident pattern. Hospitals, 22:39, 1948.

Wolf, P. A., Kannel, W. B., et al.: The role of impaired cardiac function in atherosclerotic brain infarction. The Framingham study. Am. J. Public Health 63:52, 1973.

EPIDEMIOLOGIC CONCEPTS AND MODELS

2

THE SCOPE OF EPIDEMIOLOGY

The definition of epidemiology given in the previous chapter, *the study of the distribution and determinants of diseases and injuries in human populations*, is quite inclusive. For many years the province of epidemiology was generally considered to be restricted to the infectious diseases, an understandable focus since the major scourges of man in the past were epidemics of infectious disease. Only after such epidemics had come under some satisfactory control did investigation shift toward the diseases of later life — the vascular diseases, arthritides, and malignant neoplasms.

However, even centuries ago some epidemics were traced to noninfectious causes. In the latter half of the eighteenth century colic among cider drinkers in Devonshire, England, was traced to intoxication with lead (Baker, 1767). This developed because the cider in that area was transported in leaden pipes or processed in presses which contained lead. Due to the acidity of the cider, enough lead was leached into the liquid to cause acute lead toxicity.

Another example of the application of epidemiology to a noninfectious disease relates to scurvy. The occurrence of scurvy in epidemic proportions on board British ships during long sea voyages was correctly traced to a nutritional deficiency (Lind, 1753) which could be prevented by a ration of limes. It is worth noting that effective prevention did not depend on a full understanding of the dietary lack; vitamin C was not isolated until 1928.

It is now generally accepted that epidemiologic study can appropriately be applied to all diseases, conditions, and health-related events, including mental illness, suicide, drug addiction, and injury. Further, since epidemiology aims for a comprehensive view of the dynamics of disease, it is concerned not only with epidemics but also with interepidemic periods and with sporadic and endemic occurrences of disease. *Endemic* occurrence is defined as "the habitual presence of a disease or infectious agent within a geographic area . . . or the usual prevalence of a given disease within such area." The term is used in contrast with *epidemic*, "the occurrence in a community or region of a group of illnesses . . . of similar nature, clearly in excess of normal expectancy" (Benenson, 1970).

Examination of this definition indicates that the term *epidemic* itself is defined quite broadly.

1. It includes any kind of disease (or injury).

2. There is no universally applicable number of cases which constitutes an epidemic. Rather, an epidemic exists whenever the number of cases exceeds that *expected* on the basis of past experience for a given population. Clearly this level of expectation varies for different diseases and in different circumstances. In the United States in the last 25 years one case of smallpox would exceed expectancy, whereas the occurrence of 100 cases in a single year might be under the "expected" number in Ethiopia or India.

3. There is no specification of geographic extent; an epidemic may cover a few city blocks or an entire nation, or may even be worldwide in distribution, as is true in "pandemics" of influenza.

4. An epidemic may encompass any time period; it may last a few hours (chemical intoxication or bacterial food poisoning), a few weeks (influenza or hepatitis), or several years (drug addiction). Many countries, including the United States, have been experiencing a lung cancer epidemic for the past forty years.

VARIATIONS IN SEVERITY OF DISEASE

The discussion of natural history of disease in Chapter 1 outlined progression of disease primarily in terms of chronic disease. At this point, we will shift our focus to acute short-term disease, particularly infectious disease, and consider the consequences of the fact that infectious processes can result in a variety of effects, ranging from no clinically detectable disease to fulminating symptoms and death.

Infections differ in characteristic, or modal, severity of manifestation. Some infections tend to be mostly inapparent; others typically are characterized by pronounced symptomatology. Figure 2–1 is a schematic drawing which illustrates this point. The figure presents three classes of infectious agents. Each produces infections with a range of manifestations, but the relative distribution differs.

The first bar chart (Class A) describes infections in which a high proportion are *inapparent*, i.e., the infection does not become manifest at any stage. Only a small fraction are clinically evident, an even smaller proportion severe or fatal. This type of infection has been likened to an iceberg whose visible tip represents only a small fraction of the whole. For example, the number of people with positive tuberculin tests (an indication of infection with tubercle bacilli at some time in the past) far exceeds the number who develop clinical tuberculosis. Other examples would be infections with poliovirus or hepatitis virus in early childhood and with the meningococcus. Only a small fraction of the total number of infections can be identified without special diagnostic tests.

The second horizontal bar (B) represents infections in which the inapparent component is relatively small. Most of the cases are clinically apparent and readily diagnosable (i.e., they present as "classic" cases); only a small fraction are severe or fatal. Examples are measles and chickenpox.

The last bar (C) portrays infections in which the outcome is typically severe or fatal illness. Rabies is the outstanding example since virtually 100 per cent of infections with rabies virus end in

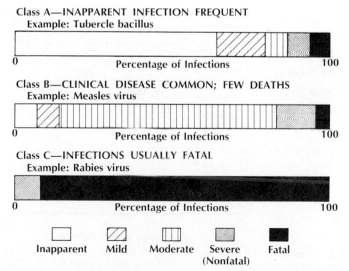

Figure 2–1   Distribution of clinical severity for three classes of infection (not to scale).

death. Another infection less uniformly fatal but still very severe is produced by *Salmonella choleraesuis.*

The analysis of severity of infections just presented is an over-simplification since it implies, incorrectly, that variation depends entirely on the infecting organism. In actuality, severity of manifestation also depends on the nature of the response to the organism. The importance of host factors will be discussed later in this chapter.

Even within one genus of bacteria there can be great variability in the severity of disease produced by different types or groups of the organism. It is well known, for example, that one specific group of hemolytic streptococci, Group A organisms, are responsible for most of the streptococcal disease of man. Similarly, the various serotypes of Salmonella differ in their tendency to produce disease. Figure 2–2 presents data from a five-year period in Poland which show that the proportion of symptomatic infections varied widely for different serotypes, from 86 per cent for S. *choleraesuis* to 7 per cent for S. *give.**

Of course, as mentioned above, for any given serotype the extent of reaction will also be influenced by characteristics of the host. The same serotype would produce symptoms in a higher

---

*Part of this variability may be due to differences in intensity of search for inapparent infections.

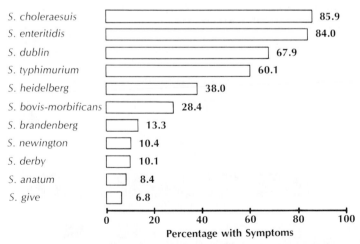

Salmonella Serotype

Serotype	Percentage with Symptoms
S. choleraesuis	85.9
S. enteritidis	84.0
S. dublin	67.9
S. typhimurium	60.1
S. heidelberg	38.0
S. bovis-morbificans	28.4
S. brandenberg	13.3
S. newington	10.4
S. derby	10.1
S. anatum	8.4
S. give	6.8

Figure 2–2 Common Salmonella serotypes isolated in Poland, 1957–1962, by percentage of positives with symptoms. (From Salmonella Surveillance Report No. 31, CDC, USPHS, U.S. Govt. Printing Office, Washington, D.C., 1964.)

proportion of persons in a home for the aged than in a school or military installation. The severity of response to Salmonella infection tends to be increased in persons with sickle cell disease or with previous gastric surgery.

In contrast to overt disease, which can be detected by clinical evaluation alone, inapparent infection cannot be diagnosed without such procedures as tuberculin tests or throat cultures for diphtheria organisms. The number of human infections with rabies virus may be adequately estimated by clinical examination, but infections with poliovirus or meningococci will largely go undetected. For accurate estimates of the extent of inapparent infection in a population, epidemiologic surveys are needed in which apparently well persons are tested for direct or indirect evidence of the presence of specific organisms. Such information on inapparent infection is important for practical reasons as well as academic curiosity. The implications of inapparent and mild infection for the **control** of disease and for interpretation of morbidity **statistics** will now be discussed.

Inapparent Infection and Control of Disease

Procedures for control must be directed toward all infections capable of being transmitted to others. Since many inapparent infections can be transmitted and produce disease in others, it is insufficient to direct procedures solely to clinically apparent cases. Before inapparent infection was well understood, control measures were directed mainly toward persons known to be ill. Emphasis was placed on isolation of patients, disinfection of their belongings and excreta, and quarantine of exposed persons (e.g., household contacts) who might be incubating disease. While isolation is still an essential part of control procedures for many diseases, the focus on isolation and disinfection has been replaced by a more general concern with the spread of organisms through a community. The current focus on detection and treatment of asymptomatic carriers of gonorrhea illustrates the importance of inapparent infection in control of disease. In fact, efforts at control may include deliberate spread of inapparent infections, such as the administration of live, attenuated oral polio vaccine.

Inapparent Infection and Disease Statistics

The impact of inapparent infection upon disease statistics is shown in Figure 2–3 for Class A infections (see Figure 2–1). Only

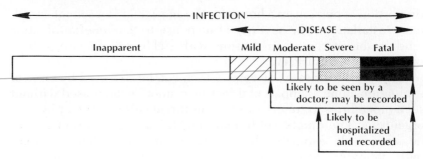

Figure 2–3 Relation of severity of illness to disease statistics (Class A).

the small fraction of infections which cause obvious disease or severe symptoms will come to medical attention; an even smaller fraction will find their way into hospital records. Therefore, statistics on infections with this kind of gradient are likely to be inaccurate. The number of infections diagnosed and reported will be smaller than the true number, i.e., understated, while the severity of the disease will be overstated. Thus, where the discrepancy between "infection" and "disease" is large, it is particularly important to know the criteria used for diagnosis. Many more infections will be recorded if those detected by laboratory methods or skin tests are included than if only clinically diagnosed cases are tabulated.

A frequently used measure of the severity of a disease is the *case fatality rate*, which indicates the probability of death among diagnosed cases.

Case fatality rate =

$$\frac{\text{number of deaths from a disease}}{\text{number of cases of that disease}} \text{ (usually expressed as percentage)}$$

MODELS OF DISEASE: MULTIPLE CAUSATION

In medicine we focus on man and the forces within him and within the environment which influence his state of health. From this viewpoint man is the *host* organism; other organisms are considered only as they relate to human health. In veterinary medicine the term "host" might refer to cats, dogs, or horses. However, many of the principles presented in this text apply equally to the study of health and disease in human and animal populations.

The egocentrism implicit in man's view of the universe has been noted in the following poignant paragraph from Zinsser's

Rats, Lice and History (1943). Epidemic typhus fever is a disease of man likely to develop in cold climates when people are crowded together in unsanitary conditions. Zinsser points out that it may be equally reasonable to view typhus as a disease of the louse or as a disease of man.

Man is too prone to look upon all nature through egocentric eyes. To the louse, *we* are the dreaded emissaries of death. He leads a relatively harmless life—the results of centuries of adaptation; then, out of the blue, an epidemic occurs; his host sickens and the only world he has ever known becomes pestilential and deadly; and if, as a result of circumstances not under his control, his stricken body is transferred to another host, whom he, in turn, infects, he does so without guile, from the uncontrollable need for nourishment, with death already in his own entrails. If only for his fellowship with us in suffering he should command a degree of sympathetic consideration.

Man and the louse inhabit the same world. Although the term "ecology" has been overused in the popular press, it is still useful to think of men and lice as parts of one ecological system. *Ecology may be defined as the study of the relationship of organisms to each other as well as to all other aspects of the environment.*

Since disease arises within an ecological system, a basic tenet of epidemiology is that an ecological approach is necessary to explain the occurrence of disease; disease cannot be attributed to the operation of any **one** factor. The requirement that more than one factor be present for disease to develop is referred to as *multiple causation* or *multifactorial etiology.*

At first glance it might seem that the introduction of an organism into a community would be enough to explain the development of an epidemic.

Organism ⟶ Man ⟶ Disease

However, the organism alone is not sufficient to account for the outbreak and cannot therefore be considered *"the* cause." The level of immunity of the population is also crucial. This can be seen from the sequence of events following introduction of measles or mumps into a *virgin population,* i.e., one in which an organism has not been present for many years, if ever. When this occurs, adults as well as children are affected. The upper age limit is determined by the number of years since the virus last circulated in the community. For example, Christensen and his colleagues (1953) found that when measles was introduced into Greenland for the first time in 1951, over 4200 cases developed in a total population of 4320 people. Those who escaped included abortive cases, patients who died without a definitive diagnosis, and some persons who either had had the disease previously in Denmark or had received prophylactic gamma globulin. Only five unprotected persons in the entire population appeared to have escaped infection entirely.

An additional set of factors, environmental conditions, also determines whether effective transmission of disease can occur in any given situation. These factors include degree of contact, level of hygienic practices, and presence of other organisms.

When a factor **must** be present (a *sine qua non*) for a disease to occur, it is called the *agent* of that disease. For example, influenza virus is the agent of influenza. Many, but not all, of the known agents of disease are located in the biological environment. Examples of agents from the physical environment are lead, asbestos, beryllium, carbon monoxide in the inspired air, and ionizing radiation. A possible agent in the social environment is maternal deprivation. Numerous studies have demonstrated that the quality of parental care in the early years of life is intimately related to normal physical, emotional, and mental development (Bowlby, 1952). In keeping with the ecological view presented above, an agent is considered to be a **necessary but not sufficient cause** of disease because suitable conditions of the host and environment must also be present for disease to develop.

It is customary to divide factors affecting the development of disease into two groups, *host factors* (intrinsic) and *factors in the environment* (extrinsic). Host factors affect susceptibility to disease; factors in the environment influence exposure and sometimes indirectly affect susceptibility as well. The interactions of these two sets of factors determine whether or not disease develops.

Host Factors (Intrinsic)

The state of the host at any given time is a result of the interactions of genetic endowment with environment over the entire life span (see Figure 2–5). For some conditions the relative contributions of genetic and environmental factors are quite clear; for others it is difficult to arrive at an assignment of weights.

An increasing number of genetically determined factors have been identified as related to either an increased or decreased susceptibility to certain diseases. ABO blood type is associated with several diseases. Persons with type A blood have an increased risk of gastric cancer (Aird et al., 1953), while those with type O are more likely to develop duodenal ulcer (Clarke et al., 1955). Deficiency in one specific enzyme, alpha-1-antitrypsin, is associated with one type of chronic obstructive lung disease (Erikkson, 1965). Sickle cell trait is associated with a decreased risk of malaria due to *Plasmodium falciparum* (Allison, 1954).

Other attributes are primarily the result of past environmental exposures. Thus, one of the major components in resistance to infectious disease is *specific immunity,* a state of altered responsiveness to a specific substance acquired through immunization or natural infection. For certain diseases (e.g., measles, chickenpox) this protection generally lasts for the life of the individual.

Personality is one host factor for which separation of intrinsic and extrinsic variables is difficult (Mischel, 1968). It is beyond our scope to explore systematically the relation between personality and illness. However, we should note that, quite apart from relations between specific traits and disease, personality variables do influence the course of illness, if only through their effect on tendency to seek medical care and to comply with medical advice. One well-documented association between personality traits and disease is that relating to coronary heart disease. Rosenman and his colleagues (1970) have noted that coronary heart disease rates are high for individuals they have labelled "Type A." These are people characterized by aggressiveness, competitiveness, ambition, restlessness, and a sense of time urgency. Type B individuals, who do not exhibit these characteristics, have lower rates of coronary heart disease. Using somewhat different terminology, other investigators have made similar observations on the differences between persons with and without coronary heart disease (Jenkins, 1971).

Social class membership is a host attribute which strongly reflects environmental influences. Because developmental experiences and life style are intimately tied to social class, some diseases show a differential frequency among persons of different social classes. For example, the social class gradient in carcinoma of the cervix (i.e., rates inversely related to social class) is compatible with class differences (Kinsey et al., 1953) in age at which heterosexual activity is initiated.

There are many unanswered questions about the role of host factors in disease. We do not know, for example, why only some of the people exposed to large doses of x-rays develop leukemia, or why all heavy smokers do not develop lung cancer. Nevertheless, at least for certain diseases, our current state of knowledge does permit us to identify individuals with more than average likelihood of developing the disease and to concentrate preventive efforts on this group.

Environmental Factors (Extrinsic)

Extrinsic or environmental factors can be classified as biological, social, and physical.

Biological Environment. This sector of the environment includes (1) infectious agents of disease, (2) reservoirs of infection (other human beings, animals, and soil), (3) vectors which transmit disease (e.g., flies and mosquitoes), and (4) plants and animals (as sources of food, antibiotics, and other drug principles or as antigens). Most of these topics will be elaborated further in Chapter 12.

Social Environment. The social environment may be defined in terms of the overall economic and political organization of a society and of the institutions by which individuals are integrated into the society at various stages in their lives. All of these factors are relevant to health. Broadly speaking, overall socioeconomic and political organization affect the technical level of medical care, the systems by which that care is delivered, the extent of support for medical care and biomedical research, and the adequacy and level of enforcement of codes and laws controlling health-related environmental hazards (pollution, housing, occupational safety, and so on).

Particular social customs may affect health. The types of foods eaten and the thoroughness of cooking determine whether there will be exposure to parasites, such as fish tapeworm and trichinae. The practice of wearing shoes can prevent acquisition of hookworms in rural areas where these parasites are prevalent.

Another important aspect of social environment is the general level of receptivity to new ideas. When physicians and other health personnel try to encourage healthful practices, resistance may develop, at least in part, because these practices run counter to deeply held beliefs and values. This can apply equally to problems encountered in insuring an adequate intake of milk in the diet of pregnant Zulu women (Cassel, 1955) and those found in persuading Americans to use seat belts. A number of other illustrations of similar phenomena are recorded and discussed in *Health, Culture and Community* (Paul, 1955).

The extent to which individuals are integrated into a society is vitally significant to health. In general, a high degree of integration is protective; social isolation and alienation are productive of disease. The pioneer work in this area was done by Durkheim (1897) in his studies of suicide. More recently, schizophrenia (Faris and Dunham, 1939; Hare, 1956) and depressed mental development in children (Spitz, 1945; Widdowson, 1951) have been found to be linked to circumstances of social isolation. Damaging effects from catastrophic losses in an individual's immediate social environment have also been demonstrated. Both suicide (MacMahon and Pugh, 1965) and entry into psychiatric care (Stein and Susser, 1969) tend to cluster in the period following bereavement. Less dramatic life changes may also take a toll.

A phenomenon related to social loss is the upheaval associated with geographic mobility, particularly if it also involves a change in cultural milieu, such as a move from a rural to an urban area. Studies in North Dakota (Syme et al., 1964) and North Carolina (Tyroler and Cassel, 1964) indicate increased rates of coronary heart disease in persons exposed to cultural discontinuities. Similarly, an excess of hypertension in urban as compared with rural Zulus has been interpreted as related to stress inherent in the process of urbanization (Scotch, 1963; Gampel et al., 1962).

Physical Environment. The physical aspects of the environment include heat, light, air, water, radiation, gravity, atmospheric pressure, and chemical agents of all kinds. In the technically developed areas of the world man has a great deal of control over the physical environment through provision of adequate shelter against extremes of weather, purification of drinking water, treatment of sewage, and year-round control of indoor temperature and humidity. Yet new environmental problems continue to arise as old ones are solved. Currently the rapid growth of population, the increase in industrial wastes of all kinds, and the ever increasing number of motor vehicles interact to produce air, water, noise, and other types of pollution of the environment.

Air pollution, for example, has recently emerged as an urgent threat to health. When weather conditions are unfavorable, masses of polluted air can be trapped and hang over a city for several days at a time, exposing the inhabitants to a variety of noxious substances. A number of acute air pollution episodes have been documented. The largest, associated with a four-day fog in London in 1952, led to some 4000 deaths in excess of the usual number (as shown in Figure 12–5). Long-term exposure to pollution probably also produces damage. There are still many unanswered questions about the role of air pollution in certain chronic diseases, including lung cancer. However, air pollution undoubtedly contributes to the higher rates of chronic respiratory disease in urban than rural areas in several countries.

Although the physical environment is often regarded mainly as a source of stressors, its positive as well as its negative aspects bear consideration. The range of environmental conditions (e.g., atmospheric pressure, oxygen supply, living space) compatible with human existence on earth is relatively narrow; in L. J. Henderson's words, there is a "fitness of the environment" (1913). Health-related environmental goals must be concerned with maintenance of this fitness as well as with elimination of identifiable stressors. A recently emerging science, known variously as environmental psychology or ekistics, is concerned with the design of living spaces. There is mounting interest in the effects of the arrangement of the physical environment on both physical and mental health (Proshansky et al., 1970; Wilner et al., 1962).

Interrelations of Factors (Ecologic Models)

Although three discrete sectors of the environment (biological, social, and physical) have been identified, it should be emphasized that this separation is artificial; they are closely interrelated with each other and with host factors. Several alternative models have been developed to depict the ways in which these interactions influence the occurrence of disease. Whichever model one uses, it is important to realize that the balance of forces which determines an individual's state of health at a given time is in a kind of dynamic equilibrium. A potentially harmful change in any of the components of the system may not lead to detectable disease if the other parts of the system have adequate reserve capacity. If the existing balance is precarious, disease may develop after even a small insult. For example, flying at a high altitude, which would ordinarily not lead to illness, might precipitate a thrombotic crisis in a person with sickle cell hemoglobin. Exposure to organisms which usually cause no damage can be serious for a person with impaired immunologic defenses. This is a problem of increasing importance as persons are kept alive by drastic medical and surgical therapies (treatment of leukemia and other malignancies, organ transplantation) which require interference with normal immune mechanisms. With these considerations in mind, then, we will present three ecological models, with emphasis on the third one.

The Epidemiologic Triangle. This model was widely used for many years and still is referred to frequently in the epidemiologic literature. The epidemiologic triangle is considered to consist of three components — host, environment, and agent. The model implies that each must be analyzed and understood for comprehension and predictions of patterns of a disease. A change in any of the components will alter an existing equilibrium to increase or decrease the frequency of the disease.

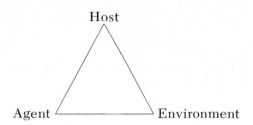

In the preceding pages we identified host and environmental factors as determining, respectively, susceptibility and exposure to disease. The epidemiologic triangle highlights as a separate component the **agent** of disease which is, of course, only one among many environmental factors.

When the focus of epidemiologic studies was limited to the infectious diseases, particularly the bacterial diseases, the infecting organisms were accorded a status separate from the other environmental factors and identified as *agents* of disease. However, with the recent application of epidemiologic concepts and methods to other categories of disease, we are dealing with conditions which have not been linked to specific agents, such as schizophrenia, coronary heart disease, and rheumatoid arthritis. Further, even for diseases with an identifiable agent, many epidemiologists prefer to regard the agent as an integral part of the total environment. Therefore, new models have been developed which deemphasize "agent" and, rather stress the multiplicity of interactions between host and environment. The two models to be presented next reflect this view.

The Web of Causation. The notion of a "web of causation" was put forth some years ago by MacMahon and his colleagues (1960). The essence of the concept is that effects never depend on single isolated causes, but rather develop as the result of chains of causation in which each link itself is the result of "a complex genealogy of antecedents." The large number of antecedents creates a condition which may appropriately be conceptualized as a "web, which in its complexity and origins lies quite beyond our understanding."*

° For a more extended explanation see MacMahon, B., Pugh, T. F., et al.: Epidemiologic Methods. Little, Brown and Company, Boston, 1960, Chapter 2.

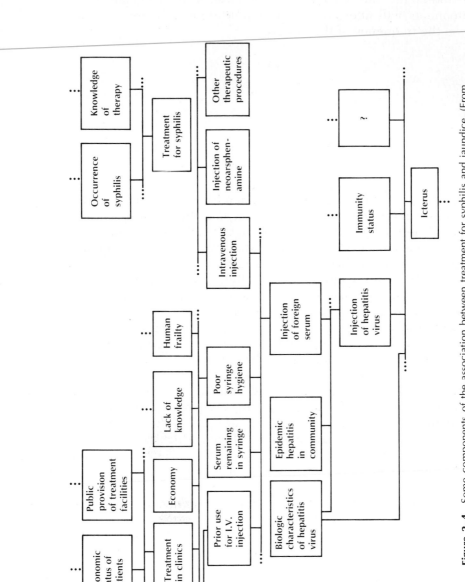

Figure 2-4 Some components of the association between treatment for syphilis and jaundice. (From MacMahon, B., Pugh, T. F., et al.: Epidemiologic Methods. Little, Brown and Company, Boston, 1960, p. 19.)

Figure 2–4 illustrates a web of causation underlying the association which existed between treatment for syphilis and the occurrence of jaundice from hepatitis virus in the days when large numbers of patients with venereal disease were treated in clinics by repeated intravenous injections of arsenicals. It is clear that this model discourages the labelling of any individual factor, including the virus of hepatitis, as **the** cause of disease.

A consequence of the multiplicity of causal chains is that it is possible to interrupt the production of disease by cutting the chains at different points. Further, as noted previously in relation to scurvy (page 21), a complete understanding of causal mechanisms is not prerequisite to development of effective measures for prevention and control. In the 1950's before an agent of hepatitis was isolated, there was some success in reducing the transmission of hepatitis virus from parenteral injections by scrupulous attention to sterilization of needles and syringes and by development of disposable equipment. The association of a specific viral antigen with one form of hepatitis (Blumberg et al., 1967) made possible new approaches to control. It is now feasible to screen potential blood donors to reduce transmission of serum hepatitis from transfused blood.

The Wheel. A model which uses the wheel (Figure 2 5) is another approach to depicting man-environment relations. The wheel consists of a hub (the host or man), which has genetic make-up as its core. Surrounding man is the environment, schematically divided into the three sectors mentioned above — biological, social, and physical. The relative sizes of the different components of the wheel depend upon the specific disease problem under consideration. For hereditary diseases, the genetic core would be relatively large. For a condition like measles, the genetic core would be of lesser importance; the state of immunity of the host and the biological sector of the environment would contribute more heavily.

Like the web of causation, the model of the wheel implies a need to identify multiple etiologic factors of disease without emphasizing the **agent** of disease. For example, the wheel model lays no greater stress on rabies virus than on the animal reservoirs of the disease. However, in contrast to the web of causation, the wheel model does encourage separate delineation of host and environmental factors, a distinction useful for epidemiologic analyses.

Since the discussion of epidemiologic models has been rather abstract, we will illustrate the application of one model, the wheel, to two different health problems.

THE IRISH POTATO FAMINE. The interrelations of these various factors can be seen clearly in the great Irish potato famine

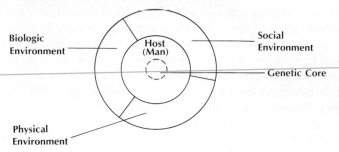

Figure 2–5 Wheel model of man-environment interactions.

of the late 1840's. In 1845 Ireland was an impoverished country with a dearth of natural resources, widespread unemployment, and a rapidly growing population largely dependent on agriculture, especially the potato, for subsistence. A wet spell in the summer of 1845 (change in the physical environment) was followed shortly by the appearance of a blight, a fungal disease, on the potato crop (biological change). The crop failure was countered with successful relief measures (social and political organization) during the winter of 1845–46 in the form of purchase of food from the United States, provision of governmental loans, and relief measures. However, at this juncture there was a change of government in the United Kingdom. The new Whig government was strongly wedded to a *laissez faire* economic policy. Thus when the crop failed again in 1846 they chose not to intervene. The famine which resulted was aggravated by a particularly severe winter. Starving mobs crowded into the towns in search of sustenance from soup kitchens and shelter in workhouses. Not surprisingly, epidemics of typhus and relapsing fever, both louse-borne diseases, broke out, adding to the miseries of dysentery, scurvy, and starvation edema. Over the five years from 1845 through 1850 Ireland lost about two million people, almost one-quarter of its population; half died, the rest emigrated.

Is it meaningful to ask about *the cause* of the starvation and of the diseases which developed during the famine, the scurvy and the typhus fever? True, the agent of typhus fever (a Rickettsia) had to be present. But the lack of response in agricultural policy, even though potato blight had appeared in other countries before it hit Ireland, the blight itself, and the malnutrition, crowding, and lack of sanitary facilities which favored the spread of louse-borne disease all contributed to one of the greatest disasters in history.

LEAD POISONING. A contemporary example of an ecological problem is afforded by lead poisoning in children, a condition of insidious onset which is sufficiently widespread that it has been referred to as a "silent epidemic." This man-made disease illustrates the concepts of natural history and levels of prevention presented in Chapter 1, as well as the interactions of factors in host and environment which lead to disease (Alpert, 1969).

Lead-based paints were commonly used for interior surfaces in this country until the 1940's when they were replaced by titanium-based paint because of the realization that lead in paint could be a source of danger for children. However, elimination of lead from interior paints did not eliminate the hazard of exposure from deteriorating houses built prior to the 1940's nor from improper use of exterior paint on interior surfaces.

In the decaying houses and apartments typical of urban slums, flaking and peeling paint may be ingested by young children with pica. Pica is defined as a tendency to eat nonedible materials. The concurrence of lead in the environment and a child with pica creates the conditions for lead poisoning *(stage of susceptibility)*. If lead is in fact ingested and if the exposure is not overwhelming, there may be a period in which the child appears well despite accumulation of lead in his tissues *(stage of presymptomatic disease)*. If this accumulation is not checked, symptoms eventually appear *(stage of clinical disease)*. The effects of chronic lead poisoning are varied. Characteristic symptoms include hyperirritability, incoordination, loss of appetite, vomiting, and abdominal pain. Finally, lead encephalopathy with brain edema and outright convulsions may ensue. Untreated, the disease may progress to death or evolve into a chronic condition in which there is permanent residual damage in the form of depressed intellectual development and difficulty in learning *(stage of disability)*.

Lead poisoning is preventable. The ideal approach, of course, is primary prevention so that the child does not become exposed to lead. If there is lead in the environment, it should be removed. Theoretically, at least, prevention of pica would also interrupt the chain of events leading to lead poisoning.

In the current state of affairs in which children are still being exposed to lead, preventive measures at a secondary level are needed. Screening efforts include testing the blood for lead and checking houses and apartments to detect lead in the environment. When elevated blood levels are found, treatment consists of deleading with chelating agents. If this is done early enough it can lessen permanent damage. It is not sufficient just to treat a child for accumulation of lead. His environment should be checked and corrected so that he is not again subjected to an excessive exposure.

Further, identification of a child with a high blood lead level or actual lead poisoning should be a signal for further case-finding efforts in that child's family and neighborhood.

Tertiary measures of prevention consist of rehabilitative efforts for all children seen after permanent damage has occurred, including special education classes and similar community facilities. It is to be hoped that tertiary and even secondary therapeutic measures will assume decreasing importance as communities move to combat the problem of lead poisoning.

To what extent does this problem exemplify the complexity of host-environment interactions extending beyond the harmful effects of a single agent, lead? As in the discussion of the Irish potato famine, we will use the wheel as a model to examine this question.

The susceptible host is a child between one and five years of age, usually one to three, in a stage of development when he needs oral gratification and has a real but limited degree of mobility, coupled with an unlimited desire to explore his environment. However, in the face of similar exposures to lead in the environment (flaking paint, peeling window ledges, and so on) not all children are equally likely to develop lead poisoning; only some children exhibit pica. If the tendency to pica is coupled with a substantial environmental exposure, the stage is set for lead poisoning to develop. The tendency to pica is only incompletely understood, but it seems to reflect the quality of parent-child interactions. There is often a background of inadequate mothering, supervision, and stimulation in children with pica. Cultural patterns may also play a role in some cases of pica. The eating of clay by Southern Blacks and of starch by pregnant Black women in Northern cities are cultural patterns which may predispose young children to pica. Thus the social environment contributes importantly to the problem.

In addition to the microlevel indicated above, i.e., the family, the social environment also determines the extent of the problem on a macrolevel through legislation governing availability of paints with lead, through economic patterns which encourage the continued use of substandard housing, and through local housing codes and their enforcement or lack of enforcement. Once excessive exposure has occurred, the availability of organized screening programs and skilled medical care are also important determinants of the outcome.

Finally, aspects of the physical environment other than the load of lead it imposes are also germane. There is a definite seasonal trend in lead poisoning, with a disproportionate number of cases becoming manifest during the summer months. The seasonality of onset is related to the fact that exposure to sunlight increases production of vitamin D, which in turn influences the metabolism of calcium and lead; there may be additional factors as well.

Ecologic Models and the Control of Disease

The multifactorial nature of disease has been emphasized because of its importance for prevention and control. Several implications of an ecologic perspective should be noted.

A full knowledge of etiologic mechanisms is not necessary for effective control measures. We have already pointed out that this was true of scurvy in the eighteenth century. Goldberger quickly came to the conclusion that pellagra was related to nutritional deficiency; very shortly after he began his investigations he suggested on an empiric basis that diet be supplemented by fresh meat, eggs, and milk in areas where pellagra was prevalent. This principle is equally applicable today. It may be possible to achieve significant reductions in the mortality from heart disease and stroke even before the interrelations among factors leading to these conditions are fully understood.

Because of the multiplicity of ecological interactions, it is often possible to affect disease, even that with a known agent, by altering other aspects of man-environment interactions. In diseases in which an organism is carried by flies or mosquitoes, successful control efforts have focussed on the insect, not the agent.

Because ecological relationships are complex, measures for disease control almost inevitably have far-reaching consequences. A striking example of this is the impact of malaria control through DDT spraying after World War II. The elimination of this disease from large areas of the world led to an unchecked growth of population and hence a new cycle of problems related to overpopulation and inadequate food supplies. This principle actually pertains to any environmental manipulation. The effects of the substitution of detergents for soap on water quality are only now becoming fully apparent. We are now coming to appreciate the costs in increased delinquency and other antisocial behavior of the decisions made in the 1950's to build high-rise housing projects rather than units close to the ground. Thus any proposed measure for control of disease should be evaluated in terms of the totality of effects it is likely to have on the ecosystem, at least as far as these can be estimated in advance. A forceful exposition of this thesis has been presented by Barry Commoner in *The Closing Circle* (1971).

SUMMARY

This chapter has delineated the broad scope of epidemiology as covering infectious and noninfectious diseases. Further, epidemiology embraces not only the occurrence of epidemics but also endemic and sporadic occurrence of diseases and conditions.

Infections were noted to differ in their characteristic severity of expression. The fact that some infections tend to be primarily inapparent has consequences for both the control of disease and morbidity statistics.

The interrelation of host and environmental factors in an ecosystem and consequent implications for control of disease were presented in terms of several models—the epidemiologic triangle, the web of causation, and the wheel. The latter was applied to the analysis of two problems, the Irish potato famine and the modern problem of lead poisoning.

STUDY QUESTIONS

2–1 Define the following terms and give an example when appropriate:

Endemic (page 22)
Epidemic (page 22)
Inapparent infection (page 23)
Case fatality rate (page 26)
Ecology (page 27)
Multiple causation of disease (multifactorial etiology) (page 27)
Agent (page 28)
Host factors (page 28)
Specific immunity (page 29)
Environmental factors of disease (biological, social, physical) (page 30 ff.)
Ecological model (page 32)

2–2 In the prevaccine era, cases of measles were more frequent than cases of poliomyelitis. For example, in Maryland for the 27 years from 1916 through 1943, there were approximately 100,000 cases of measles and 1200 cases of poliomyelitis reported. For both diseases most of the reported infections occurred in children.

Does it necessarily follow from the difference in reported number of cases that a higher proportion of young adults were immune to measles than to polio? Explain your answer.

Answer on page 343.

2-3 A. Analyze the problem of injuries from motor vehicle crashes in terms of one of the ecological models presented in this chapter.

B. Indicate some applications of the model to control measures to reduce injuries and deaths.

Answer on page 343.

2-4 Select an infectious disease (e.g., tetanus) which could seem on first thought to be simply related to one causal factor. Indicate how the concept of multiple causation is applicable to this condition.

REFERENCES

Aird, I., Bentall, H. H., et al.: Relationship between cancer of stomach and ABO blood groups. Br. Med. J., *1*:799, 1953.

Allison, A. C.: Protection afforded by sickle-cell trait against subtertian malarial infection. Br. Med. J., *1*:290, 1954.

Alpert, J. J., Breault, H. J., et al.: Subcommittee on accidental poisoning, American Academy of Pediatrics. Prevention, diagnosis and treatment of lead poisoning in childhood. Pediatrics, *44*:291, 1969.

Baker, G.: An essay on the cause of the endemic colic of Devonshire, 1767. Reprinted by Delta Omega Society, American Public Health Association, New York, 1958.

Benenson, A. S. (ed.): Control of Communicable Diseases in Man, 11th ed. American Public Health Association, New York, 1970.

Blumberg, B. S., Gerstley, B. J. S., et al.: A serum antigen (Australia antigen) in Down's syndrome, leukemia and hepatitis. Ann. Intern. Med., *66*:924, 1967.

Bowlby, J.: Maternal Care and Mental Health, 2nd ed. WHO, Geneva, 1952.

Cassel, J.: A comprehensive health program among South African Zulus. In Paul, B. D. (ed.), Health, Culture and Community. Russell Sage Foundation, New York, 1955.

Christensen, P. E., Schmidt, H., et al.: An epidemic of measles in Southern Greenland, 1951. Measles in virgin soil. II. The epidemic proper. Acta. Med. Scand., *144*:430, 1953.

Clarke, C. A., Cowan, W. K., et al.: Relationship of ABO blood groups to duodenal and gastric ulceration. Br. Med. J., *2*:643, 1955.

Commoner, B.: The Closing Circle. Alfred A. Knopf, Inc., New York, 1971.

Durkheim, E.: Suicide: A study in sociology. 1897. Reprinted by Free Press, Glencoe, Ill., 1951.

Eriksson, S.: Studies in α–antitrypsin deficiency. Acta. Med. Scand., (supp. 432) *177*:1, 1965.

Faris, R. E. L., and Dunham, H. W.: Mental disorders in urban areas: An ecological study of schizophrenia and other psychoses. University of Chicago Press, Chicago, 1939.

Gampel, B., Slome, C., et al.: Urbanization and hypertension among Zulu adults. J. Chronic Dis., *15*:67, 1962.

Hare, E. H.: Mental illness and social conditions in Bristol. Br. J. Psychiatry, *102*: 349, 1956.

Henderson, L. J.: Fitness of the Environment, MacMillan, New York, 1913. Reprinted by Beacon Press, Boston, 1958.

Jenkins, C. D.: Psychologic and social precursors of coronary disease. N. Eng. J. Med., *284*:244, 307, 1971.

Kinsey, A. C., Pomeroy, W. B., et al.: Sexual Behavior in the Human Female. W. B. Saunders Company, Philadelphia, 1953.

Lind, J.: A treatise of the scurvy. Kincaird and Donaldson, Edinburgh, 1753. Reprinted in Steward, C. P., and Guthrie, D. (eds.), Lind's treatise on scurvy. University Press, Edinburgh, 1953.

MacMahon, B., and Pugh, T. F.: Suicide in the widowed. Am. J. Epidemiol., *81*:23, 1965.

MacMahon, B., Pugh, T. F., et al.: Epidemiologic Methods. Little, Brown and Company, Boston, 1960.

Mischel, W.: Personality and assessment. John Wiley & Sons, Inc., New York, 1968.

Paul, B. D. (ed.): Health, Culture and Community. Russell Sage Foundation, New York, 1955.

Proshansky, H. M., Ittelson, W. H., et al.: Environmental Psychology: Man and His Physical Setting. Holt, Rinehart and Winston, Inc., New York, 1970.

Rosenman, R. H., Friedman, M., et al.: Coronary heart disease in the Western Collaborative Group Study. J. Chronic Dis., *23*:173, 1970.

Scotch, N. A.: Sociocultural factors in the epidemiology of Zulu hypertension. Am. J. Public Health, *53*:1205, 1963.

Spitz, R. A.: Hospitalism: An inquiry into genesis of psychiatric conditions in early childhood. The Psychoanalytic Study of the Child. I. International Universities Press, New York, 1945.

Stein, Z. A., and Susser, M. W.: Widowhood and mental illness. Br. J. Prev. Soc. Med., *23*:106, 1969.

Syme, S. L., Hyman, M. M., et al.: Some social and cultural factors associated with the occurrence of coronary heart disease. J. Chronic Dis., *17*:277, 1964.

Tvroler, H. A., and Cassel, J.: Health consequence of culture change. II. The effect of urbanization on coronary heart disease in rural residents. J. Chronic Dis., *17*:167, 1964.

Widdowson, E. M.: Mental contentment and physical growth. Lancet, *1*:1316, 1951.

Wilner, D. M., Walkley, R. P., et al.: The Housing Environment and Family Life: A Longitudinal Study of the Effects of Housing on Morbidity and Mental Health. Johns Hopkins University Press, Baltimore, 1962.

Zinsser, H.: Rats, Lice and History. Little, Brown and Company, Boston, 1943.

DESCRIPTIVE EPIDEMIOLOGY: PERSON

3

It is customary to consider epidemiologic studies as falling into two broad categories: study of the *amount* and *distribution* of disease within a population by person, place, and time (called **descriptive** epidemiology) and more focussed study of the *determinants* of disease or *reasons* for relatively high or low frequency in specific groups (called **analytic** epidemiology). This chapter and the next will focus on descriptive epidemiology. To describe the occurrence of a disease fully, three broad questions must be posed and answered. **Who** is affected? **Where** and **when** do the cases occur? In other words, it is necessary to specify **person, place,** and **time.**

Although people may be characterized with respect to an almost infinite number of variables, in practice the number must be limited according to the purposes and resources of the specific study. In epidemiologic study it is almost routine to specify three characteristics of persons—age, sex, and ethnic group or race. These demographic variables will be discussed first.

AGE

Overall, age is the most important determinant among the personal variables. Mortality and morbidity rates of almost all conditions show some relation to this variable. We will first consider relation of age to mortality. Figure 3–1 shows death rates from all causes in the United States (1968) by age, sex, and color. Compare the relative impact of these three variables on death rate.

The four curves portraying age-specific death rates for each race-sex group are quite similar; all are J-shaped. In all four groups

43

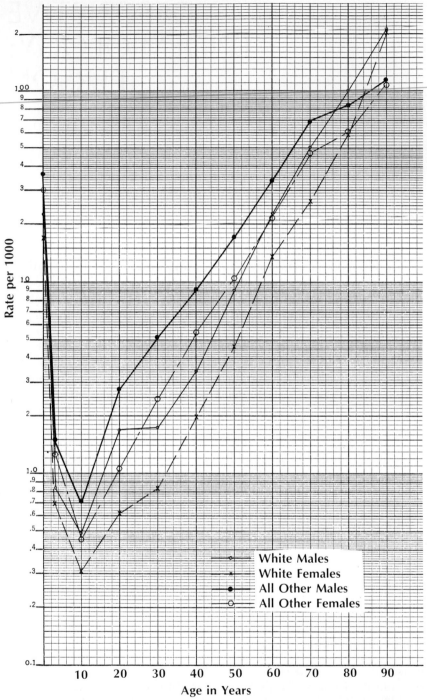

Figure 3-1 Death rates per 1000 by age, color, and sex, United States, 1968 (Semilogarithmic scale). (From National Center for Health Statistics: Vital Statistics of the United States, 1968, Vol. IIA. U.S. Govt. Printing Office, Washington, D.C., 1972.)

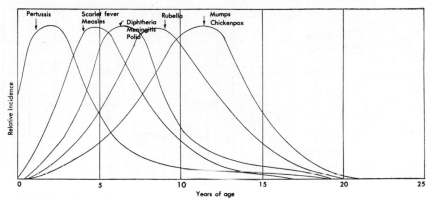

Figure 3–2 Schematized age curves for several acute communicable diseases. (Adapted from Hanlon, J. J.: Principles of Public Health Administration, 5th ed. The C. V. Mosby Company, St. Louis, 1969, p. 358.)

the death rate is fairly high in infancy, then decreases markedly, reaching its lowest point between ages 5 and 14. The rate then climbs gradually until age 40, after which it increases almost exponentially, virtually doubling with each decade. These sharp differences in death rate by age make it necessary to correct ("adjust") for any differences in age composition of population groups if their death rates are to be compared (see Chapter 7).

We will turn now to a consideration of the relation of age to patterns of morbidity. In general, chronic conditions tend to increase with age whereas the relation of age to acute infectious diseases is less consistent.

Young children readily acquire acute respiratory infections. Maternal antibodies transmitted during fetal life protect the infant for approximately the first half-year after birth. Thereafter, protection wanes and the number of respiratory infections increases, tending to peak in the period when the child starts to attend school.

The infectious diseases which confer lifelong immunity (e.g., measles, chickenpox, mumps) also occur mainly in children, varying in peak age of occurrence, as shown in Figure 3–2. For certain infections the age and sex distribution reflects occupational exposure; an example would be brucellosis or anthrax in adult males who are exposed to the agents of these diseases in the course of their work. The striking age-sex distribution of cases of brucellosis in a Midwestern agricultural state in the late 1940's is shown in Figure 3–3.

Age is related not only to the *frequency* of infectious disease

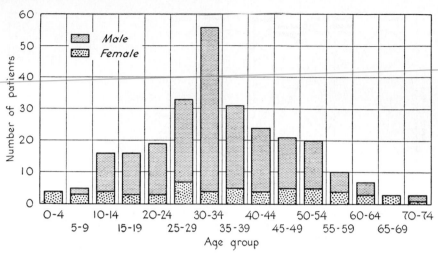

Figure 3–3 Age-sex distribution of 268 proven cases of brucellosis, Minnesota, 1945–1948. (From Magoffin, R. L., Kabler, P., et al.: An epidemiologic study of brucellosis in Minnesota. Public Health Rep., 64:1021, 1949).

but also to *severity*. Certain organisms, e.g., Pneumococcus and Salmonella, tend to produce particularly severe disease in the very young, the very old, and the debilitated. Newborns and the aged are particularly sensitive to bacteria, such as coliform organisms and *Staphylococcus aureus*, which are usually nonpathogenic in other age groups.

The tendency for chronic diseases to increase with age is

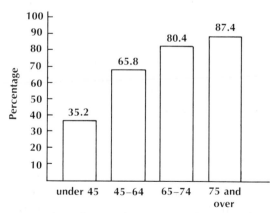

Figure 3–4 Percentage of population with one or more chronic conditions, by age, United States, July, 1963–June, 1965. (From Gleeson, G. A.: Age patterns in medical care, illness, and disability, United States, July 1963–June 1965. USPHS Pub. No. 1000, Series 10, No. 32, U.S. Govt. Printing Office, Washington, D.C., 1966.)

shown in Figure 3–4, which depicts the proportion of the general population in different age groups who, on home interviews, reported having one or more chronic conditions. The effect of age on frequency of certain diseases is especially marked. For example, "arthritis" is ten times more common among persons 45 to 64 than among those under 45 and the rate doubles again for those 65 and over. Other ills which befall people as they age are dental problems, edentia and periodontal disease. One-third of persons 65 and over have no teeth, and less than 10 per cent are free of periodontal disease.

SEX

The most striking aspect of analysis of disease and death rates by sex is the contrast between mortality and morbidity rates. Death rates are higher for males than females, but morbidity rates are generally higher in females.

TABLE 3–1 Mortality Rates from Selected Causes for Males and Females, United States, 1971 *

| Cause | Mortality Rate † | | | Ratio of Male to Female Rate |
	Total	Male	Female	
Emphysema and bronchitis	10.2	18.6	3.7	5.0
Respiratory cancer	29.4	51.8	11.0	4.7
Homicide	10.0	16.3	4.0	4.1
Buccal cavity and pharyngeal cancer	3.1	4.9	1.6	3.1
Tuberculosis	1.8	2.9	1.0	2.9
Motor vehicle accidents	26.6	39.5	14.4	2.8
Other accidents	25.3	37.6	13.8	2.7
Urinary cancer	5.6	8.5	3.2	2.7
Peptic ulcer	3.0	4.6	1.8	2.6
Suicide	11.9	17.2	7.1	2.4
Cirrhosis of the liver	14.7	20.4	9.8	2.1
Ischemic heart disease	226.8	314.8	153.9	2.0
Influenza and pneumonia	19.3	24.9	14.8	1.7
Leukemia	5.7	7.1	4.5	1.6
Digestive cancer	34.8	42.8	28.4	1.5
Nephritis and nephrosis	3.3	3.4	2.8	1.4
Cerebrovascular diseases	65.7	72.5	60.2	1.2
Diabetes mellitus	13.8	13.2	14.2	0.9

*From Division of Vital Statistics, National Center for Health Statistics, unpublished data, 1971.

†Annual rates per 100,000 population, age-standardized.

Figure 3–1 shows that death rates from all causes are higher for males than females at every age; this is true of both whites and nonwhites. *In utero* and neonatal death rates are also higher for males. The higher death rates for males throughout life may be due to sex-linked inheritance or to differences in hormonal balance, environment, or habit patterns. The differential between males and females varies greatly for specific disease entities, as shown in Table 3–1, ranging from a male to female ratio of five in respiratory disease (i.e., emphysema, bronchitis, and respiratory cancer) to slightly less than one for diabetes mellitus. The sex difference is not as large for ischemic heart disease as for certain other conditions. However, because this condition accounts for such a high proportion of deaths, the excess mortality in males from this cause alone is tremendous.

As we indicated above, the higher mortality rates for men are not paralleled by higher rates of illness. Data from several sources indicate that, in almost all age groups and for a number of different conditions, women have more episodes of illness and more physician contact than men. This is true of women past 45 as well as those in the reproductive years of life (Bauer, 1970). Possible explanations for the relatively high morbidity and low mortality in women are that women seek medical care more freely and perhaps

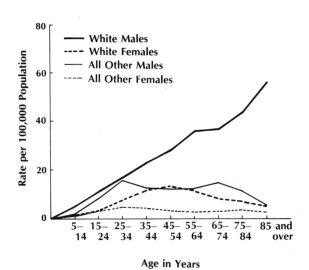

Figure 3–5 Suicide rates by age, color, and sex, United States, 1968. (From National Center for Health Statistics: Vital Statistics of the United States, 1968, Vol. IIA. U.S. Govt. Printing Office, Washington, D.C., 1972.)

at an earlier stage of disease or that the same disease will tend to have a less lethal course in women than in men.

Depression provides a good example of male-female differences in pattern of disease and death. Rates for many forms of depression are higher in women than in men (Silverman, 1968), as is the rate of attempted suicide. However, completed suicides occur with greater frequency in men, particularly among the elderly (Figure 3–5).

ETHNIC GROUP AND COLOR

The classification and recording of data by color or race present conceptual and practical difficulties. Nevertheless, even though it is controversial, such classification has been traditional in health statistics, since (1) many diseases differ markedly in frequency, severity, or both in different racial groups, and (2) statistics by race are helpful for identifying health problems. The fact that many of the observed differences are related to differences in socioeconomic status does not detract from the usefulness of color as an indicator of groups with particular deficiencies in health care.

In the United States, the Bureau of the Census classifies the population as white and "all other." In 1970 these groups comprised 87.4 per cent and 12.6 per cent of the population, respectively. The "others" consist of Negroes* (almost 90 per cent), American Indians, Japanese, Chinese, Filipinos, and all others "not classified as white." The nonwhite population in the United States is at a marked disadvantage with respect to mortality. As shown in Figure 3–1, except for those 75 and over, nonwhites had higher death rates than whites for each age-sex group. The gap has been narrowing in past years, but is far from obliterated, as seen in several important indices of health (Table 3–2).

Certain racial differences in morbidity and mortality are noteworthy. Blacks have substantially higher death rates (adjusted for differences in age composition) from hypertensive heart disease, cerebrovascular accidents, tuberculosis, syphilis, homicide, and accidental death. Whites have higher death rates from arteriosclerotic heart disease, suicide (see Figure 3–5), and leukemia. Whites and nonwhites also differ in the frequency of several neoplasms other

---

*"Negro" is Census Bureau terminology and conforms with earlier usage. The term "Black," which is more commonly used today, has not been adopted in their publications.

TABLE 3–2 Vital Statistics of the United States, 1971 *

	Total	White	All Other
Fetal mortality rate†	13.3	11.6	20.8
Neonatal mortality rate	14.2	13.0	19.6
Infant mortality rate	19.1	17.1	28.5
Maternal mortality rate (per 100,000 live births)	18.8	13.0	45.3
Expectation of life at birth (years)	71.0		
Male		68.3	61.2
Female		75.6	69.3

*National Center for Health Statistics: Vital Statistics in the United States, 1971. U.S. Govt. Printing Office, Washington, D.C., 1974.
†All rates are deaths per 1000 live births, except as noted.

than leukemia. Cancer of the cervix is markedly higher in Blacks, so much so that it is a leading site of cancer causing death in Black females. In contrast, cancer of the breast is appreciably higher in whites. As noted above, some racial differences, such as the virtual restriction of sickle cell anemia to Blacks, are genetically determined. However, most undoubtedly reflect, at least in part, differences in various environmental exposures, in life style, and in the extent and quality of medical care.

Like race, *ethnic stock* is a variable whose effect must be separated from the effects of environment. Studies of international migrants have been particularly valuable for this purpose. Any differences in rates of disease between migrants and those who remained at home must be interpreted cautiously, however, since migrants are usually self-selected. Where the differences are marked, the importance of environment in development of disease is suggested. For example, the rate of cancer of the stomach is very high in Japan. The appreciably higher rate for native Japanese than Japanese descendants in the United States suggests that an environmental factor is important in the etiology of this disease (Haenszel and Kurihara, 1968; Buell and Dunn, 1965).

While the "melting pot" effect in the United States has tended to reduce differences in style of life among the many ethnic groups in the population, there is still variation in patterns of disease, part of which may be attributed to cultural differences. For example, alcoholism is markedly less common among Jews than among many other ethnic groups, although increasing remoteness from old-world religious patterns among Jews born in this country is reducing the difference in patterns of alcohol use (Snyder, 1958).

SOCIAL CLASS

Social class is a widely used concept for ranking or stratifying a total population into subgroups which differ from each other in prestige, wealth, and power. These three dimensions are usually related; a person high in one tends to be high in the others, and vice versa. Despite some discrepancies among the dimensions of social class (e.g., in the United States university professors and skilled blue collar workers differ more in prestige than in income), the concept of "class" is a useful summarizing variable linking occupation, education, area of residence, income, and, in fact, total life style. In view of the pervasiveness of social class in so many aspects of life, it is not surprising that a marked gradient by class in morbidity and mortality is the rule rather than the exception in epidemiologic studies. For a comprehensive survey of the historical literature on life expectancy and mortality by social class Antonovsky (1972) may be consulted.

Because of practical considerations, occupation alone is often used in epidemiologic studies as a measure of overall socioeconomic status. In Great Britain for over a hundred years it has been customary to present social and health data in terms of five well defined occupational ("social") classes. A very large body of information has thus been developed. Table 3–3 shows the classification scheme, along with two indices of health, standardized mortality ratios for males, and infant mortality rates. (For a definition of standardized mortality ratio, see Chapter 7.)

TABLE 3–3 Standardized Mortality Ratios[*] for Males Aged 20–64 and Infant Mortality Rates[**] by Occupational Class of Father, England and Wales, 1949–1953[†]

Occupational Class	Standardized Mortality Ratio (Deaths from All Causes)	Infant Mortality Rate
I Professional	98	17.9
II Intermediate	86	22.2
III Skilled	101	28.1
IV Semiskilled	94	33.7
V Unskilled	118	40.7

[*]The ratio for the entire population of males aged 20–64 is 100.
[**]Deaths per 1000 live births.
[†]From Registrar General for England and Wales. Decennial Supplement–1951. Occupational Mortality, Part II. Her Majesty's Stationary Office, London, 1958.

The infant mortality rates show a distinct inverse class gradient. In contrast, mortality ratios for adult males aged 20 to 64 show an irregular pattern by class, save for an excess in Class V. The lack of a clear gradient masks opposing trends for different conditions. Tuberculosis and bronchitis, for example, are more common in the lower classes; coronary heart disease and leukemia take a greater toll in the upper classes.

Further analysis of social class differences within specific age groups does reveal a differential by class in mortality rates (Table 3–4). This differential is greater for younger than for older men.

In the United States the poorer health status of nonwhites is probably due in large part to the fact that a disproportionate number of them live in conditions of poverty. The median family income of Negroes in 1970 was $6520, about two-thirds of the median income for white families. In that year about one-third of the Black population, but only 10 per cent of the white, was living below the poverty level (Current Population Reports, 1971). A marked gradient in mortality rate among nonwhites by occupational level (Guralnick, 1962) confirms that socioeconomic status contributes importantly to apparent differentials by color.

Poverty affects utilization of medical care services for a variety of reasons. In addition to having fewer material resources and restricted access to medical care, the poor tend to underutilize available preventive services. Motivation to seek such care entails a concern about health and about future health problems. Surveys of perceived needs among the urban poor show that problems such as employment and housing are so overwhelming that health needs tend to have relatively low priority.

The relation between economic status and health care can be

TABLE 3–4   Average Annual Mortality Rates from All Causes per 100,000 Men by Social Class, England and Wales, 1949–1953[*]

Age Group	Social Class I and II	Social Class IV and V	Ratio of IV and V to I and II
25–34	124	180	1.45
35–44	226	332	1.47
45–54	712	895	1.26
55–64	2097	2339	1.12

[*]From Breslow, L., and Buell, P.: Mortality from coronary heart disease and physical activity of work in California. J. Chronic Dis., *11*:420, 1960.

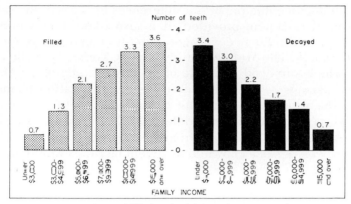

Figure 3–6 Average numbers of filled and of decayed primary and permanent teeth per child aged 6–11, by family income, United States, 1963–1965. (From The Health of Children. Selected Data from the National Center for Health Statistics. U.S. Govt. Printing Office, Washington, D.C., 1970, p. 37.)

clearly identified in Figure 3–6, which shows opposing trends for number of teeth filled and number of teeth decayed in American children 6 to 11 years of age, grouped according to family income.

In mental illness a heavy concentration of schizophrenia in the lowest social classes of urban communities has been found in a number of studies. Two conflicting hypotheses have been developed to account for this phenomenon. According to the *breeder hypothesis*, the conditions of life in lower class society contribute to the development of schizophrenia (Faris and Dunham, 1939). The other explanation, the *drift hypothesis*, states that the inverse relationship between rate of schizophrenia and social class exists not because low socioeconomic status predisposes to schizophrenia, but because the illness itself leads to a downward drift in potential for employment and hence in socioeconomic position. Strong evidence has been developed in support of the drift hypothesis (Goldberg and Morrison, 1963; Dunham, 1965), and recently Birtchnell (1971) found that downward mobility is not limited to schizophrenia, but is generally true of psychosis save for depressive psychosis. Actually both these mechanisms may contribute to a social class gradient through a complex set of interrelations to which genetic susceptibility probably contributes.

Social class is related to mental illness in other ways as well. In 1958 Hollingshead and Redlich published a study of the relation between social class and treated mental illness in New Haven. Not only did they find the social class gradient described above, but they also documented important differences by class in the setting and type of treatment provided. It is also likely that a person's social class will influence whether or not he receives care for psychiatric illness. The Midtown Study in New York City (Srole et al., 1962), which surveyed a sample of the general population, found that for persons severely impaired on a global rating of mental health, the proportion receiving treatment was 19 per cent for upper class, 4 per cent for middle class, but only 1 per cent for lower class subjects. It is clear from this that rates of mental illness based only on persons known to treatment facilities would be quite misleading.

OCCUPATION

Since people spend a substantial portion of their lives at work under widely differing conditions, it is not surprising that occupationally related experiences can exert a profound effect on health and contribute to large differences in mortality (Guralnick, 1962) and morbidity rates. This influence may occur through a variety of exposures — unfavorable physical conditions (heat, cold, changed atmospheric pressure), chemicals, noise, occupationally-induced stress. On the other hand, rates of disease among occupational groups may differ not because of the work itself but because of differential selection into various occupations.

Epidemiologic investigation has related many specific diseases to occupational exposures. Among them are pulmonary fibrosis from exposure to free silica (SiO_2) (Trasko, 1958), mesothelioma and lung and gastrointestinal cancers in asbestos workers (Selikoff et al., 1968), bladder cancer in workers exposed to aniline dyes (Case et al., 1954), and lung cancer among chromate workers (Brinton et al., 1952). It might also be justified, if unconventional, to list drug addiction among physicians, nurses, and Vietnam war veterans as an occupationally acquired condition.

Workers in mining, construction, and agriculture have high rates of injury and death from trauma. In another sense, however, the occupations which are associated with physical activity may be protective. There is some evidence (Morris and Crawford, 1958; Mann et al., 1965) that working in an occupation which demands physical exertion protects against coronary heart disease. Morris (1973) has recently demonstrated that vigorous leisure-time physical activity can serve the same function.

The occupational milieu includes not only physical surroundings but also a social and psychologic climate, an important aspect of which is the degree of stress of the job. Except for extreme conditions, stress is difficult to quantify; a situation which is extremely stressful to one individual may be emotionally neutral for another. To test possible effects of stress on health, Cobb and Rose (1973) selected for study a group incontrovertibly subject to a high level of occupational stress, air traffic controllers. The work of this group is unusually stressful because of the constant vigilance required and the potentially disastrous effects of errors in judgment. When the health records of the controllers were compared with a control group, the controllers were found to have higher rates of hypertension, peptic ulcer, and possibly diabetes.

If specific occupational risks are identified and corrective programs instituted, then successive groups of workers can be followed to determine whether the risk has been eliminated. Seltser and Sartwell (1965) studied the mortality experience of several medical specialty groups to test whether occupational exposure to radiation shortens life. Three specialty groups were selected — radiologists, internists, and opthalmologists-otolaryngologists — to provide a gradient of occupationally-related exposure to radiation. Mortality was analyzed for two time periods, 1935 to 1944 and 1955 to 1958. It could be expected that the level of occupational exposure would have declined in the interval.

In the earlier period, the predicted gradient in mortality was noted in all age groups; radiologists had the highest death rates, the opthalmologists and otolaryngologists the lowest. In the later period there was still a difference among the older physicians, but not among the younger ones. This study, which is basically analytic rather than descriptive, is cited here to illustrate the effects of occupational exposure on health and the way in which disease and death rates can be used to monitor health hazards.

In interpreting differences in morbidity and mortality among occupational groups, it must be remembered that state of health itself may determine entry into a specific occupation. Undemanding jobs may attract people in poor health, and demanding jobs selectively include only those in good health.

Occupational selection was demonstrated by Morris and his colleagues in studies done to test the hypothesis that physical activity at work protects against coronary heart disease (CHD). In one study, coronary heart disease rates were compared for drivers and conductors of the London transport system (Morris et al., 1953). The drivers spend the day sitting; the conductors are much more active. The rate of CHD was found to be lower among the conductors. However, there was also evidence that the two groups differed initially. By obtaining indirect measures of physique through records of the sizes of uniforms issued to the men, an approach labelled "the epidemiology of uniforms," Morris demonstrated that drivers were more corpulent than conductors even in their twenties (Morris et al., 1956).

MARITAL STATUS

It has been observed repeatedly over the past hundred years that marital status is associated with level of mortality for both sexes. Death rates, for most specific diseases and from all causes combined, have generally been found to vary from lowest to highest in the following order: married, single, widowed, and divorced. Although better health of the married may be attributed in part to the psychologic and physical support provided by the spouse, the more favorable health record may not be due entirely to the effects of being married. Selective factors also influence marital status; people who get married may be more robust physically or emotionally than those who remain single. Misclassification of marital status on death certificates or in the census (Sheps, 1961; Berkson, 1962) may also contribute to the reported differences.

For women, marital status may also be related to health through differences in sexual exposure, pregnancy, childbearing, and lactation. These etiologic factors differ in relative importance in different diseases. For example, in cancer of the cervix, a disease more common in married than single women, early sexual experience and multiple partners appear to be decisive factors (Martin, 1967). In contrast, for carcinoma of the breast, which is more common among single than married women, hormonal balance is probably of crucial importance. Factors associated with *lower* risk of breast cancer are early age at first pregnancy (MacMahon et al., 1970a, b) and artificial menopause before the age of 40 years (Feinleib, 1968). Sexual activity probably is important only as it affects the risk of pregnancy.

The old idea that prolonged lactation protects against breast cancer was tested recently through an international collaborative study (MacMahon et al., 1970a, b). No support for this hypothesis was found. Large series of cases and controls in 7 countries did not differ significantly with respect to history of lactation.

Pregnancy and childbearing also entail special risks aside from any possible effects on subsequent development of cancer. In early pregnancy the woman is subject to various risks from abortion (either spontaneous or induced) and its complications and from rupture of an ectopic (nonuterine) pregnancy. Toward term toxemia, although decreasing in frequency, still accounts for some mortality. Parturition itself is associated with hazards which include hemorrhage and anesthetic accidents. Complications of the puerperium include sepsis and thromboembolic phenomena, as well as postpartum psychosis. Another aspect of pregnancy is its effect on preexisting disease. Pregnancy tends to exacerbate some conditions (hypertension and rheumatic heart disease) and to unmask certain latent problems (diabetes), while it often leads to remission of others (rheumatoid arthritis).

OTHER FAMILY VARIABLES

The preceding section dealt with differentials in death and disease associated with a person's own marital condition. In the terminology of the anthropologist, we have looked at the *family of procreation,* the family during the reproductive years when the person is the actual or potential head of a household. We move now to a consideration of the effects on health of the *family of origin or orientation,* the family into which a person is born or with which he spends his formative years. Numerous aspects of the family of orientation may be examined: the number of generations represented in the household; whether both parents are present; the number of children; the position of the "index person" in the sibship; the age of both parents at the child's birth; religion of the parents; presence of any marked discrepancy in age, religion, or social class of origin of the two parents, and so on. Although it is difficult to establish an etiologic significance for these variables separately since they tend to be interrelated, it is worth considering a few factors individually.

Family Size

Family size is associated with social class, large families being more common among the poor. In large families, especially if they are poor, children may be at a disadvantage since many persons have to share the family's limited resources. The current trend toward a lowered birth rate and smaller families has important implications for changes in life style and hence changes in health.

Birth Order

A variety of findings relating to birth order have been reported, from an increased representation of first-borns among eminent and highly educated persons, to association of birth order with diverse diseases—asthma, schizophrenia, peptic ulcer, and pyloric stenosis. There is no doubt that birth order does play a part in a person's life experiences. The first-born in particular receives a kind of attention from his family which is not duplicated for his younger sibs. However, studies of birth order are fraught with danger of bias. Schooler (1972) has stressed the biassing effects of trends in family size over time. Others have emphasized the errors inherent in studies based on incomplete sibships. For example, by reanalyzing the data from several widely quoted studies which had shown a predominance of first-borns among infants with pyloric stenosis, Huguenard and Sharples (1972) found no such excess.

Maternal Age

Maternal age is known to be of distinct etiologic importance in a number of congenital malformations. Figure 3–7 shows that several malformations have a J- or U-shaped incidence curve, with high rates at one or both extremes of maternal age, particularly the upper end of the age range. The outstanding example is Down's syndrome (mongolism). In European populations the risk of this anomaly is less than 1 in 1000 births for women under the age of 30. It then increases. For women between 40 and 44 years of age it is close to 1 in 100, and at ages 45 and above it is about 1 in 50.*

Parental Deprivation

Effective loss of one or both parents by death, divorce, or separation has been found to be particularly high among certain types of patients—those with psychiatric and psychosomatic disorders, persons with tuberculosis, those who have attempted suicide, and accident repeaters (Chen and Cobb, 1960). This suggests a particular need for intensified health supervision for children who have lost one or both parents. Unfortunately, this group is very large; the 1970 census revealed that one-sixth of all children under 18 in the United States were living with neither or only one parent. Com-

---

*Several forms of chromosomal abnormality are associated with Down's syndrome. Only one, that associated with trisomy-21, is related to maternal age.

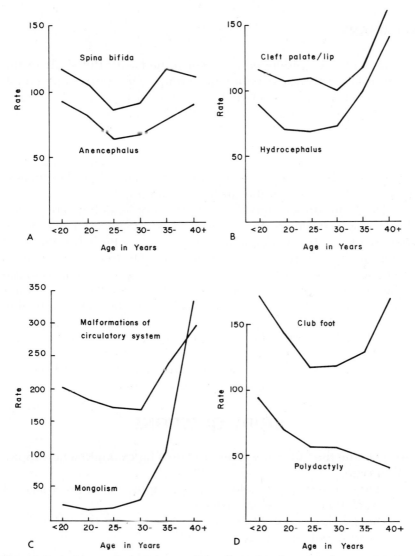

Figure 3–7 Incidence of selected congenital malformations by maternal age, upstate New York, 1950–1960 (cases per 100,000 total births). (From Gittelson, A. M., and Milham, S., Jr.: Vital record incidence of congenital malformations in New York State. In Neel, J. V., Shaw, M. W., et al. (eds.), Genetics and the Epidemiology of Chronic Diseases. USPHS Pub. No. 1163, U.S. Govt. Printing Office, Washington, D.C., 1965.)

pounding the problem is the fact that a large proportion of these children are concentrated in lower class families.

SUMMARY

Descriptive epidemiology is concerned with the study of the distribution of disease in population groups. Descriptive epidemiology summarizes in systematic fashion the basic data on health and the major causes of disease and death. The objectives are (1) to permit evaluation of trends in health and comparisons among countries and among subgroups within countries; (2) to provide a basis for the planning, provision, and evaluation of health services; and (3) to identify problems to be studied by analytic methods and to suggest areas which may be fruitful for investigation.

The major dimensions of descriptive epidemiology are person (host), place, and time. In this chapter we reviewed a number of host characteristics which affect health status. Probably the most important are the attributes of age and sex. Despite the egalitarian aspirations of the country, socioeconomic status and color continue to be important predictors of health status throughout life. Other factors pertinent to health are occupation, marital status, and other family variables.

Although this chapter focussed to a great extent on each host variable separately, it should be remembered that these factors do interact with each other and with environmental factors (discussed in the previous chapter under ecological models).

STUDY QUESTIONS

3–1 Define the following terms and give an example when appropriate:
Descriptive epidemiology (demographic variables) (page 43)
Analytic epidemiology (page 43)
Social class (page 51)
Drift hypothesis (page 53)

3–2 A. Indicate an implication for prevention of suicide that may be drawn from the age-sex-color-specific curves shown in Figure 3–5.
B. List other demographic and social factors which might contribute to observed patterns of suicide? Indicate how knowledge of such risk factors could be used for suicide prevention.

Answer on page 345.

3–3   In a longitudinal study of 800 children in Newcastle, England, it was found that the total incidence of respiratory disease was unrelated to social class. However, the incidence of severe respiratory disease was strongly correlated, with a tenfold difference between children of Class V and those of Class I (Figure 3–8).

List factors which might contribute to the social class differences.

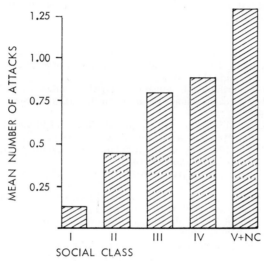

Figure 3–8   Severe respiratory disease in relation to social class in the Newcastle upon-Tyne survey, 1947–1952. (From Court, S. D. M.: Epidemiology and natural history of respiratory infections in children. J. Clin. Pathol., *21*(supp. 2):31, 1968.)

REFERENCES

Antonovsky, A.: Social Class, Life Expectancy and Overall Mortality in Jaco, E.G. Patients, Physicians and Illness. A Source Book in Behavioral Science and Health, 2nd ed. The Free Press, New York, 1972.

Bauer, M. L.: Current Estimates from the Health Interview Survey United States–1968. USPHS Pub. No. 1000, Series 10, No. 60, U.S. Govt. Printing Office, Washington, D.C., 1970.

Berkson, J.: Mortality and marital status. Am. J. Public Health, 52:1318, 1962.

Birtchnell, J.: Social class, parental social class, and social mobility in psychiatric patients and general population controls. Psychol. Med. *1*:209, 1971.

Brinton, H. P., Frasier, E. S., et al.: Morbidity and mortality experience among chromate workers. Public Health Rep., 67:835, 1952.

Buell, P., and Dunn, J. E., Jr.: Cancer mortality among Japanese Issei and Nisei of California. Cancer, *18*:656, 1965.

Case, R. A. M., Hosker, M. E., et al.: Tumors of the urinary bladder in workmen engaged in the manufacture and use of certain dyestuff intermediates in the British chemical industry. Br. J. Ind. Med., *11*:75, 1954.

Chen, E., and Cobb, S.: Family structure in relation to health and disease. J. Chronic Dis. *12*:544, 1960.

Cobb, S., and Rose, R. M.: Hypertension, peptic ulcer, and diabetes in air traffic controllers. J.A.M.A., *224*:489, 1973.

Current Population Reports. Special Studies. The Social and Economic Status of Negroes in the United States, 1970. Bureau of the Census, Series P23, No. 38, U.S. Govt. Printing Office, Washington, D.C., 1971.

Dunham, H. W.: Community and Schizophrenia; An epidemiological analysis. Wayne State University Press, Detroit, 1965.

Faris, R. L., and Dunham, H. W.: Mental Disorders in Urban Areas: An Ecological Study of Schizophrenia and Other Psychoses. University of Chicago Press, Chicago, 1939. Reprinted by Hafner Publishing Company, New York, 1965.

Feinleib, M.: Breast cancer and artificial menopause: A cohort study. J. Natl. Cancer Inst., *41*:315, 1968.

Goldberg, E. M., and Morrison, S. L.: Schizophrenia and social class. Br. J. Psychiatry, *109*:785, 1963.

Guralnick, L.: Mortality by occupation and industry among men 20 to 64 years of age, United States, 1950. Vital Statistics Special Reports 52:2, U.S. Govt. Printing Office, Washington, D.C., 1962.

Haenszel, W., and Kurihara, M.: Studies of Japanese migrants: I. Mortality from cancer and other diseases among Japanese in the United States. J. Natl. Cancer Inst., *40*:43, 1968.

Hollingshead, A. B., and Redlich, F. C.: Social Class and Mental Illness: A Community Study. John Wiley & Sons, Inc., New York, 1958.

Huguenard, J. R., and Sharples, G. E.: Incidence of congenital pyloric stenosis in birth series. J. Chronic. Dis., *25*:727, 1972.

MacMahon, B., Cole, P., et al.: Age at first birth and breast cancer risk. Bull. WHO, *43*:209, 1970a.

MacMahon, B., Lin, T. M., et al.: Lactation and cancer of the breast. A summary of an international study. Bull. WHO, *42*:185, 1970b.

Mann, G. V., Shaffer, R. D., et al.: Physical fitness and immunity to heart disease in Masai. Lancet, *2*:1308, 1965.

Martin, C. E.: Marital and coital factors in cervical cancer. Am. J. Public Health, *57*:803, 1967.

Morris, J. N., Chave, S. P. W., et al.: Vigorous exercise in leisure-time and the incidence of coronary heart-disease. Lancet, *1*:333, 1973.

Morris, J. N., and Crawford, M. D.: Coronary heart disease and physical activity of work. Br. Med. J., *2*:1485, 1958.

Morris, J. N., Heady, J. A., et al.: Coronary heart-disease and physical activity of work. Lancet, *2*:1053, 1111, 1953.

Morris, J. N., Heady, J. A., et al.: Physique of London busmen. Epidemiology of uniforms. Lancet, *2*:569, 1956.

Schooler, C.: Birth order effects: Not here, not now. Psychol. Bull., *78*:161, 1972.

Selikoff, I. J., Hammond, E. C., et al.: Asbestos exposure, smoking and neoplasia. J.A.M.A., *204*:106, 1968.

Seltser, R., and Sartwell, P. E.: The influence of occupational exposure to radiation on the mortality of American radiologists and other medical specialists. Am. J. Epidemiol. *81*:2, 1965.

Sheps, M. C.: Marriage and mortality. Am. J. Public Health, *51*:547, 1961.

Silverman, C.: Epidemiology of Depression. John Hopkins University Press, Baltimore, 1968.

Snyder, C. R.: Alcohol and the Jews. A Cultural Study of Drinking and Sobriety. Free Press, Glencoe, Ill., 1958.

Srole, L., Langner, T. S., et al.: Mental Health in the Metropolis, the Midtown Manhattan Study. Vol. I. McGraw-Hill, Inc., New York, 1962.

Trasko, V. M.: Silicosis, a continuing problem. Public Health Rep., 73:839, 1958.

DESCRIPTIVE EPIDEMIOLOGY: PLACE AND TIME

4

In these considerations lie the germs of a science, which . . . will give: firstly, a picture of the occurrence, the distribution and the type of diseases of mankind, in distinct epochs of time, and at various points of the earth's surface; and secondly, will render an account of the relations of these diseases to the external conditions surrounding the individual and determining his manner of life (Hirsch, 1883).

Hirsch's statement, although written almost a century ago to define the science he called geographic and historical pathology, embodies current thinking about the importance of place and time to disease. It states explicitly that the frequency of disease often varies by geographic location and period of time. It implies that these variations in frequency provide etiologic clues. In this chapter we will explore some sources, manifestations, and implications of variations in frequency of disease by place and time.

PLACE

Frequency of disease can be related to place of occurrence in terms of areas set off either by natural barriers, such as mountain ranges, rivers, or deserts, or by political boundaries.

Natural Boundaries

Natural boundaries are likely to be more useful than political lines for understanding the etiology of disease. An area defined by natural boundaries may have a high or low frequency of certain diseases because it is characterized by some particular environmental or climatic condition, such as temperature, humidity, rainfall, altitude, mineral content of soil, or water supply. Moreover, the physical boundaries separating the region from neighboring areas may have led to the isolation of a population group distinguished by genetic inheritance or social custom. Natural contours also affect economic activities and patterns of transportation, including access to medical care facilities.

Characteristics of the physical and biological environment (Chapter 2) can cause certain diseases to be particularly prevalent in certain areas. Diseases which depend upon specific environmental conditions may be considered *place diseases.* Parasitic and other infectious diseases, which exhibit marked differences in occurrence between tropical and temperate areas, exemplify such place diseases. Other examples are endemic goiter in iodine-deficient inland regions and certain fungus diseases, or mycoses. One of the mycoses, coccidiodomycosis, also known as "San Joaquin Valley fever," is found in the hot, arid southwest portion of the United States. Another, histoplasmosis, is found along the inland river valleys where humidity is high. Figure 4–1 shows the pronounced geographic variation in histoplasmin sensitivity (i.e., positive skin test to an extract of the organism *Histoplasma capsulatum*) among United States naval recruits who were lifetime residents of one county. The percentage of reactors was found to vary from less than 5 per cent in many areas to over 80 per cent along the river valleys in the central portion of the country.

Another example of "place" epidemiology is the irregular geographic distribution of mottled dental enamel, a condition found to be related to the fluoride content of drinking water. Knowledge of this association led first to an identification of the role of fluoride in preventing dental caries, and subsequently to artificial fluoridation of drinking water supplies.

Two other conditions with distinctive geographic distribution are Burkitt's lymphoma and multiple sclerosis. Burkitt's lymphoma (Burkitt, 1962) is a malignant neoplasm endemic to New Guinea and equatorial Africa. The localization of this neoplasm to specific low-lying areas of high temperature and rainfall, as well as its peak incidence in early childhood, suggested that a vector-borne organism could be the etiologic agent. Further evidence of an infectious etiology has been achieved by the repeated recoveries of a virus known as Epstein-Barr (EB) virus from cultures of Burkitt tumor cells and by the regular finding of high titers to EB virus in African patients with Burkitt's lymphoma (Epstein, 1971).

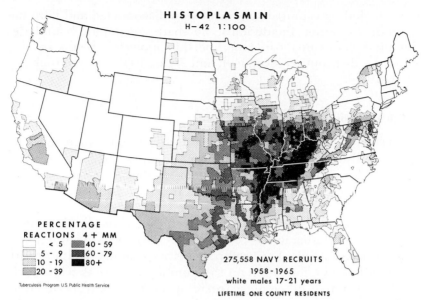

Figure 4-1 Geographic variation in the frequency of reactors to histoplasmin. (From Edwards, L. B., Acquaviva, F. A., et al.: An atlas of sensitivity to tuberculin, PPD-B, and histoplasmin in the United States. Am. Rev. Resp. Dis., 99(supp.):1, 1969.)

Multiple sclerosis, a remitting but progressive neurologic disease which typically develops in young adults, shows a different type of geographic pattern. The disease is rare between the equator and 30 to 35° latitude. It then increases with increasing distance from the equator in both northern and southern hemispheres.

In contrast to the above are two examples of geographically localized phenomena which depend largely on social and cultural influences. The first concerns intellectual development in children living in isolated areas in the southeastern portion of the United States. In comparison with children of similar ethnic background living in less isolated villages with better schools, the mountain children demonstrate appreciably lower IQ's, especially on verbal tests. Apparently their physical isolation limits the educational and cultural exposures necessary for normal development.

The second illustration relates to kuru, a progressive, rapidly fatal neurologic disease localized to one area of New Guinea mainly among one tribal group, the Fore natives. This condition apparently results from cannibalistic practices which lead to exposure to an infective agent with a long latent period. As the area has come under control of the Australian government, various tribal practices, including cannibalism, have been discouraged and kuru has been disappearing. Incidentally, no sharp geographic boundaries delimit the kuru area; tribal membership appears to be the key factor in the distribution (Gajdusek and Zigas, 1957; Hornabrook and Moir, 1970).

Political Subdivisions

Despite the relation of natural boundaries and climate to occurrence of disease, it is often more convenient to deal with disease statistics by political units since data for these are more readily available. The political units may vary in size from entire nations to counties, towns, and boroughs. Not only do political subdivisions provide denominators for rates from census data, but local agencies often collect information on cases (numerator) because of their own administrative needs. For example, a city or county health department will need information on the number of persons with newly diagnosed, active tuberculosis residing in its area of jurisdiction, the number of premature infants who may require supervision by public health nurses, or the number of handicapped children unable to attend school.

Natural and political boundaries may be coterminous. Thus, the Mississippi River establishes state borders and the Andes mountains separate Argentina and Chile. Often, however, political boundaries are arbitrary, and either bisect homogeneous areas or join disparate ones. The latter problem is exemplified by the variation in health and socioeconomic indicators within almost any large city. In Philadelphia, for example, the infant mortality rate of 23.0 per 1000 in 1971 masked a more than twofold variation in rates, from 13.6 to 31.5 for different health districts of the city.

Where political boundaries join heterogeneous areas, it is necessary to examine the data by subdivisions in order to appreciate the distribution of disease and to plan appropriately for health services. Conversely, where political subdivisions separate units which perhaps should be joined, there is a great advantage in regionalization. This concept is coming to the fore increasingly as communities grapple with such problems as water supply, air pollution, vector control, and provision of emergency medical care. In accordance with the concept of providing statistics useful for regional planning, the census now presents data in terms of large urban conglomerates known as standard metropolitan statistical areas (Chapter 10).

For all large cities, geographic units called census tracts have been designated. At least initially, these were homogeneous in character. Over time some tracts have tended to become diversified in income, racial composition, and so on. Nevertheless, such heterogeneity has not significantly impaired the usefulness of census tracts as ecological units. Because of the wealth of social and economic data available from the United States census, classification by census tract continues to yield information on social and economic factors as well as on geographic distribution of disease. Of course, numbers of cases of disease for a census tract or other designated area must be converted to rates before the frequency of disease can be interpreted; without this information differences in population density alone could make a disease appear prevalent or rare in a given area.

Mapping of Environmental Factors

To examine distribution of disease even more specifically, it is common practice to plot individual cases by census tract or block on maps. Superimposed representation of such environmental factors as water supply, milk routes, direction of prevailing winds, school buses, and so on may sometimes provide a clue about mode of spread.

The following example illustrates the usefulness of such environmental analysis. Early in the summer of 1960, an outbreak of hepatitis occurred in two small communities in Connecticut (Rindge et al., 1962). There were 21 cases in July of that year and 9 cases in August. Investigation revealed that all but one of the 20 children in the initial wave of cases attended a consolidated school. The school went from kindergarten through grade six, but illness was confined to grades three through six. There were no cases among children who attended a nearby parochial school.

Localization of the cases to grades three through six ruled out person-to-person spread on school buses as well as transmission by food and milk in the cafeteria, since all children shared such exposure. Study of the water supply (Figure 4–2) provided an explanation. Ever since a valve had been shut a few months earlier, there were essentially two separate water supplies in the school. One well, the east well, supplied three fountains used by children in kindergarten through grade two; none of these children developed hepatitis. Water from the other two wells, which intercommunicated, supplied the upper grades. On examination during the subsequent school year, the west well repeatedly showed bacterial contamination.

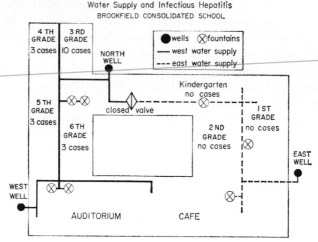

Figure 4-2 Diagram of water supply and cases of infectious hepatitis in a grade school in Connecticut, 1960. (From Rindge, M. E., Mason, J. O., et al.: Infectious hepatitis. Report of an outbreak in a small Connecticut school due to water-borne transmission. J.A.M.A., *180*:36, 1962.)

Urban-Rural Differences

In describing trends in urban-rural distribution of the United States population, probably the central fact is the extensive migration from the farms to the cities over the past 100 years. Underlying factors have been the mechanization of farm work and consequent decreased number of jobs on the farms, coupled with the availability of jobs and other attractions in the cities. Whereas 50 years ago the population was almost evenly split between rural and urban areas, today the population is largely urbanized (73.5 per cent in the 1970 census). A significant proportion of those who have remained in the rural areas are disadvantaged through illiteracy, lack of job opportunities, malnutrition, disease, and a shortage of medical personnel and facilities. Some rural areas in particular—Appalachia, the bayou country of Louisiana, the more remote Indian reservations—maintain an isolation which has kept their residents apart from many of the advances of the twentieth century.

There are a number of health problems peculiar to working farms. Farm accidents remain a serious cause of disability and death; they are the result of the use of mechanized equipment without the benefit of the training and supervision that are standard in industrial operations. Other potential hazards related to agricultural work include silo-filler's disease, skin cancers from repeated exposure to ultraviolet radiation, and exposures to pesticides and to a variety of microorganisms (e.g., anthrax, tetanus, actinomyces).

One group found in rural areas in many parts of the country consists of migrant workers who shuttle from one community to another following the crops. Although the appalling circumstances in which they live have been publicized widely, their health problems remain serious. As recently as 1972 a massive outbreak of typhoid fever (over 200 cases) occurred in a migrant labor camp in Florida because of pollution of the camp's water supply.

On the other hand, cities also pose a variety of hazards to health. One of the chief problems is air pollution. The concentration of industrial plants and large numbers of automobiles has led to a critical deterioration of the quality of air in urban areas. The Environmental Protection Agency and its counterparts in state and local governments have sketched in broad outline the extensive changes needed to reverse environmental deterioration. Despite some partial successes, translation of their proposals into a comprehensive program of action faces grave obstacles.

In addition to environmental problems, the big cities continue to be faced with the consequences of anomie and social disorganization, including homicide and other acts of violence, as well as patterns of behavior which favor the spread of venereal disease and drug abuse. As an incidental note, these problems are not limited to big cities. Smaller communities are experiencing similar troubles. Other effects on health of the change from a rural to an urban setting have been noted previously (page 31).

In earlier days the life patterns of rural and urban dwellers probably differed more than they do today. The isolation of rural residents has decreased because of improved transportation and communication. Similarly, rural areas have become more accessible to city dwellers. Further, with the development of extensive suburban areas around big cities, large numbers of working people are exposed to the hazards of an urban setting by day and then come home to an environment which holds some of the dangers typical of rural areas, such as exposure to rickettsial disease from tick bites, to mosquito-borne encephalitides, and, occasionally, to rabies from feral animals. Other factors have also reduced rural-urban differences in patterns of occupational disease. The programs to cradicate bovine tuberculosis and brucellosis in herds of animals have decreased the risk of these diseases for farm workers.

International Comparisons

One of the most important political boundaries for epidemiologic purposes is that between nations. Disease and death rates for each country provide information needed to monitor the country's health status. International comparisons of these health indices are widely used to assess relative progress in control of disease. (See, for example, the discussion in Chapter 9 on infant mortality rates.) They are also of interest because they may provide clues to causation of disease. Contrasts in the frequency of a particular disease can be utilized for studies of possible association with climatic and ecological factors as well as with socioeconomic indices, customs, and genetic constitution.

In making comparisons of disease frequency among countries, one should be aware that apparent differences can be created by confounding factors, such as variation in accuracy of diagnosis, in

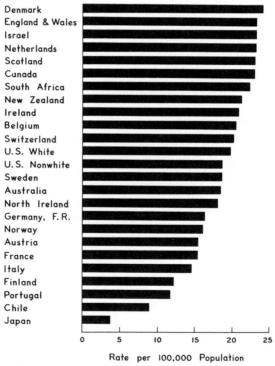

Figure 4–3 Age-adjusted death rates for malignant neoplasm of the breast for females, selected countries, 1962–1963. (From Lilienfeld, A. M., Pedersen, E., et al.: Cancer Epidemiology: Methods of Study. Johns Hopkins University Press, Baltimore, 1967, p. 58.)

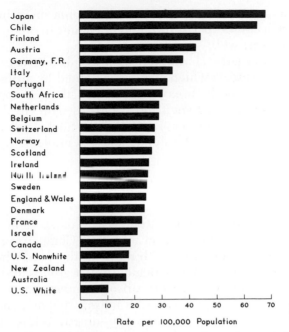

Japan
Chile
Finland
Austria
Germany, F.R.
Italy
Portugal
South Africa
Netherlands
Belgium
Switzerland
Norway
Scotland
Ireland
North Ireland
Sweden
England & Wales
Denmark
France
Israel
Canada
U.S. Nonwhite
New Zealand
Australia
U.S. White

0   10   20   30   40   50   60   70
Rate per 100,000 Population

Figure 4-4 Age-adjusted death rates for malignant neoplasm of stomach for males, selected countries, 1962–1963. (From Lilienfeld, A. M., Pedersen, E., et al.: Cancer Epidemiology: Methods of Study. Johns Hopkins University Press, Baltimore, 1967, p. 57.)

completeness of reporting, and in classification and statistical processing of data.

One example of differences in diagnostic labelling comes from the field of respiratory disease. For many years there was debate over apparently major differences in the nature of the chronic, obstructive respiratory disease seen in Great Britain and the United States, Great Britain having higher rates of bronchitis, the United States of emphysema. After conducting a study which applied a standardized questionnaire and examination protocol to "typical" patients in both countries, Fletcher and his collaborators (1964) concluded that "the distinction between British bronchitis and American emphysema is largely semantic."

Similarly, an extensive series of cross-national studies of psychiatric diagnosis (Cooper et al., 1970; Cooper, 1972) demonstrated differences in psychiatric labelling by psychiatrists in New York and London. This can explain in part the markedly higher rates of schizophrenia in the United States and of manic-depressive psychosis in the United Kingdom. The New York psychiatrists were found to apply the diagnosis of schizophrenia more broadly than their London counterparts (or their colleagues in other parts of the United States as well).

Many international differences are substantively large and exceed discrepancies which may be explained by artifacts. For example, for cancer of the breast and stomach, there is approximately a sixfold difference between the countries with the highest and lowest death rates (Figures 4–3 and 4–4). Such marked contrasts provide opportunities to formulate and test etiologic hypotheses.

Study of Migrants

One type of study which attempts to separate genetic from environmental factors focusses on migrants. Comparison of disease and death rates for migrants with those for their kin who remained at home permits study of genetically similar groups under different environmental conditions. Comparison of migrants with residents of the new country or area provides information on genetically different groups living in a similar environment. While such studies are helpful in separating factors of place from those of person, selective factors in migration must always be kept in mind during interpretation of findings.

Several groups of migrants have been particularly valuable sources of epidemiologic information. Death rates of Japanese migrants to the United States have been studied intensively because the patterns of death from cancer and cardiovascular disease are very dissimilar in the two countries (Haenszel and Kurihara, 1968). Figures 4–3 and 4–4 illustrate differences observed in cancer of the breast and cancer of the stomach (see also page 50).

The great influx of Jews from all over the world to Israel has been useful for epidemiologic study. For example, the peculiar geographic distribution of multiple sclerosis was noted earlier in this chapter. When the rates of this disease were studied in immigrants to Israel (Alter et al., 1962), they were found to reflect the rates characteristic of the country of origin. Groups whose rates were high originally remained at high risk even years after migration. It is possible that this may reflect exposure to an infectious agent early in life.

Cancer of the colon provides an interesting contrast to the pattern described for multiple sclerosis. For reasons which are still obscure, death rates from cancer of the colon are higher in urban than rural areas in the United States and elsewhere. In evaluation of death rates by current and previous area of residence, Haenszel and Dawson (1965) found that death rates from cancer of the colon tend to reflect the type of residence (i.e., urban or rural) at death rather than residence in early life.

TIME

Study of disease occurrence by time is a basic aspect of epidemiologic analysis. Occurrence is usually expressed on a monthly or annual basis. As mentioned earlier, decennial years (e g , 1960, 1970) are particularly useful because they provide a census count rather than an estimated population for calculation of rates. If there are not enough cases of a particular disease annually for stable rates, cases for several years around a census may be combined (e.g., 1969 to 1971).

Three major kinds of change with time may be identified. The first consists of long-term variations called *secular trends*. The second are periodic fluctuations on an annual or other basis, *cyclic changes*. Finally, there are short-term fluctuations, such as are found in epidemics of infectious disease. Secular trends and cyclic changes will be discussed here. Short-term fluctuations will be discussed in Chapter 12.

Secular Trends

This term refers to changes over a long period of time, years or decades. Such trends may occur in both infectious and noninfectious conditions.

Figure 4–5 shows the trends in the leading causes of death for several age groups between 1900 and 1964. Diphtheria, tuberculosis, gastrointestinal infections, pneumonia, and influenza all showed a marked drop in frequency over this time period. As a consequence of the decline in infectious causes of death, accidents emerged as the leading cause of death over the time period despite the absence of any marked trend in death rates from accidents.

An interesting example of a secular trend from the field of growth and development is the change in age at menarche (i.e., onset of menstruation) in northwest Europe between 1840 and 1970 (Figure 4–6). Changes in nutrition probably account for the striking decline in menarchal age.

Secular trends in this century have occurred in death rates from cancer of several sites. In Figures 4–7 and 4–8 note the declining

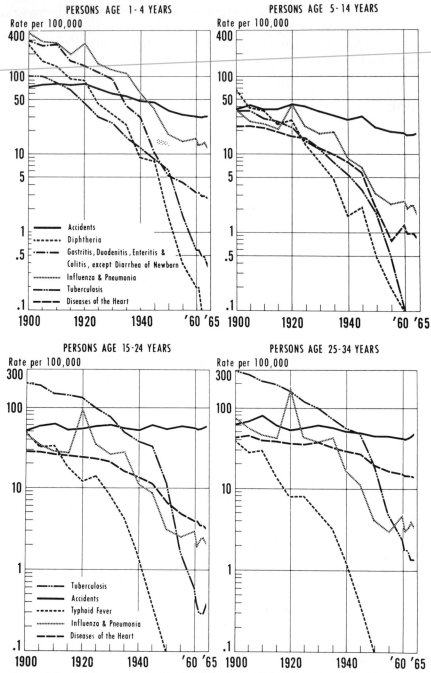

Figure 4–5 Death rates for the five leading causes of death for persons aged 1–4, 5–14, 15–24 and 25–34 years, United States, 1900–1964. (From Iskrant, A. P., and Joliet, P. V.: Accidents and Homicide. Harvard University Press, Cambridge, Mass., 1968.)

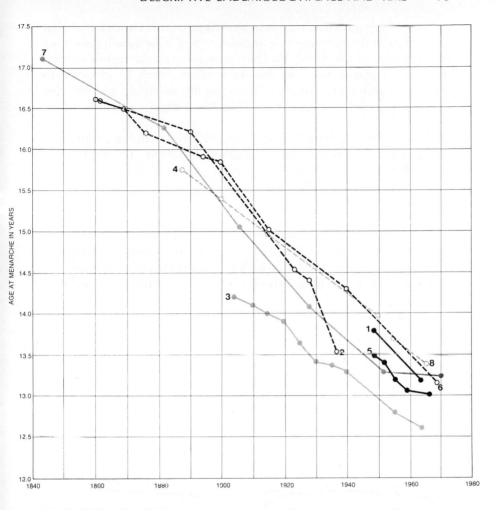

death rate from cancer of the stomach and the rise in cancer of the lung and pancreas. In contrast, there has been little change in the death rate from breast cancer over this time. The secular trend in death rates from lung cancer is discussed further in Chapter 5. Other examples of secular trends are presented in Figures 1–3 (emphysema) and 4–16 (rheumatic fever and chorea).

In assessing secular trends in *deaths* one must consider to what extent they reflect changes in *incidence* and how much they may reflect changes in *survival*. Further, apparent secular trends in morbidity or mortality may be due to artifacts, such as changes in physicians' index of suspicion, in diagnostic methods, and in rules for reporting and coding cause of death on death certificates (see Chapter 8).

In general, the larger an observed difference the more likely it is to be real. But even with substantial apparent change, such as that which occurred in mortality from stomach and lung cancer, improved diagnostic ability should be ruled out as a possible explanation. A study of the decrease in death rates from cancer of the stomach (Pedersen and Magnus, 1961) indicated that the change appeared to exceed the possible effect of a shift in diagnostic fashion from one form of abdominal cancer to another. Similarly, Gilliam (1955) found evidence for a true increase in lung cancer, although he concluded that early misdiagnosis of some lung cancer as

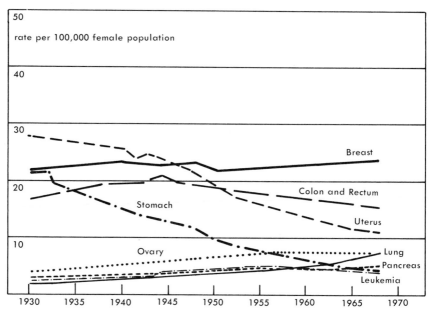

Figure 4–7 Age-adjusted death rates* per 100,000 population, by selected sites of cancer for females, United States, 1930–1968. (From National Vital Statistics Division and Bureau of the Census, United States.)

---

*Rate for the female population standardized for age on the 1940 United States population.

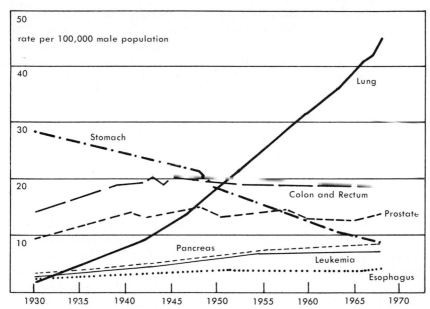

50

rate per 100,000 male population

40

Lung

30

Stomach

20

Colon and Rectum

Prostate

10

Pancreas

Leukemia

Esophagus

1930   1935   1940   1945   1950   1955   1960   1965   1970

Figure 4–8   Age-adjusted death rates* per 100,000 population, by selected sites of cancer, United States, 1930–1968. (From National Vital Statistics Division and Bureau of the Census, United States.)

*Rate for the male population standardized for age on the 1940 United States population.

tuberculosis probably inflated the apparent magnitude of the increase over time.

One consequence of marked secular trends is their effect on the age distribution of a disease at a given point in time. For full understanding of the dynamics underlying a secular change, it may, therefore, be necessary to analyze the disease in terms of the experience of *birth cohorts* (i.e., groups of people born within defined periods of time). This will be discussed at greater length in Appendix 4–1.

Cyclic

Cyclic change refers to recurrent alterations in the frequency of disease. Cycles may be annual (seasonal) or have some other periodicity. For example, measles epidemics used to occur every two or three years (see Figure 12–9). Influenza A epidemics tend to occur in two- to three-year cycles, whereas epidemics of Influenza B are more widely spaced, recurring every four to six years (see Figure 12–13).

Seasonal fluctuations in frequency of disease and death are observed in many conditions, both infectious and noninfectious. The overall death rate (all causes) fluctuates markedly by season, with rates higher in winter than summer. Figure 4–9 shows this seasonal fluctuation as well as two brief periods of excess mortality associated with epidemics of influenza in January and February of 1970 and 1972.

Seasonal analysis has been particularly useful for evaluation of the possible role of insect vectors since temperature and humidity provide the limiting conditions for this kind of transmission. Seasonal variation in infectious diseases may also be related to differences in people's activity. For example, bathing and fishing provide exposure to Leptospira, a type of spirochete, in water contaminated with the urine of infected animals. However, the seasonal occurrence characteristic of many infections remains puzzling. Explanations such as congregation of children indoors with the opening of school (e.g., for influenza epidemics) and changes in host resistance due to drying of mucosal surfaces by central heating are not entirely satisfactory. The seasonal nature of some diseases spread largely by the enteric route has also not been explained fully.

Certain presumably noninfectious conditions also show seasonal variation. The seasonal occurrence of drownings and skiing injuries could easily be predicted, but other seasonal relations remain relatively obscure.

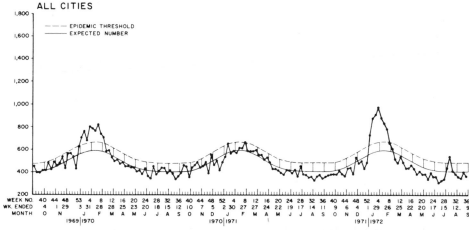

Figure 4–9 Pneumonia-influenza deaths in 122 United States cities. (From Morbidity and Mortality Weekly Report, CDC, USPHS, *21*:37, 1972.)

Knobloch and Pasamanick (1958) related season of birth to subsequent childhood course. When they studied rates of first admission to a school for the mentally retarded over a 35-year period in relation to month of birth, they found that admission rates varied by season of birth; the rates were highest for the winter months, with a peak in February. The authors proposed poor nutrition of mothers early in pregnancy during the hot summer as an explanation for these findings.

Clusters in Time and Place

In the past few years there has been considerable interest in several apparent "clusters" of leukemia. Hitherto, cases of this rare condition have been considered unrelated to each other. If it could be demonstrated that cases occurred in *clusters* linked in time and space more often than could be expected by chance, this would provide strong evidence in support of a common etiology.

Where very low levels of epidemic concurrence are suspected, the usual statistical procedures for demonstrating an excess number of cases are not adequate. Special techniques have been developed to analyze cases for possible space-time clustering (Mantel, 1967). With such techniques several apparent clusters of leukemia have not been confirmed, but a few appear to represent valid findings (Knox, 1971).

A recent report of interest was that of an "extended epidemic" of Hodgkin's disease (Vianna et al., 1972) In this outbreak, more than 30 socially-linked persons in Albany, New York, most of them graduates of one high school, were found to have developed Hodgkin's disease or a solid lymphoma between 1948 and 1971. Determination of the statistical significance of the linkages between the cases could not be accomplished because of the lack of a defined denominator. In a subsequent study, the same investigators found further evidence for person-to-person transmission of Hodgkin's disease among teachers and students attending the same schools (Vianna and Polan, 1973). In view of the fact that other investigators have not confirmed time-place clustering in Hodgkin's disease (MacMahon, 1973), further studies are indicated.

SUMMARY

Population medicine requires that the boundaries of an area under study be specified. Implicit in the term "place" are such considerations as climatic conditions and natural as well as political boundaries. Political subdivisions are useful primarily for the planning and administration of health services, while classification by natural conditions tends to be more useful in the search for clues to etiology of disease. Whatever the objective, the concept of place, i.e., a clearly defined geographic area with its related population, is central to epidemiologic study.

Epidemiologic analysis also requires that cases be located in time. The major types of variation over time — secular, cyclic, and short-term fluctuations — were outlined and the first two discussed briefly. We noted the value of studies of migrants for delineating the relative contributions of genetic inheritance and environment to the etiology of disease. We concluded by reference to current epidemiologic studies designed to test the occurrence of possible clusters of disease in time and space.

COHORT ANALYSIS OF MORTALITY

When the frequency of a disease is changing over time (see page 73), it may be helpful to analyze the data by grouping the patients according to date of birth. The resulting groups are called birth cohorts.

A *cohort* is a group of persons who share a common experience

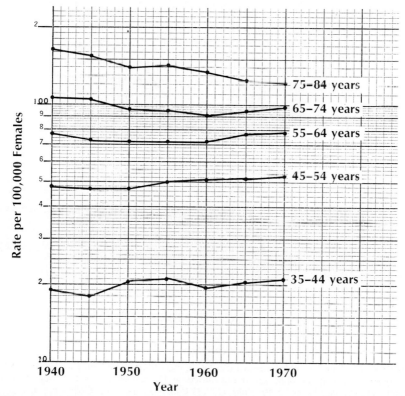

Figure 4–10 Death rates from breast cancer, by age group, white females, United States, 1940–1968 (calendar year on abscissa). (From Grove, R. D., and Hetzel, A. M.: Vital Statistics Rates in the United States, 1940–1960. USPHS Pub. No. 1677, U.S. Govt. Printing Office, Washington, D. C., 1968; National Center for Health Statistics: Vital Statistics of the United States, Vol. IIA. U.S. Govt. Printing Office, Washington, D.C., annual.)

within a defined time period. For example, a *birth cohort* consists of all persons born within a given period of time. A marriage cohort would consist of all persons married within a certain time period. In studies of chronic disease, a cohort of diseased persons (e.g., with stomach cancer or rheumatic fever) could be defined as all whose disease was first diagnosed during a given time period. The advantage of using a cohort approach to study mortality in a disease of changing frequency was first pointed out for tuberculosis (Frost, 1939).

Information about disease is usually presented as curves of age-specific morbidity or mortality rates for specific calendar years. For example, Figure 4–10 presents age-specific death rates for a

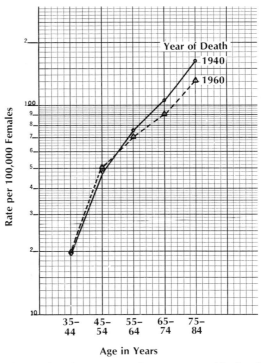

Figure 4–11 Death rates from breast cancer, by age group, white females, United States, 1940 and 1960 (age on abscissa). (From Grove, R. D., and Hetzel, A. M.: Vital Statistics Rates in the United States, 1940–1960. USPHS Pub. No. 1677, U.S. Govt. Printing Office, Washington, D.C., 1968; National Center for Health Statistics: Vital Statistics of the United States, Vol. IIA. U.S. Govt. Printing Office, Washington, D.C., annual.)

disease without a pronounced secular trend, cancer of the breast, over the period 1940 to 1968. A portion of the same information is rearranged in a less usual manner, with age rather than time on the x-axis (Figure 4–11).

This latter method of presentation can also be applied to a disease of changing frequency, such as tuberculosis. In Figure 4–12 the age-specific death rates from tuberculosis are seen to have declined in each successive time period from 1900 to 1960. In addition, there is an apparent shift in the age pattern. The second peak in rates (following a peak in early childhood and trough for children of school age) appears to have occurred at successively older ages.

All of the curves presented thus far are called *cross-sectional curves* because they cut across birth cohorts at a given point in time. They thus provide a "snapshot" of mortality experience at that time. The information on death rates from tuberculosis can also be arranged (Figure 4–13) so that the lines, instead of connecting age-specific death rates by year of *death*, as in Figure 4–12, connect age-specific death rates by year of *birth*. This creates a family of

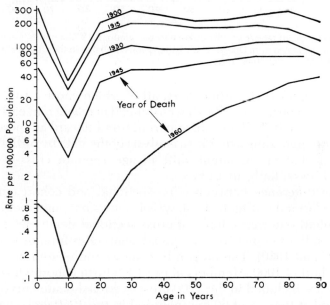

Figure 4–12 Death rates from tuberculosis, by age group, United States, selected years. (Adapted from Doege, T. C.: Tuberculosis mortality in the United States, 1900 to 1960. J.A.M.A., *192*:1045, 1965.)

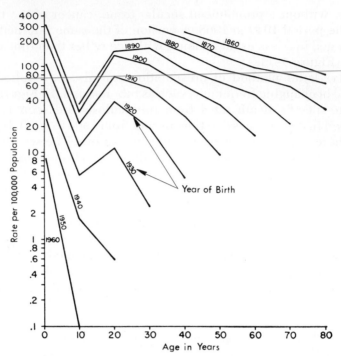

Figure 4–13 Death rates from tuberculosis, by age group, for birth cohorts, United States, 1860–1960. (Adapted from Doege, T. C.: Tuberculosis mortality in the United States, 1900 to 1960. J.A.M.A., *192*:1045, 1965.)

curves, one for each birth cohort, all of which show a similar age pattern. The peak rate following childhood is reached in early adult life, and there is no longer an apparent trend toward an increase in rates with increasing age. Thus, analysis of the data by birth cohorts indicates that the apparent shift in age seen in cross-sectional curves is essentially an artifact.

The difference between cross-sectional and cohort curves is further clarified in Figure 4–14, which shows how members of one birth cohort enter into different cross-sectional death curves. Two unbroken lines depict cross-sectional death rates from tuberculosis (in 1900 and 1960). The broken line shows the death rates for the birth cohort of 1900. Members of the 1900 birth cohort who died in infancy are included in the 1900 cross-sectional death curve; those who died at the age of 60 are included in the 1960 cross-sectional death curve. The same principle would apply to the intervening decades between 1900 and 1960. (We have omitted these curves on the graph but have noted in the cohort curve where the intersections with cross-sectional curves would have occurred.)

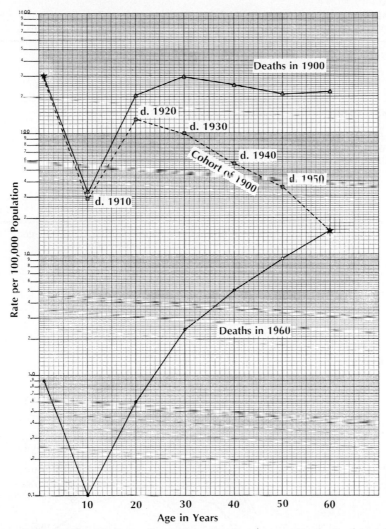

Figure 4-14 Relation between cohort and cross-sectional curves. Death rates from tuberculosis, by age group, for 1900 birth cohort and for calendar years 1900 and 1960. (Adapted from table provided through the courtesy of Dr. T. C. Doege.)

Table 4-1, which presents age-specific death rates by decade for 1900 through 1960, further illustrates how the members of one birth cohort enter into different cross-sectional curves. The age-specific death rates for the cohort of 1900 are shown in bold type on the diagonal and correspond to the intersecting points shown in Figure 4-14.

When death rates are decreasing with time, as is true of

TABLE 4–1 Death Rates Per 100,000 Population from Tuberculosis, by Age Group, for Selected Years, United States Death Registration States*

Year	Age Group							
	under 1	1–4	5–14	15–24	25–34	35–44	45–54	55–64
1900	**311.6**	101.8	36.2	205.7	294.3	253.6	215.6	223.0
1910	212.9	84.6	**29.7**	152.0	217.6	214.9	188.1	192.9
1915	168.6	68.0	26.9	146.1	198.0	196.9	176.8	177.0
1920	106.5	45.4	22.4	**136.1**	164.9	147.4	137.2	141.3
1930	51.6	25.9	11.9	77.3	**102.8**	92.4	93.2	97.0
1940	24.6	12.3	5.5	38.2	56.3	**59.4**	66.3	76.1
1945	16.3	8.7	3.6	34.1	49.3	49.8	58.1	66.0
1950	8.5	6.3	1.8	11.3	19.1	26.1	**35.9**	47.7
1960	.9	.6	.1	.6	2.4	5.1	9.3	**15.5**

*Adapted from table provided through the courtesy of Dr. T. C. Doege.

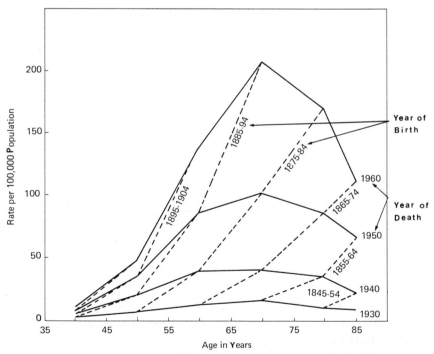

Figure 4–15 Relation between cohort and cross-sectional curves. Death rates from lung cancer, by age, for selected birth cohorts (broken lines) and for selected calendar years (solid lines), white males, 40 years and older, United States. (From NCI Monograph No. 6, 1961; USPHS Pub. No. 113, U.S. Govt. Printing Office, Washington, D.C., 1963.)

tuberculosis, the older groups appear to have higher death rates than younger people on cross-sectional curves. This occurs because the elderly come from earlier birth cohorts who are at greater risk. Conversely, when death rates are increasing with time, as is true of lung cancer (Figure 4–15), cross-sectional curves show apparently decreasing rates with increasing age.

STUDY QUESTIONS

4–1 Define the following terms and give an example when appropriate:

Place disease (page 64)
Secular trend (page 73)
Cyclic changes (page 77)
Time-place cluster (page 79)
Cohort analysis of mortality (page 81 ff.)
Cohort (page 81)
Birth cohort (page 82)

4–2 A. Name the anatomic site with the largest number of deaths from cancer in the United States in the following years: males: 1930, 1968; females: 1930, 1968.
B. Indicate the nature of the trend in death rates (increasing, stationary, decreasing) from cancer of the following sites in the United States between 1930 and 1968: (1) stomach, (2) breast, (3) uterus, (4) pancreas, and (5) colon and rectum.

Answer on page 345.

4–3 Figure 4–16 shows mortality rates from rheumatic fever and chorea in England and Wales from 1921 to 1966. Rheumatic fever is a condition associated with altered sensitivity to Group A streptococci. Chorea is a neurologic manifestation of rheumatic fever.

A. Comment on the mortality trend from 1921 to 1966.
B. To what extent can chemotherapy and antibiotics account for the changes shown here?
C. Note that the graph is drawn on semi-logarithmic paper. That is, the y-axis is on a logarithmic scale. List two advantages of a logarithmic over an arithmetic scale.

Answer on page 345.

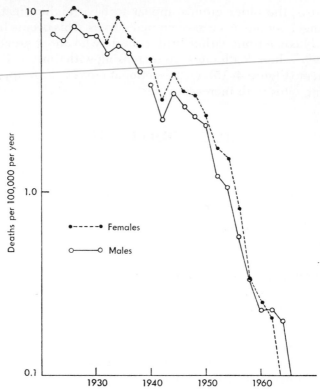

Figure 4–16 Mortality rates from rheumatic fever and chorea, boys and girls aged 5–14 years, England and Wales, 1921–1966. Gaps in the curves indicate point at which a change in the disease classification occurred. (From Reid, D. D., and Evans, J. G.: New drugs and changing mortality from non-infectious disease in England and Wales. Br. Med. Bull., 26: 191, 1970.)

4–4 Age-adjusted* mortality rates for cancer of the lung in several time periods are shown below and in Figure 4–17.

Rates per 100,000	T_1			T_2
	1939–1942	1947–1950	1954–1957	1962–1965
Males	13.0	23.4	33.7	41.1
Females	3.5	4.5	4.7	6.4

A. Compare the relative change in death from cancer of the lung over the two time periods, T_1 and T_2. Comment on any difference in trend for the two sexes.
B. Can the increase in lung cancer death rates be attributed to growth of the United States population between 1940 and 1965? Explain your answer.
C. List two other possible explanations for the marked secular trend in rates shown in Figure 4–17.

Answer on page 346.

*Age-adjustment of rates is discussed in Chapter 7.

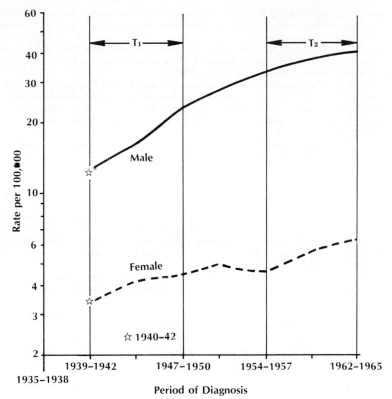

Figure 4–17 Age-adjusted mortality rates per 100,000 for cancer of the lung and bronchus* by sex and period of diagnosis; Connecticut, 1939–1965. (Adapted from Sullivan, P. D., Christine, B., et al.: Analysis of trends in age-adjusted incidence rates for 10 major sites of cancer. Am. J. Public Health, 62:106, 1972.)

---

*Includes trachea and deaths unspecified primary or secondary.

4–5 The health officer of a large city is planning to initiate a screening and treatment program for individuals with hypertension in his community. What demographic variables should be considered in estimating the number of persons to be served by this program?

REFERENCES

Alter, M., Halpern, L., et al.: Multiple sclerosis in Israel: Prevalence among immigrants and native inhabitants. Arch. Neurol., 7:253, 1962.

Burkitt, D.: A tumor syndrome affecting children in tropical Africa. Postgrad. Med. J., 38:71, 1962.

Cooper, J. E.: The use of a procedure for standardizing psychiatric diagnosis. In

Hare, E. H., and Wing, J. K. (eds.), Psychiatric Epidemiology. Proceedings of the International Symposium held at Aberdeen University, July, 1969. Oxford University Press, London, 1970.

Cooper, J. E., Kendall, R. E., et al.: Psychiatric diagnosis in New York and London: A comparative study of mental hospital admissions (Maudsley Monographs, No. 20). Oxford University Press, London, 1972.

Epstein, M. A.: The possible role of viruses in human cancer. Lancet, *1*:1344, 1971.

Fletcher, C. M., Jones, N. L., et al.: American emphysema and British bronchitis. A standardized comparative study. Amer. Rev. Respir. Dis., *90*:1, 1964.

Frost, W. H.: The age selection of mortality from tuberculosis in successive decades. Am. J. Hyg., *30*(A):91, 1939.

Gajdusek, D. C., and Zigas, V.: Degenerative disease of the central nervous system in New Guinea. The endemic occurrence of "Kuru" in the native population. N. Engl. J. Med., *257*:974, 1957.

Gilliam, A. G.: Trends of mortality attributed to carcinoma of the lung: Possible effects of faulty certification of deaths due to other respiratory diseases. Cancer, *8*:1130, 1955.

Haenszel, W., and Dawson, E. A.: A note on mortality from cancer of the colon and rectum in the United States. Cancer, *18*:265, 1965.

Haenszel, W., and Kurihara, M.: Studies of Japanese migrants. I. Mortality from cancer and other diseases among Japanese in the United States. J. Natl. Cancer Inst., *40*:43, 1968.

Hirsch, A.: Handbuch der historisch geographischen pathologie, 1883.

Hornabrook, R. W., and Moir, D. J.: Kuru. Epidemiologic trends. Lancet, *2*:1175, 1970.

Knobloch, H., and Pasamanick, B.: Seasonal variation in the births of the mentally deficient. Am. J. Public Health, *48*:1201, 1958.

Knox, E. G.: Epidemics of rare diseases. Br. Med. Bull., *27*:43, 1971.

MacMahon, B.: Is Hodgkin's disease contagious? N. Engl. J. Med., *289*:532, 1973.

Mantel, N.: The detection of disease. Clustering and a generalized regression approach. Cancer Res., *27*:209, 1967.

Pedersen, E., and Magnus, K.: Gastro-intestinal cancer in Norway. Acta Un. Int. Cancer, *17*:373, 1961.

Rindge, M. E., Mason, J. O., et al.: Infectious hepatitis. Report of an outbreak in a small Connecticut school due to water-borne transmission. J.A.M.A., *180*:33, 1962.

Vianna, N. J., Greenwald, P., et al.: Hodgkin's disease; Cases with features of a community outbreak. Ann. Intern. Med., *77*:169, 1972.

Vianna, N. J., and Polan, A. K.: Epidemiologic evidence for transmission of Hodgkin's disease. N. Engl. J. Med., *289*:499, 1973.

THE SEARCH FOR CAUSAL RELATIONS: OBSERVATIONAL STUDIES

5

In Chapters 3 and 4 we have indicated the dimensions along which one may describe the distribution of disease in population groups by person, place, and time. A logical question is: what is the ultimate purpose of such efforts at description? Aside from their value for the planning and programming of health services, descriptive data provide a first step in elucidating the causes of disease by identifying groups with high or low rates of a specific disease. Once such identification has been made, the next step is an attempt to determine **why** the rate is high or low in a particular group. Observations of differences in occurrence of disease between populations lead to the formulation of *hypotheses*, i.e., testable propositions, which can then be accepted or rejected through more searching epidemiologic studies. In turn, the results of these analytic studies generate ideas for additional descriptive studies as well as new hypotheses. This sequence of events may be schematized as a feedback system or an *epidemiologic study cycle* (Figure 5–1).

In determination of etiology, the usual progression is from study of the association of a factor and a disease in groups to study of their association in individuals. For example, on the basis of international differences in death rates from lung cancer, tobacco consumption in different countries might be studied for a relation to death rates from lung cancer. If one were to find such a correlation

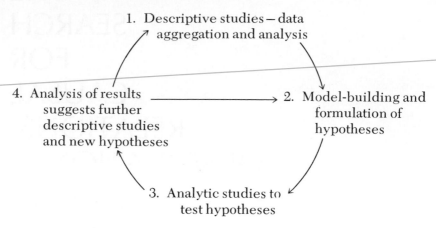

Figure 5–1 Schema for an epidemiologic study cycle.

for population groups, an appropriate next step would be to study the smoking habits of individuals in a country having a high rate. This step would demonstrate whether it is, indeed, the smokers and not the nonsmokers in that country who were contributing to the high death rate from lung cancer.

OBSERVATIONAL VS. EXPERIMENTAL STUDIES

Basically there are two approaches to testing hypotheses about etiology, experimental and observational. The experimental approach is perhaps more familiar, since it provides the basic model for investigation in other sciences. In an *experiment* the investigator studies the impact of varying some factor which is under his control. For example, he may take a litter of rats, expose one of two randomly selected halves to a supposedly carcinogenic agent, and then record the frequency with which cancer develops in the two groups. The translation of this animal experiment into a study of the etiology of disease in human beings would entail selecting a number of individuals alike in specified characteristics, subjecting a randomly chosen subgroup to an hypothesized disease-producing factor, and then comparing the occurrence of disease in this subgroup with the control group. Patently, this is not possible in human subjects except in rare instances.

In the more usual approach the investigator can only observe the occurrence of disease in people who are already segregated into groups on the basis of some experience or exposure (e.g., married vs. single or smoker vs. nonsmoker). In this kind of study, allocation into groups on the basis of exposure to a factor is not under the control of the investigator. The study is *observational* since contrasts between study groups in outcome are observed, not created experimentally.

The difficulty with observational studies is that the observed groups usually differ in some characteristics in addition to the specific factor under study. Thus, people in various occupations differ not only in exposure to occupational hazards but also in prior life experiences. That is, different occupations may recruit different kinds of people. In part this may be a matter of self-selection, but it can also reflect prior education as well as fitness for a particular occupation and the selective effects of hiring practices. Because of these confounding factors the role of a specific factor under investigation is more difficult to demonstrate.

While experimentation can establish the causal association of a factor with a disease more conclusively than observation, observational studies have provided and continue to provide the major contribution to our understanding of many diseases. Upon rare occasions, by chance, groups may exist which are similar in every respect save for degree of exposure to a specific environmental factor. In such circumstances the conditions for drawing conclusions about the cause of disease may be so favorable that a *natural experiment* is said to exist.

Natural Experiments

Perhaps the most famous natural experiment is that reported by John Snow (1855), a British physician, over a hundred years ago. On the basis of extensive studies on the epidemiology of cholera, Snow had formulated the hypothesis that cholera could be transmitted by discharge of fecal wastes into water supplies. Some preliminary analyses by the Registrar General during an outbreak of cholera in 1853 suggested that among people living in the same area of London, those served by one water company, the Lambeth Company, had a lower death rate from cholera than those served by another company, Southwark and Vauxhall. The latter received water drawn from the Thames River at points where the water was already contaminated by sewage from London. Snow reported that nature had devised an

...experiment, ... on the grandest scale (in that) no fewer than three hundred thousand people of both sexes, of every age and occupation, and of every rank and station, from gentlefolks down to the very poor, were divided into two groups without their choice, and, in most cases, without

TABLE 5–1 Deaths from Cholera by Company Supplying Water to the Household*

Water Company	Number of Houses	Deaths from Cholera	Deaths in Each 10,000 Houses
Southwark and Vauxhall Company	40,046	1263	315
Lambeth Company	26,107	98	37
Rest of London	256,423	1422	59

*From Snow, J.: On the Mode of Communication of Cholera (2nd ed.). Churchill, London, 1855. Reproduced in Snow on Cholera, Commonwealth Fund, New York, 1936. Reprinted by Hafner Publishing Company, New York, 1936.

their knowledge; one group being supplied with water containing the sewage of London, and, amongst it, whatever might have come from the cholera patients, the other group having water quite free from such impurity.

To turn this grand experiment to account, all that was required was to learn the supply of water to each individual house where a fatal attack of cholera might occur.

Snow's subsequent investigations, which showed an eightfold difference in the death rates for the households supplied by the two companies (Table 5–1), gave clear evidence of an association between cholera death rate and source of water supply to the household.

More recently, the close juxtaposition of areas quite similar except for the fluoride concentration in the drinking water provided another fortuitous experiment. Contrasts in the amounts of dental mottling and dental caries in these areas led to a series of actual experiments which will be described further in the next chapter.

Another natural experiment was afforded by the atomic bombing of Japan in World War II. It was possible to observe the subsequent course of survivors who were classified by the estimated dose of radiation they had received. The effects of radiation traced to this exposure include an increased incidence of leukemia and cancer of the thyroid, as well as small head circumference associated with mental retardation in infants exposed in utero (Brill, 1962; Miller, 1969).

THE CONCEPT OF CAUSALITY AND STEPS IN THE ESTABLISHMENT OF CAUSAL RELATIONSHIPS

The determination of the cause of a disease through either natural or manipulated experiments may be fairly straightforward. The problem of identifying causal relations in the more usual observational studies is much more difficult. Nevertheless, it is of central importance. Detection of causal associations may indicate key points at which a chain of disease production can be interrupted. On the other hand, it is important not to mislabel an association as causal if it is not, since that could initiate fruitless control efforts and deflect attention from more profitable approaches to prevention. Therefore, before any association is accepted as causal, all alternative explanations should be considered. How then do we decide if a **factor is causally linked to a disease?** What chain of logic can we follow to determine whether a specific exposure is related to a specific disease entity?

Let us say, for example, that each year a certain proportion of the general population develops a certain disease. If there were no difference in risk for subgroups in the population one would expect that essentially the same proportion of any subgroup would develop the disease in a given time period. However, if a higher proportion of a subgroup evidenced disease in an observational study, one could not conclude from this alone that there is a causal relation between some factor in the subgroup and the disease. Several questions must be considered and answered first.

The first question to ask about a difference between groups in frequency of disease is whether it is statistically significant. If it is not, the problem may either be dismissed or pursued further through studies on a larger sample. If the difference is significant, a *statistical association* is said to exist. This may be positive or negative. It is positive if the proportion of individuals with both the factor and the disease is higher than expected, negative if the proportion is lower.

Another question is whether the subgroup with the high (or low) rate of disease has any characteristics (e.g., age distribution, urban vs. rural residence, and so on) other than the one being studied which might influence this rate. If there are evidences of such "noise" in the system, analytic procedures can be employed to determine the effect of such factors and to neutralize them. Of course, one cannot insure that all relevant variables have been considered, merely those judged to be important on the basis of existing knowledge.

Let us assume, then, that a statistical association between a factor and a disease has been demonstrated in groups which are similar or for whom differences have been erased by adjustment. Such an association may be of three types: (1) artifactual (or spurious), (2) indirect, or (3) causal.

Artifactual (Spurious) Association

As the name implies, an *artifactual association* is a false or fac-
titious association which can be due to chance occurrence or to
some bias in study methods. One implication of decision theory
based on concepts of probability is that in a certain proportion of
trials an outcome will be declared statistically significant even
though it actually results from random fluctuation (so-called Type I
error). In order not to be misled into premature acceptance of an association, one should attempt to confirm a positive finding by
replication. One can suspect that an association is spurious if it does
not hold up on such attempts.

As we have indicated, bias can also give rise to artifactual associations through the methods used to conduct the study or the
selection of the study group. (Bias is defined and discussed more
fully in Chapter 7.) First, an example of bias arising from a defect in
methods is presented. Let us assume that a study is being conducted to test whether a given disease (X) is associated with alcohol
intake. If an interviewer knew whether he were dealing with a case
(i.e., a person with disease X) or a control and if he believed in the
hypothesis linking alcohol and disease, he might probe more intensively for a history of drinking for a case than for a control.Even if
one were to guard against this by holding the interviewer to a fixed
interview schedule, there might still be subtle differences in facial
expression or tone of voice that could influence the replies. The
solution to this kind of problem is to keep the interviewer unaware
of the status of his respondent as case or control (i.e., blind interview).

Another source of bias lies in the selection of the study group.
The group chosen for comparison with the cases, the *controls,* can
easily be a source of bias, particularly if they consist of patients attending a treatment facility for some disease other than the one
under study. Where this is true, there may be characteristics
peculiar to the control group which would not be present if it were
truly representative of the population.

The following illustrates the importance of choice of control
group. In a study of the role of early socialization experiences and
intrafamilial environment in the development of mental illness in
children (Oleinick et al., 1966), two controls were selected for each
case seen in a psychiatric clinic. One was a *hospital* control, a child
who had attended the pediatric or ophthalmology (refraction) clinic
or had had an appendectomy or a tonsillectomy during the same
time period. The other was a *population* control drawn from Baltimore public school children.

The cases consistently showed more problem behavior and symptoms than the controls. However, the two control groups differed on a number of parameters. Hospital controls had more fears, problems with temper, and more frequent nightmares than the population controls. The hospital controls also were intermediate (as compared with cases and population controls) with regard to possible etiologic factors, such as frequency of disruption of the parents' marital relationship and separation of father and child. This finding is not surprising when we consider that emotional problems could lead to hospitalization and various types of operative procedures.

If only hospital controls had been used, the results would have been misleading. In this example, the study would have understated the difference between cases and controls. It is also possible for differences to be exaggerated as, for example, when more medical information is available about the cases than the controls.

Thus, whenever a statistically significant association is found, it must be scrutinized carefully to be sure that it is not attributable to some artifact or bias. Further discussion of bias may be found in the next two chapters.

Indirect Association

By *indirect association* we mean that a factor and a disease are associated only because both are related to some common underlying condition. This is a noncausal type of association. Alteration in an indirectly associated factor will not produce alteration in the frequency of disease unless the change also affects the common underlying condition as well. Many associations which at first appeared to be causal in nature have been found upon further study to be due to indirect association, as will be shown in the following two examples.

Altitude and Cholera. In studying the statistics on cholera in nineteenth-century England, William Farr, the Registrar General, noted an inverse relation between altitude and deaths from cholera. He interpreted this as support for the then popular theory that miasma, i.e., bad air, was responsible for causing the disease. According to this theory one would expect high cholera rates in areas of low altitude because the air is more dangerous and, conversely, low rates in regions with pure air. Indeed, the observed mortality (Figure 5–2) is remarkably close to that predicted on the basis of the miasma theory. According to current knowledge, however, cholera death rates were high in areas of fetid air because they were areas of low

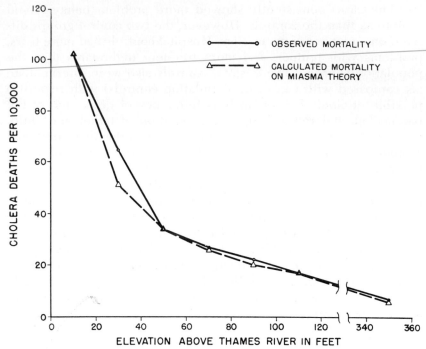

Figure 5-2 Correlation of cholera mortality and elevation above the Thames River, London, 1849. (From Langmuir, A. D.: Epidemiology of airborne infection. Bacteriol. Rev., 25:3, 1961.)

altitude where water supplies were also less pure. It was the impure water, not the fetid air, which led to the high death rate from cholera. Figure 5-2 demonstrates that classes of events which are indirectly, rather than causally, related can nonetheless yield an impressive correlation.*

Sucrose and Coronary Heart Disease. Some years ago Yudkin (1964) hypothesized that sucrose consumption plays an important role in the development of coronary heart disease. To test this hypothesis he determined dietary intake for three groups: patients with a recent first myocardial infarction (heart attack); patients with peripheral arterial disease of atheromatous origin; and controls, patients hospitalized because of an accident as well as healthy per-

---

*Parenthetically, it may be noted that the nineteenth-century studies of cholera draw heavily on *mortality* statistics. At that time mortality closely paralleled incidence because the case fatality rate was so high, probably over 50 per cent. With current practices of rapid rehydration, fatalities can be virtually eliminated if treatment is initiated promptly.

sons interviewed at home. The sugar intake was found to be substantially higher for the two groups with arteriosclerotic disease than for the controls, as seen in Table 5-2. Yudkin interpreted these findings as evidence that a high sugar intake "is an important factor in the causation of myocardial infarction and peripheral arterial disease."

However, other investigators (Bennett et al., 1970; Elwood et al., 1970) undertook studies to test whether consumption of sucrose was associated with other variables, such as cigarette smoking, which might be causally related to coronary heart disease. Indeed, it was found that nonsmokers used less sugar than current smokers and ex-smokers, and, further, that heavy smokers tended to use more sugar than light smokers. The relation of each of these variables to atherosclerotic heart disease was then examined in two series of patients from Central Middlesex Hospital in London. In both series, patients with a number of different diseases were questioned about their smoking habits and sugar consumption, as shown in Table 5-3.

In both series the proportion of patients with myocardial infarction was higher among the smokers than the nonsmokers at each level of sugar consumption; within smoking categories there was no increase in the proportion of patients with myocardial infarction as sugar consumption increased. These data, together with the information that smokers use more sugar than nonsmokers, suggest that the association between sucrose consumption and myocardial infarction found earlier by Yudkin was indirect and due to the independent association of each variable with a third, cigarette smoking. The association of smoking with coronary heart disease has also been found in many other studies.

TABLE 5-2 Sugar Intake of Subjects with Myocardial Infarction and Peripheral Arterial Disease and Control Subjects, Men Aged 45-65 Years*

| | | | Sugar Intake (Grams per Day) | |
| | | Mean Age | | |
Group	Number	in Years	Mean	Median
Myocardial infarction	20	56.4	132	113
Peripheral arterial disease	25	56.5	141	128
Control	25	56.0	77	56

*From Yudkin, J., and Roddy, J.: Levels of dietary sucrose in patients with occlusive atherosclerotic disease. Lancet, 2:6, 1964.

TABLE 5–3 Relation between Smoking Status, Intake of Sugar, and Diagnosis of Myocardial Infarction in Two Series of Hospitalized Patients*

	Smoking Category	Percentage with Myocardial Infarction According to Sugar in Hot Drinks Per Day		
		Less Than 9 Teaspoons	9–12 Teaspoons	13 or More Teaspoons
Series I	Nonsmokers or ex-smokers	9	10	0
	Current smokers	14	17	9
Series II	Nonsmokers or ex-smokers	18	23	13
	Current smokers	38	37	43

*From Bennett, A. E., Doll, R., et al.: Sugar consumption and cigarette smoking. Lancet, *1*:1011, 1970.

Causal Association

Although the word "cause" is part of everyday speech, it is, nonetheless, difficult to define. Different philosophers have assigned different meanings to the term. With due recognition that philosophic differences exist, we will define *cause* by saying that two variables are causally related if a change in one is followed by a change in the other.

The set of rules known as *Koch's postulates* represents an attempt to develop criteria for establishing causal relations for one class of agents, microorganisms. These rules, as translated in Susser (1973), require that the following conditions be fulfilled before an organism is accepted as the agent of a disease.

... first, the organism is always found with the disease, in accord with the lesions and clinical stage observed; second, the organism is not found with any other disease; third, the organism, isolated from one who has the disease and cultured through several generations, reproduces the disease (in a susceptible experimental animal). . . . Even where an infectious disease cannot be transmitted to animals, the "regular" and "exclusive" presence of the organism proves a causal relationship.

That is, if the first two postulates are satisfied, a causal relation has been demonstrated.

Upon close inspection these postulates are somewhat less helpful than one might wish. Even when all three postulates are fulfilled, animal studies provide only indirect evidence that the organism can be introduced and propagated in a human host. Further, the existence of inapparent infection interferes with a one-to-one relationship between the presence of the organism and the existence of disease.

Without the artificial conditions of a rigidly controlled experiment, it is generally not easy to determine that a causal relationship exists. In real life any relationship is likely to be obscured by a large number of confounding variables. Since decisions about causality can have far-reaching practical consequences, a rigorous set of criteria for evaluation of evidence about causality is needed. Such criteria will be presented in the next section of this chapter.

FURTHER CRITERIA FOR JUDGING WHETHER AN ASSOCIATION IS CAUSAL

The following set of formal criteria are widely used to evaluate the likelihood that an association is causal.

Strength of the Association.   This criterion refers to the ratio of disease rates for those with and those without the hypothesized causal factor. The larger the ratio, the greater is the likelihood that the factor is causally related to the outcome. Furthermore, the likelihood of a causal relation is strengthened if a dose-response effect (gradient) can be demonstrated. That is, with increasing levels of exposure to the factor, a corresponding rise in occurrence of disease is found.

Consistency of the Association.   This criterion requires that an association uncovered in one study persist on testing under other circumstances, with other study populations, and with different study methods. The more often the association appears under diverse circumstances, the more likely it is to be causal in nature. One should be aware, however, that the same bias (i.e., systematic error) occurring in multiple studies could produce an apparent but spurious consistency.

Temporally Correct Association.   Exposure to the putative factor must antedate the onset of disease and allow for any necessary period of induction and latency. Temporal relations between environmental factors and outcomes are easy to demonstrate for events such as a food-borne epidemic or the London fog of 1952. They are more difficult to establish in many chronic conditions, especially those with a long latent interval.

Specificity of the Association.   This criterion refers to the extent to which the occurrence of one variable can be used to predict the

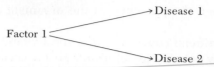

Figure 5–3 Model in which one factor is shown to lead to more than one disease.

occurrence of another. To quote Susser (1973):

... the ideal is a one-to-one relationship, where a cause is both necessary and sufficient. The more closely the relationship meets these conditions, the more specific it will be. Specificity is complete where one manifestation follows from only one cause.

The requirement of specificity is less satisfactory than the first three criteria for two reasons. The first relates to the fact that a single factor can cause more than one disease (Figure 5–3).

The second derives from the multifactorial nature of disease. Two models of multifactorial causation are shown in Figure 5–4. In one model (A) there are alternative causal factors; in the other (B) the causal factors act cumulatively. None of the factors alone is sufficient to produce disease.

While one-to-one specificity would add to the total weight of evidence supporting causal association, lack of specificity is of less significance. This will be illustrated later in the chapter by reference to the role of cigarette smoking in producing lung cancer.

Coherence with Existing Information (Biological Plausibility). Finally, additional support for the causal nature of an association exists if a causal interpretation is plausible in terms of current knowledge about the factor and the disease (e.g., its pathology, natural history, and so on). This, of course, is dependent upon the state of scientific information at a given time. Certainly a proposed explanation which conflicted with the existing body of knowledge would have to be examined with particular care.

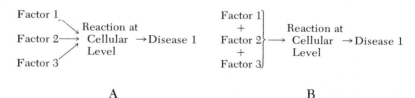

Figure 5–4 Two models of multifactorial etiology of disease. (Adapted from Lilienfeld, A. M., Pedersen, E., et al.: Cancer Epidemiology: Methods of Study. Johns Hopkins University Press, Baltimore, 1967.)

On the other hand, major advances in knowledge have resulted from findings which could not be incorporated into the existing body of knowledge and therefore were regarded at the outset with extreme skepticism. Apparently Minot's Nobel prize-winning work on the use of liver to treat pernicious anemia was accomplished in the face of repeated dissuasion from people who felt that liver had already been "proven" ineffective for that condition (Williams, 1954).

Application to a Specific Problem: Cigarette Smoking and Lung Cancer

Let us now apply these five criteria to a specific problem, the nature of the relationship between cigarette smoking and lung cancer. In doing this we will cover territory explored in depth in the early 1960's by an official committee composed of experts from various biomedical fields. The report of this committee is widely known as the Surgeon General's Report (Smoking and Health, 1964).

For illustration we will draw on data from several major epidemiologic studies which were used by the Surgeon General's committee in their deliberations. In the section on biological plausibility we will also cite evidence which has been developed since publication of the report. Table 5–4 summarizes the major facts from three so-called prospective studies. In each study the mortality experience of nonsmokers was set at 1.0 and the experience of smokers compared to that of the nonsmokers. This is an indirect method of age-adjustment (see page 137).

STRENGTH OF THE ASSOCIATION. Table 5–4 shows that in all three studies the death rates from lung cancer were higher for smokers than for nonsmokers. The mortality ratio for heavy smokers was approximately 20 to 1 in two of the studies and 40 to 1 in the third. Furthermore, there is a dose-response effect. Death rates from lung cancer are higher with each successive increment in amount smoked. Thus the criterion of strength of association is fulfilled.

CONSISTENCY OF THE ASSOCIATION. The association between cigarette smoking and lung cancer has been found in several countries among diverse study groups. Moreover, the association was demonstrated by studies which followed different designs, so-called retrospective and prospective studies (Chapter 13). In the *retrospective* studies patients with lung cancer and controls were identified and then compared as to smoking history. In the *prospec-*

TABLE 5-4 Lung Cancer Mortality Ratios for Current Smokers of Cigarettes* by Amount Smoked from Three Prospective Studies †

Study	Doll and Hill (1956)	Hammond and Horn (1958)	Dorn (1958)
Types of subjects	British doctors	United States men, nine states	United States veterans
Number of subjects	34,000	188,000	248,000
Age range	35–75 and over	50–69	30–75 and over
Months followed	120	44	78
Mortality Ratios			
Nonsmokers	1.0	1.0	1.0
Smokers (cigarettes per day)			
Less than 10	4.4	5.8	5.2
10–20	10.8	7.3	9.4
21–39	43.7	15.9	18.1
40 and over		21.7	23.3

*Excludes persons who smoked pipes or cigars in addition to cigarettes.

†Adapted from Smoking and Health. Report of the Advisory Committee to the Surgeon General of the Public Health Service, U.S. Dept. of Health, Education, and Welfare. USPHS Pub. No. 1103, U.S. Govt. Printing Office, Washington, D.C., 1964, pp. 83, 164.

tive studies (Table 5–4) people were classified with respect to smoking habits and then followed to observe the occurrence of lung cancer and other diseases. These various studies were consistent not only with respect to the existence of an association, but also, in general, with regard to the magnitude and gradient of the effect.

It is true that the mortality ratio was higher in the Doll and Hill study of British doctors than in the studies done in the United States. This may be explained by factors in addition to the number of cigarettes smoked—greater air pollution or other differences in smoking habits, such as age at starting, or differences in the proportion of smokers who use filtered cigarettes or who inhale. It is known that the British tend to smoke cigarettes down to a tiny stub.

TEMPORALLY CORRECT ASSOCIATION. This criterion too is satisfied by the known facts about cigarettes. Lung cancer tends to develop late in life, many years after the inception of cigarette smoking. This is compatible with the known, long latent period characteristic of carcinogenesis.

Another type of temporal evidence is found in the Hammond and Horn study (Table 5–5). For both light and heavy smokers (i.e., less than and more than one pack per day, respectively) the death rate from lung cancer decreases with increasing duration of time off cigarettes. The rate for heavy smokers remains elevated even years after cessation of smoking, but is appreciably reduced in comparison with the rate for those who continue to smoke.

SPECIFICITY OF THE ASSOCIATION. Most of the controversy over the cigarette-cancer hypothesis has centered around this criterion. One statistician, Berkson (1958), cited the wide range of diseases (Table 5–6) claimed to be associated with smoking as evidence against the causal role of cigarette smoking in lung cancer.

Actually this argument is not tenable. It is true that smoking is associated with many diseases other than lung cancer. This is not surprising since tobacco smoke is a complex substance containing not only benzpyrene and other known carcinogens but also nicotine, particulates, carbon monoxide, and other ingredients. Its different components might be expected to relate independently to different disease states. Moreover, there is specificity in the *strength* of the association, as shown in Table 5–6. For cancer of the lung, the difference in death rates of smokers and nonsmokers far exceeds that found in any other condition. The ratio in lung cancer is about 10 to 1 whereas in coronary heart disease, for example, it is 1.7 to 1.

Under the heading of specificity two further observations require comment: (1) not every one who smokes develops lung cancer; (2) not every one who develops this kind of cancer has smoked. The first apparent paradox is related to the multifactorial nature of disease. It may well be that there are other factors as yet unidentified which must be present in conjunction with smoking for lung cancer to develop. As for lung cancer in nonsmokers, we

TABLE 5–5 Death Rates from Lung Cancer among Current Smokers and Ex-smokers by Length of Time since Smoking Had Stopped and by Heaviest Consumption*

	Age Standardized Death Rates per 100,000	
	Less than 1 Pack a Day	*1 or More Packs a Day*
Still smoking in 1952	57.6	157.1
Stopped smoking less than 1 year	56.1	198.0
Stopped smoking 1–10 years	35.5	77.6
Stopped smoking 10 or more years	8.3	60.5

*From Hammond, E. C., and Horn, D.: Smoking and death rates—report on forty-four months of follow-up on 187,783 men. II. Death rates by cause. J.A.M.A., *166*:1294, 1958.

TABLE 5–6 Expected and Observed Deaths for Smokers of Cigarettes*
Compared to Nonsmokers, with Mortality Ratio; Seven Prospective Studies
Combined, For Selected Causes of Death †

Underlying Cause of Death	Expected Deaths (E)	Observed Deaths (O)	Mortality Ratio (O/E)
Cancer of lung	170.3	1,833	10.8
Bronchitis and emphysema	89.5	546	6.1
Cancer of larynx	14.0	75	5.4
Cancer of esophagus	37.0	152	4.1
Stomach and duodenal ulcer	105.1	294	2.8
Cancer of bladder	111.6	216	1.9
Coronary artery disease	6430.7	11,177	1.7
General arteriosclerosis	210.7	310	1.5
Cancer of the rectum	207.8	213	1.0
All causes of death	15,653.9	23,223	1.7

*Excludes those who smoked pipes or cigars in addition to cigarettes.
†Adapted from Smoking and Health. Report of the Advisory Committee to the Surgeon General of the Public Health Service, U.S. Dept. of Health, Education, and Welfare. USPHS Pub. No. 1103, U.S. Govt. Printing Office, Washington, D.C., 1964, p. 102.

know that there are factors other than smoking which increase the risk of lung cancer, including occupational exposure to chromates, asbestos, nickel, chloromethyl methyl ether (Figueroa et al., 1973), and, possibly, exposure to air pollution. Deviations from a one-to-one relation between cigarette smoking and lung cancer therefore cannot be said to rule out a causal relationship.

COHERENCE WITH EXISTING KNOWLEDGE. This criterion is amply met by cigarette smoking. For one thing, cigarette smoke, as noted, contains a number of carcinogens. Inhalation draws hot smoke into the lungs, bringing these carcinogens into intimate contact with tissues. Secondly the temporal trends in lung cancer are consistent with what is known of cigarette consumption in the population. The increase in use of cigarettes preceded by about 30 years the increase in death rates from lung cancer. Male-female differences in trends of lung cancer death rates are also consonant with the more recent adoption of cigarette smoking by women. Death rates rose first in males, but are now increasing relatively more rapidly in females, as shown in the top portion of Figure 5–5.

Finally, there is coherence in terms of anatomic evidence of tissue changes. In extensive autopsy studies Auerbach (1961) identified epithelial change (i.e., loss of cilia, increase in number of cell rows, and presence of atypical cells) in the tracheobronchial trees of smokers; these changes were present to a much lesser extent in nonsmokers. A series of ex-smokers (Auerbach, 1962) showed epithelial changes intermediate in extent between those of smokers and nonsmokers.

The anatomic evidence includes the induction of pulmonary tumors similar to those of human beings in beagle dogs trained to smoke through tracheostomy tubes (Auerbach, 1970) and in hamsters and rats treated by intratracheal instillation of components of cigarette smoke condensate (Health Consequences of Smoking, 1973).

In summary, the association between cigarette smoking and occurrence of lung cancer essentially meets all the criteria proposed for judging such relations. Nevertheless, we must also ask if an alternative hypothesis could be invoked to explain these findings. We can rule out a spurious association on the basis of the massive and generally consistent evidence. The association does not appear to be an artifact. However, could the explanation be an indirect association? Is there a common factor underlying both cigarette smoking and lung cancer which might produce the results shown? The opponents of the cigarette hypothesis have adopted this position. They have posited constitutional differences between smokers and nonsmokers to explain these apparent effects of cigarette

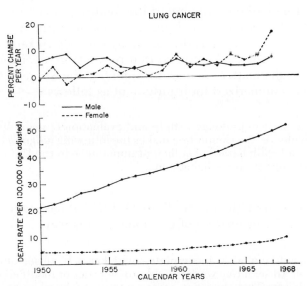

Figure 5–5 Male and female age-adjusted, lung-cancer death rates, and the yearly percentage change in male and female lung cancer death rates, United States, 1950–1968. (Adapted from Burbank, F.: U.S. lung cancer death rates begin to rise proportionately more rapidly for females than for males: A dose response effect. J. Chronic Dis., 25:473, 1972.)

smoking (Fisher, 1958; Seltzer, 1968). Against this hypothesis is the convergence of the several lines of evidence already cited.

As we have noted before, the only indisputable way to settle this matter would be to put the effect of smoking to experimental test in human beings. Since this is impossible we cannot disprove the constitutional hypothesis. However, the weight of evidence for a causal role of cigarettes is so massive that most scientists find it totally persuasive. In their report (1964) the Surgeon General's committee concluded that:

... cigarette smoking is causally related to lung cancer in men; the magnitude of the effect of cigarette smoking far outweighs all other factors. The data for women, though less extensive, point in the same direction.

As we have pointed out, the rate of lung cancer in women is now increasing more rapidly than it was at the time of the initial report.

This brings us to the critical point. When should one make a decision that a causal relation has been established? It is unlikely that we will ever have incontrovertible experimental proof that cigarette smoking is a causal factor in lung cancer in human beings. Nevertheless, health officials have to make practical decisions (i.e., support of antismoking programs, control over cigarette advertising) based on acceptance or rejection of the cigarette hypothesis. There is no absolute rule which can guide such decisions; rather, they must be based on review of the totality of evidence in accordance with the criteria which have just been outlined.

Each factor under scrutiny as being causally linked to a health problem deserves evaluation so that responsible decisions can be reached. In the matter of cigarette smoking, the Surgeon General's committee summarized their judgment as follows:

On the basis of prolonged study and evaluation of many lines of converging evidence, the Committee makes the following judgment: Cigarette smoking is a health hazard of sufficient importance in the United States to warrant appropriate remedial action.

On a more general level, Bradford Hill (1965) has summed up the problem of the evaluation of evidence in this way:

All scientific work is incomplete — whether it be observational or experimental. All scientific work is liable to be upset or modified by advancing knowledge. That does not confer upon us a freedom to ignore the knowledge we already have, or to postpone the action that it appears to demand at a given time.

SUMMARY

The descriptive epidemiology presented in earlier chapters has led us to the ultimate goal of epidemiology, the search for causes (determinants) of disease as the key to identifying effective preventive measures. Although experimental studies can provide definitive proof of the causes of disease, they are rarely possible in human beings. Therefore, we are often limited to observational studies for evidence of causal relations.

The concept of causality and the steps in establishing causal associations from observational studies were outlined. Five criteria were presented for judging the evidence for causal association: strength of the association, consistency, temporal relations, specificity, and coherence with existing knowledge. These criteria were illustrated by application to the hypothesis linking cigarette smoking to lung cancer.

Unfortunately the widespread public dissemination of information linking cigarette smoking to lung cancer, and to other diseases as well, has led to only a moderate degree of reduction in smoking levels. Cigarette smoking provides only too poignant an illustration of the lag which can occur between the development of knowledge and its application in the prevention of disease.

STUDY QUESTIONS

5–1 Define the following terms and give an example when appropriate:
Hypothesis (page 91)
Experiment (page 92)
Observational study (page 93)
Natural experiment (page 93)
Statistical association (page 95)
Types of association (artifactual, indirect, causal) (page 95ff.)
Controls (control group) (page 96)
Cause (page 100)
Koch's postulates (page 100)
Criteria for judging an association (strength, consistency, temporal relation, specificity, coherence) (page 101)

5–2 Following is the annual death rate per 100,000 population from certain chronic respiratory diseases for selected states in two regions of the United States:

Southwest		Northeast	
Arizona	27.8	New Jersey	10.8
Colorado	20.6	New York	12.0
New Mexico	19.1	Pennsylvania	15.6

Do these figures indicate a causal association between climate and death from bronchopulmonary disease? If not, indicate other possible explanations.

Answer on page 346.

5–3 In Table 5–5 note that among those who smoked one pack or more per day the death rate from lung cancer was higher for those who had stopped smoking within the year than for current smokers. Suggest an explanation for this paradoxical finding.

Answer on page 347.

REFERENCES

Auerbach, O., Hammond, E. C., et al.: Effects of cigarette smoking on dogs. II. Pulmonary neoplasms. Arch. Environ. Health, 21:754, 1970.

Auerbach, O., Stout, A. P., et al.: Bronchial epithelium in former smokers. N. Engl. J. Med., 267:119, 1962.

Auerbach, O., Stout, A. P., et al.: Changes in bronchial epithelium in relation to cigarette smoking and in relation to lung cancer. N. Engl. J. Med., 265:253, 1961.

Bennett, A. E., Doll, R., et al.: Sugar consumption and cigarette smoking. Lancet, 1: 1011, 1970.

Berkson, J.: Smoking and lung cancer: Some observations on two recent reports. J. Amer. Stat. Assn., 53:28, 1958.

Brill, A. B., Tomonaga, M., et al.: Leukemia in man following exposure to ionizing radiation: A summary of the findings in Hiroshima and Nagasaki, and a comparison with other human experiences. Ann. Intern. Med., 56:590, 1962.

Burbank, F.: U.S. lung cancer death rates begin to rise proportionately more rapidly for females than for males. A dose response effect. J. Chronic Dis., 25:473, 1972.

Doll, R., and Hill, A. B.: Lung cancer and other causes of death in relation to smoking. Br. Med. J., 2:1071, 1956.

Dorn, H. F.: The mortality of smokers and non-smokers. Proc. Soc. Stat. Sect. Amer. Stat. Assn., 1958, pp. 34–71.

Elwood, P. C., Moore, S., et al.: Sucrose consumption and ischaemic heart-disease in the community. Lancet, 1:1014, 1970.

Figueroa, W. G., Raszkowski, R., et al.: Lung cancer in chloromethyl methyl ether workers. N. Engl. J. Med., 288:1096, 1973.

Fisher, R. A.: Lung cancer and cigarettes? Nature, 182:108, 1958.

Hammond, E. C., and Horn, D.: Smoking and death rates—report on forty-four months of follow-up on 187,783 men. II. Death rates by cause. J.A.M.A., 166: 1294, 1958.

Health consequences of smoking: U.S. Dept. of Health, Education, and Welfare

Pub. No. 73–8704, U.S. Govt. Printing Office, Washington, D.C., 1973, pp. 79–80.

Hill, A. B.: The environment and disease: Association or causation? Proc. R. Soc. Med., 58:295, 1965.

Lillienfeld, A. M., Pedersen, E., et al.: Cancer Epidemiology: Methods of Study. Johns Hopkins University Press, Baltimore, 1967.

Miller, R. W.: Delayed radiation effects in atomic bomb survivors. Science, 166:569, 1969.

Oleinick, M. S., Bahn, A. K., et al.: Early socialization experiences and intrafamilial environment. A study of psychiatric outpatient and control group children. Arch. Gen. Psychiatry, 15:344, 1966.

Seltzer, C. C.: Morphological constitution and smoking. A further validation. Arch. Environ. Health, 17:143, 1968.

Smoking and Health. Report of the Advisory Committee to the Surgeon General of the Public Health Service. U.S. Dept. of Health, Education, and Welfare, USPHS Pub. No. 1103, U.S. Govt. Printing Office, Washington, D.C., 1964.

Snow, J.: On the Mode of Communication of Cholera (2nd ed.). Churchill, London, 1855. Reproduced in Snow on Cholera, Commonwealth Fund, New York, 1936.

Susser, M.: Causal Thinking in the Health Sciences. Concepts and Strategies in Epidemiology. Oxford University Press, New York, 1973.

Williams, R. H.: The clinical investigator and his role in teaching, administration, and the care of the patient. J.A.M.A., 156:127, 1954.

Yudkin, J., and Roddy, J.: Levels of dietary sucrose in patients with occlusive atherosclerotic disease. Lancet, 2:6, 1964.

PROPHYLACTIC AND THERAPEUTIC TRIALS: EXPERIMENTAL STUDIES

6

Experiments provide the strongest evidence for testing any hypothesis, whether related to etiology, control of disease, or any other scientific question. If among randomly selected groups of individuals exposed to a noxious factor, a higher proportion consistently develop a specific disease than do groups not so exposed, we have strong evidence for causation. Obviously, such experiments to test the causation of a disease are rarely possible in human populations. However, experiments to reduce the frequency of disease are possible. These can consist of trials either to prevent disease (*prophylactic trials*) or to treat established disease processes (*therapeutic trials*). They may involve whole communities or selected groups of individuals.

We will begin the discussion by outlining some basic principles which should govern the conduct of trials and will then cite several examples of experimental trials conducted with individual subjects and with whole communities. Finally, we will discuss some ethical issues related to human experimentation.

PRINCIPLES OF CONDUCTING EXPERIMENTAL TRIALS

The essence of an experiment is that, under the control of the investigator, some system is subjected to a manipulation. This manipulation creates an *independent variable* whose effect is then determined through measurement of a subsequent event in the system. The subsequent event constitutes the *dependent variable.* Application of this abstract formulation to experiments with human beings will be illustrated later in the chapter.

The Protocol

Prerequisite to any experimental trial is the development of a standard *study protocol* which defines the question or questions to be answered and specifies all details of the selection of subjects and of procedures. The protocol should include an explicit statement of the characteristics of the subjects to be recorded at the start of the trial. Since there are necessarily restrictions on the number of measurements which can be made in advance of the experiment, the characteristics to be recorded should be selected with careful attention to the issues in the study. In therapeutic trials, for example, staging of disease is of crucial importance.

Part of the preparation for conducting a trial is determination of the number of subjects needed.* At times it would take an excessively long time to enroll the desired study group if the investigation were limited to one institution or one area. Under these circumstances, it is usual to set up a multicenter trial. Other advantages of a multicenter trial include the opportunity for greater variety in the types of subjects enrolled and the fact that it may be easier to keep the results unknown to the investigators. In trials in which a number of investigators are cooperating to carry out the study, it is especially important that a rigorously defined protocol be developed and adhered to. Obviously, maintaining standard procedures under such circumstances is far from easy.

Reference and Experimental Populations

Studies are generally carried out only if the results can be applied to a larger group than the one actually studied. There would be little interest in carrying out a test of pertussis vaccine, for example, if one could not apply the findings of the trial to subsequent groups of children. The group of ultimate interest is called the *reference population,* the group actually studied the *experimental population.*

---

*A technique which eliminates the need for fixing sample size in advance of the trial is the sequential trial (page 122).

There may be difficulty in deciding the extent to which results from a study are generalizable. Possibly some specific characteristic of the experimental population — geographic location, socioeconomic status, or other characteristic — may have affected the outcome. In addition, the investigator may deliberately have limited his subjects to a particular age-sex group to reduce the number of host variables. Because most studies are conducted with limited populations, results from a single study are usually not accepted unless the findings are confirmed in other, somewhat different study groups.

Having selected an experimental population, the investigator must then recruit its members for his study. The issues of informed consent and other rights of subjects have recently received a great deal of attention as absolute prerequisites to ethically sound research. Many professional organizations have adopted codes of ethics to guide human experimentation. The National Institutes of Health have a firm rule that no research supported by them may be funded until a disinterested committee in the investigator's institution has studied and approved the procedures proposed for protecting the rights of subjects.

Allocation of Subjects

Once recruited, the population of subjects is divided by random allocation into subgroups. In the simplest model, two groups are formed. One, the experimental or study group, receives a drug, vaccine, or other procedure; the other group, often referred to as the control group, receives either no treatment, a placebo (dummy) procedure, or a standard form of therapy.

Random allocation is the process of permitting chance to determine assignment of subjects to subgroups. A table of random numbers is usually employed to accomplish this. With random allocation, the groups formed can be expected to be generally alike at the beginning of the trial. This should be true for risk factors as well as other characteristics, all within the limits of sampling variability. However, it is always wise to check that the groups formed initially are, in fact, basically similar in composition.* Randomization prevents subjects from determining their assignment to

---

*Where response to a treatment is likely to differ markedly for subgroups in the study population (e.g., patients with different stages of cancer), the population may be stratified according to the relevant clinical characteristic either before or after random allocation.

a specific study group. Therefore, the effect of the intervention program can be measured without the confounding influences of self-selection often present in observational studies.

The steps in the conduct of an experimental trial are shown in Figure 6–1 (adapted from MacMahon and Pugh, 1970). We have already commented on the relation between the experimental (study) and reference populations. The figure makes it very clear that assignment of the experimental population to study and control groups is done **after** those who have agreed to participate have been identified. That is, the nonparticipants should have been eliminated from the pool of potential subjects before experimental and control groups are formed.

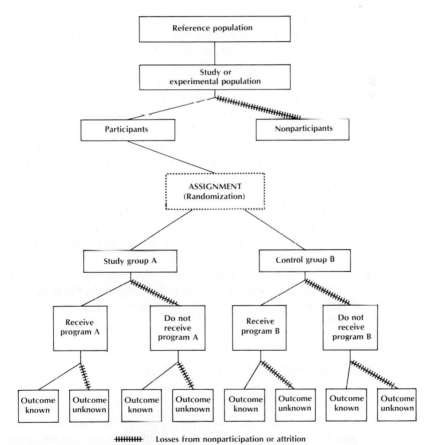

Figure 6–1 Steps in the selection of participants in a controlled intervention study. (Adapted from MacMahon, B., and Pugh, T. F.: Epidemiology Principles and Methods. Little, Brown and Company, Boston, 1970.)

Attrition During the Study

Figure 6–1 also serves to emphasize that attrition may occur throughout the study. In addition to those who do not enter the study initially, some of those assigned to the study and control groups do not complete the study protocol. Lastly, not all of those who complete the program may be available for the final evaluations. If there is a substantial amount of nonparticipation and attrition, it may be difficult to generalize from the results of the trial to the total experimental population since nonparticipants tend to differ from participants (page 140). Generalization to the reference population may be even more hazardous.

Elimination of Bias

Finally, an important consideration in any trial is the possible introduction of bias in assessment of outcomes from the expectations of either the investigator or the participant. The best protection against this source of bias is to have neither experimenter nor subject know the group to which the subject has been assigned. Such a trial is called *double blind.* If only the experimenter knows the assignment, it is said to be *single blind.*

A double-blind trial provides the least opportunity for bias to enter, but it is not always feasible. For one thing, the active substance may produce side effects which are not mimicked by the placebo. In addition, the setting in which care is given (e.g., home vs. hospital) may be the crucial experimental variable. Lastly, the physician may need information about the patient's assignment in the trial to monitor his clinical status. At times the latter problem can be circumvented if a physician not involved in the evaluation of results can take over the management of the patient's condition. Where the study is not conducted blind, it is important that the experimental and control groups be followed with equal intensity for evaluation of the outcome.

EXAMPLES OF EXPERIMENTAL TRIALS

With this general background we will now illustrate the range of problems to which the method of experimental trials has been applied. On the whole, the results of experimental trials have formed the basis for accepted modes of prophylaxis and therapy; full implementation of the findings of other trials, such as fluorida-

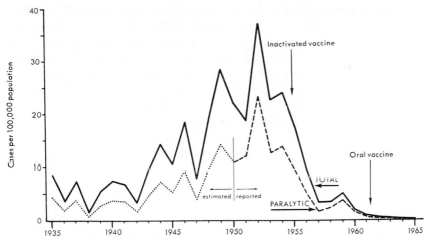

Figure 6–2 Annual poliomyelitis incidence rates, United States, 1935–1965. (From Morris, L., Witte, J. J., et al.: Surveillance of poliomyelitis in the United States, 1962–65. Public Health Rep., 82:417, 1967.)

tion of water, and even immunization, remains to be achieved in the future.

There have been numerous trials to test the efficacy and safety of vaccines. Generally, vaccines, once tested and licensed, have found ready acceptance in practice. For example, virtual elimination of poliomyelitis in the United States was achieved within a decade of the introduction of vaccine against the disease (Figure 6–2).*

The WHO trial of typhoid vaccine in Yugoslavia in the mid-1950's (Yugoslav Typhoid Commission, 1962) is interesting because it demonstrates that effectiveness of a vaccine in the field cannot always be predicted from laboratory studies. In this trial, some persons received a heat-killed, phenol-preserved vaccine, others an alcohol-killed and preserved vaccine. Better protection was expected from the latter because a substance known as Vi antigen is better preserved in it. However, the actual trial showed that only the phenol-preserved vaccine gave substantial protection. The mechanism for the difference in effectiveness of the two vaccines is not clear.

Experimental trials have also been applied to prophylactic modalities other than vaccines. Hammon's controlled trial of the ef-

---

*Study question 6–2 contrasts the two study plans that were used in the 1954 field tests of the Salk vaccine against poliomyelitis.

ficacy of gamma globulin for the prevention of poliomyelitis (1952) is a classic investigation of this kind. Although the trial gave clear evidence of the efficacy of this substance in preventing polio, the temporary nature of the effect and the development of long-acting vaccines shortly thereafter decreased the potential applicability. In contrast to the unequivocally good results obtained in poliomyelitis and hepatitis A is the lack of clear evidence of the effectiveness of gamma globulin in preventing hepatitis following transfusion, despite data from controlled trials. Chemoprophylaxis has also been studied experimentally. Since 1955, the United States Public Health Service has conducted a series of trials of isoniazid in the prophylaxis of tuberculosis. The efficacy of this drug has been demonstrated in children with primary tuberculosis, in household contacts of cases, in mental patients, and in Alaskan villagers (Ferebee, 1964).

On the whole, there has been less willingness to apply the principles of randomized clinical trials to therapy than to prophylaxis. Nevertheless, a number of such trials in diverse fields can be cited, e.g., the trials of chemotherapeutic agents in tuberculosis, of antimetabolites for ulcerative colitis, of steroids and immunosuppressive agents for chronic active hepatitis, and of different modes of surgery for portal hypertension. In the field of cancer, trials have centered principally on chemotherapeutic agents, especially for nonsolid tumors, such as leukemia, and for disseminated disease from solid tumors.

In mental illness, the effectiveness of psychoactive drugs has been demonstrated through controlled trials, mainly in institutional settings. In a unique clinical trial, Pasamanick and his associates (1967) evaluated the feasibility of home care for psychiatric patients. They randomly assigned acutely ill schizophrenics to one of three alternative forms of care: hospital treatment, home care on drugs, or home care on placebo. The study demonstrated that where there was a family member or other person willing to provide supervision at home, drug therapy together with adequate attention from public health nurses did reduce the frequency of hospitalization. Unfortunately, the trial was terminated after two and a half years. A follow-up study at the end of five years (Davis et al., 1972) found that the previous differences between groups had been gradually erased. Thus the ultimate potential of a continued aggressive program of home care in combination with psychoactive medication is not known.

Sometimes the results of a trial can challenge established concepts of therapy. An example is afforded by the recent collaborative trial known as the University Group Diabetes Program (UGDP) (Klimt et al., 1970; Meinert et al., 1970). This multicenter trial was set up in 1961 to evaluate the efficacy of oral hypoglycemic agents (i.e., tolbutamide and later phenformin) for preventing vascular complications in patients with mature onset, non–insulin-dependent diabetes. Approximately 800 patients in 12 centers were enrolled and followed for at least four years. The trial of oral agents had to be terminated because of the unexpected finding that the patients on these agents had higher death rates from cardiovascular disease than the comparison groups. The controversy over the findings (Feinstein, 1971; Schor, 1971) led to further analysis by Cornfield (1971) which demonstrated that small initial differences between groups could not have accounted for the significant differences in outcome.

Community Trials

In most trials, allocation to treatment groups is carried out on an individual basis. However, at times the unit of allocation may be an entire community or political subdivision, as in the trials of artificial fluoridation. It had been observed that residents of areas with water naturally high in fluoride had considerably less dental caries than residents of low-fluoride areas (Dean, 1942). Shortly thereafter, trials to test the prophylactic effectiveness of artificial fluoridation of water were proposed (Ast, 1943). Several pairs of neighboring cities were chosen, all with a naturally low level of fluoride in the drinking water. Following baseline measurements of fluoride content and of dental caries, the water of one city in each pair was left unchanged, the other treated by the addition of approximately one part per million (ppm.) of fluoride.

All the trials gave evidence of protection against caries by fluoride. For example, Figure 6–3 shows data from the Kingston-Newburgh trial in New York State 11 years after the start of fluoridation. Children aged 6 to 12 years in Newburgh, the city with fluoridated water, were found to have approximately 50 per cent less caries than children in Kingston. When the analysis was refined to exclude the older children who had not been exposed to fluoridated water in their earliest years, even greater evidence of protection was found; the amount of caries in Newburgh was 60 per cent less than that in Kingston.

Despite strong evidences of benefit from fluoridation and absence of significant toxic effects, a vigorous antifluoridation movement has impeded the widespread acceptance of this public health

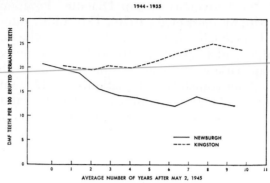

Figure 6–3 Permanent tooth caries experience of children aged 6–12 years, based on clinical examinations only, Newburgh and Kingston, New York, 1944–1955. Sodium fluoride was added to Newburgh's water supply beginning May 2, 1945. The DMF index, a count of decayed, missing and filled teeth, is used as a measure of the impact of caries experience, especially in children. (From Ast, D. B.: Dental public health. In Sartwell, P. E. (ed.): Maxcy-Rosenau Preventive Medicine and Public Health. Appleton-Century-Crofts, New York, 1965, p. 571.)

measure (McNeil, 1957). It is estimated that even now approximately 70 million people in the United States who live in low-fluoride areas with central water supplies still do not have fluoridated water.

THE NEED FOR EXPERIMENTALLY DERIVED INFORMATION: ETHICAL ISSUES

The need for sound, experimentally derived data on which to base public health programs and the medical care of individual patients cannot be emphasized too strongly. The medical literature is a virtual graveyard for inadequately tested preparations which die ignominiously after a brief moment of glory. Williams (1954) has aptly charted (Figure 6–4) the life history of the typical introduction of a drug into clinical use. After initial skepticism, uncontrolled trials lead to uncritical acceptance by hopeful investigators and desperate patients; this then gives way to a period of equally unbalanced negativism as the "miracle" drug proves to have its quota of complications and side effects. Finally, an equilibrium position is reached in which the drug reaches a level of acceptance appropriate to the benefits and risks associated with its use. At least part of this seesaw effect could be eliminated if a controlled trial were set up to test the drug at the outset.

Unfortunately, controlled trials are a relatively new arrival on the clinical scene and are not used to the extent that they should be even today. Many standard medical and surgical practices used currently antedate the development of controlled trials and now enjoy an acceptance not supported by decisive evidence of their superiority over other forms of treatment. For example, only recently has the evaluation of drugs for effectiveness received adequate attention. The Food, Drug, and Cosmetic Act of 1938 required that drugs be proven safe before they were marketed. Not until 1962 did amendments to that act mandate that efficacy be demonstrated as well. This led to extensive review first of prescription drugs, then of preparations sold over the counter. In the study of prescription drugs, panels of experts found that only 23 per cent of some 16,000 drugs could be classified unequivocally as "effective"; 13 per cent were considered "probably effective," 43 per cent "possibly effective," and 21 per cent "lacking substantial evidence of effectiveness" either alone or in fixed combinations (Bryan, 1972).

With the growing emphasis on "scientific" medicine in the past two decades one might expect that drugs introduced during this period would all have been subjected to careful clinical trials to evaluate their effectiveness and dangers. Unhappily this has not been true. As a result, "physicians are today treating seriously ill patients with powerful compounds whose therapeutic efficacy is unproved." Skinner and Schwartz (1972) voiced this complaint about drugs used in the treatment of chronic renal disease, but it applies with equal force to others—to certain anticancer drugs and to steroids and anticoagulants employed in the treatment of acute myocardial infarction.

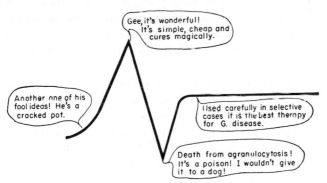

Figure 6–4 Oscillations in the development of a drug. (From Williams, R. H.: The clinical investigator and his role in teaching, administration, and the care of the patient. J.A.M.A., 156:131, 1954.)

Similarly, a number of surgical procedures introduced without adequate testing through controlled trials have also become the "accepted" or standard treatment for certain diseases. In this country thousands of women are subjected to radical mastectomy each year for breast cancer despite the fact that we do not know securely whether any defined subgroup or subgroups of the entire number might be more effectively treated with less radical surgery, such as simple mastectomy (Fisher, 1973). A collaborative trial is now underway to provide definitive evidence on this point. Another procedure widely employed, especially in previous years, has been tonsillectomy. As recently as 1969, Bolande estimated that 20 to 30 per cent of the children in most communities still undergo this operation. Yet here too controlled trials to test the benefits and dangers of this procedure have been conspicuously absent.

Experimental trials can detect evidence of harm as well as benefit. There is usually no reason to assume *a priori* that a new form of prophylaxis or therapy can have only positive effects. Several of the examples we have cited illustrate this point. This reasoning applies equally to surgical therapy and to drugs. Since lymphoid tissues participate in immunologic defenses, their removal by tonsillectomy or radical mastectomy should be considered carefully to make sure that the benefits outweigh the disadvantages.

In summary, while ethical problems in experimental trials must not be brushed aside, the basic question would seem to be not **whether** experimental trials with human subjects are needed but rather **how** they should be conducted. As Bradford Hill has noted (1971), the ethical problems underlying a decision about undertaking a clinical trial are "eased more often than not by the state of our ignorance. (If) we have no acceptable evidence that a particular established treatment does benefit patients ... whether we like it or no, we are then experimenting upon them." The question then is under what safeguards should trials be conducted to yield a maximum amount of information from the minimum number of study subjects.

One technique developed to minimize the ethical problems of withholding possibly beneficial agents is the *sequential trial*. The essence of this type of trial is an ongoing monitoring of results; the study is continued and new patients admitted to the trial only until statistical significance is achieved. In this way the number of patients in the trial is held to a minimum.*

---

*For a discussion of the difficulties in deciding when to call a halt to a controlled trial and of other scientific and ethical issues related to clinical trials, see Chalmers, T. C., Block, J. B., et al.: Controlled studies in clinical cancer research. N. Engl. J. Med., 287:75, 1972.

SUMMARY

This chapter outlined the principles underlying the conduct of prophylactic and therapeutic trials. An experimental trial requires that there be a carefully designed protocol which specifies the criteria for selection of subjects, the procedures for allocation into study and control groups, the use of blind techniques, and any other measures to reduce bias in the collection and analysis of the data. Random allocation is essential to ensure that study and control groups are alike.

The chapter concluded with a discussion of some of the ethical issues inherent in trials on human subjects. The need for experimentally derived data to provide a scientific basis for choosing among alternative modes of prevention and therapy was emphasized.

STUDY QUESTIONS

6–1 Define the following terms and give an example when appropriate:
Independent variable (page 113)
Dependent variable (page 113)
Study protocol (page 113)
Reference population (page 113)
Experimental population (page 113)
Random allocation (randomization) (page 114)
Double-blind trial (page 116)
Single-blind trial (page 116)
Sequential trial (page 122)

6–2 In the United States, the first vaccine (Salk) available against poliomyelitis was inactivated virus, administered parenterally. In 1954, two large-scale trials were designed to evaluate this newly developed product. In both trials parents of school children were asked to give permission for their children to be enrolled in the trial. The study designs are described below.

   1. *Observed control study.* According to this plan, which was developed by the National Foundation for Infantile Paralysis, vaccine was administered to second grade children only. First and third graders in the same schools were not inoculated but were observed for the development of poliomyelitis (hence the name, "observed" control study). The

study group included over one million children in grades one through three in several areas of the country.

2. *Placebo control study.* In this plan the subjects were approximately 750,000 children in grades one through three. The children whose parents gave permission were randomized into two groups. One-half received vaccine; the other half received an inert solution of similar appearance. Both materials were labelled only by code, the key to which was held by the Evaluation Center at the University of Michigan.

    A. Is either of the two study plans superior to the other? If so, in what way?
    B. List any advantages of the other plan.

Answer on page 347.

6–3 A new drug has been developed for home use in incipient attacks of asthma among children. You have been asked to design a study to determine the safety and efficacy of this product.

    A. What is the independent variable in the study?
    B. By what process should a control group be set up?
    C. What is the dependent variable or variables to be selected? Are different measures needed to determine safety and efficacy?
    D. What are the major ethical problems in such a study and how would you attempt to meet them?

REFERENCES

Ast, D. B.: The caries-fluorine hypothesis and a suggested study to test its application. Public Health Rep., 58:857, 1943.

Bolande, R. P.: Ritualistic surgery—circumcision and tonsillectomy. N. Engl. J. Med., 280:591, 1969.

Bryan, P. A.: DESI who? FDA Consumer, 6:11, 1972.

Chalmers, T. C., Block, J. B., et al.: Controlled studies in clinical cancer research. N. Engl. J. Med., 287:75, 1972.

Cornfield, J.: The University Group Diabetes Program. A further statistical analysis of the mortality findings. J.A.M.A., 217:1676, 1971.

Davis, A. E., Dinitz, S., et al.: The prevention of hospitalization in schizophrenia: Five years after an experimental program. Am. J. Orthopsychiatry, 42:375, 1972.

Dean, H. T., Arnold, F. A., Jr., et al.: Domestic water and dental caries. Public Health Rep., 57:1155, 1942.

Feinstein, A. R.: Clinical biostatistics 8. An analytic appraisal of the University Group Diabetes Program (UGDP) study. Clin. Pharmacol. Ther., 2:167, 1971.

Ferebee, S. H.: United States Public Health Service trials of isoniazid prophylaxis. Bull. Int. Union Tuberc., 35:108, 1964.

Fisher, B.: Cooperative clinical trials in primary breast cancer. A critical appraisal. Cancer, 31:1271, 1973.

Hammon, W. McD., Coriell, L. L., et al.: Evaluation of Red Cross gamma globulin as a prophylactic agent for poliomyelitis. J.A.M.A., 150:739, 1952.

Hill, A. B.: Principles of Medical Statistics, 9th ed. Lancet Ltd., London, 1971, p. 245.

Klimt, C. R., et al.: A study of the effects of hypoglycemic agents on vascular complications in patients with adult-onset diabetes. I. Design, methods and baseline results. Diabetes 19(supp.):747, 1970.

McNeil, D. R.: The Fight for Fluoridation. Oxford University Press, New York, 1957.

Meinert, C. L., et al.: A study of the effects of hypoglycemic agents on vascular complications in patients with adult-onset diabetes. II. Mortality results. Diabetes 19(supp.):789, 1970.

Pasamanick, B., Scarpitti, F., et al.: Schizophrenics in the community: An experimental study in the prevention of hospitalization. Appleton-Century-Crofts, New York, 1967.

Schor, S.: The University Group Diabetes Program. A statistician looks at the mortality results. J.A.M.A., 217:1673, 1971.

Skinner, M. D., and Schwartz, R. S.: Immunosuppressive therapy. 2. N. Engl J Med., 287:281, 1972.

Williams, R. H.: The clinical investigator and his role in teaching, administration, and the care of the patient. J.A.M.A., 156:127, 154.

Yugoslav Typhoid Commission: A controlled trial of the effectiveness of phenol and alcohol typhoid vaccines (final report). Bull. WHO 26:357, 1962.

MEASURES OF MORBIDITY AND MORTALITY

7

Early in this text we established that the underlying measure of disease frequency in epidemiology is the *rate*, a measure of some event, disease, or condition in relation to a unit of population, along with some specification of time. A number of different measures of *morbidity*, i.e., illness, are used in public health and epidemiology. Since all fall into two basic types, measures of incidence and measures of prevalence, it is desirable to discuss in some detail the meaning of these terms.

This chapter has three parts, each related to the measurement of disease. In the first, we will discuss incidence and prevalence. The second part will distinguish between rates which describe a total population and rates used to describe specific subgroups. The final section will deal with sources of error in measurement of disease. Following this we will devote a chapter to the sources of data on health and then, in Chapter 9, discuss the most commonly used health indices.

INCIDENCE AND PREVALENCE RATES

Incidence rates are designed to provide a measure of the rate at which people without a disease develop the disease during a specified period of time, i.e., the number of *new* cases of a disease in a population over a period of time. The *prevalence rate** measures the number of people in a population who *have* the disease at a given point in time. These rates are defined as follows:

$$\text{Incidence rate} = \frac{\text{number of } new \text{ cases of a disease}}{\text{population at risk}} \text{ over a period of time}$$

$$\text{Prevalence rate}† = \frac{\text{number of } existing \text{ cases of a disease}}{\text{total population}} \text{ at a point in time}$$

Thus, incidence tells us the rate at which new illness occurs, whereas prevalence measures the "residual" of such illness, the amount existing at a given point in time in a community. Prevalence depends on two factors: how many people have become ill in the past (i.e., previous incidence) and the duration of their illnesses. Even if only a few people in a group become ill each year, if the disease is chronic the number will mount and the prevalence will be relatively large in relation to incidence. On the other hand, if the illness under consideration is of short duration (acute) because of either recovery or death, or if there is migration of ill persons from the area, then prevalence will be relatively low.

The fact that prevalence (P) is related to both incidence (I) and duration (d) of disease is expressed in the formula P ~ I × d, which states that prevalence varies directly with both incidence and duration. If the incidence and duration have both been stable over a long period of time, then this formula becomes P = I × d. Under these circumstances, if prevalence and duration are known, it is possible to derive incidence.

Prevalence is important in determining work load, particularly in chronic diseases, in which it is a useful tool for the planning of facilities and manpower needs. Prevalence, however, is not the ideal measure for studies of etiology of disease. In contrast, incidence is the fundamental tool for studying the etiologic factors of both acute and chronic illness. Incidence rates are important because they provide a direct measure of the rate at which individuals in a given population become ill and thus provide a basis for statements about

---

*Although prevalence aims to measure disease at a **point** in time (e.g., on a specific day), the actual collection of data pertaining to that reference point may take longer than just that day. For example, the census refers to the population as of April 1 on a given year, even though the actual enumeration takes approximately three months.

†Some epidemiologists refer to prevalence at a point in time as a ratio, reserving the term rate for events or cases over a period of time. We will use the more general concept of rate to include any specification of time, instantaneous as well as interval. The terms "rate" and "ratio" are discussed further on page 184.

probability or risk of illness. By comparing incidence rates of a disease among population groups varying in one or more identified factors, one can get some notion about whether a factor affects the risk of acquiring a disease and, if so, about the magnitude of the effect. This is not true for prevalence data.

As an example, let us suppose we wished to see if heavy drinking contributes to peptic ulcer. Surveys of the prevalence of ulcer among those who consume large amounts of alcohol and among those who abstain might give a misleading impression. A prevalence count would not include as cases of disease people who had already developed and then recovered from peptic ulcer, including any who had stopped drinking specifically because of the ulcer. Further, persons who had succumbed to ulcer disease prior to the study would not be included in the survey. Therefore, incidence rates of peptic ulcer in drinkers and nondrinkers would provide a more valid measure of the impact of drinking on the development of ulcer disease than would prevalence rates. This is true of any "cross-sectional" survey, since it does not provide the opportunity for studying the antecedents of a condition.

In summary, prevalence is affected by factors which influence the duration of a disease as well as its development. Incidence reflects only factors which affect the development of disease. Thus, introduction of a treatment which prolongs life (e.g., as in diabetes or childhood leukemia) might lead to an increase in prevalence. Since incidence reflects only the development of disease, it would remain unchanged by the new treatment.

Prevalence: Point vs. Period Prevalence

The prevalence measure we have discussed so far, and the one usually referred to by the term prevalence, is actually *point prevalence*. There is another less commonly used measure of prevalence, *period prevalence*.

$$\text{Period prevalence} = \frac{\begin{array}{c}\text{number of existing cases of illness}\\ \text{during a period or interval}\end{array}}{\text{average population}^\circ}$$

Period prevalence is constructed from prevalence at a point in time plus new cases (incidence) and recurrences during a succeeding

---

°When the interval is a calendar year, the midyear estimate (July 1) is generally used for the denominator.

time period (e.g., one year). An example of period prevalence is found in Hollingshead and Redlich study (page 53) of the relation between social class and mental illness in New Haven. In that study, a case was defined as a person in treatment with a private psychiatrist or under the care of a psychiatric clinic or mental hospital between May 31 and December 1, 1950. Thus it included all people ill as of May 31 (point prevalence) plus those who became ill (incidence) or in whom illness recurred during the succeeding six months.

Period prevalence is frequently preferred to point prevalence or incidence for analyzing data on mental illness because of certain problems in the measurement of mental diseases. Exact date of onset needed for incidence is often difficult to determine; similarly, it may not be possible to state whether mental illness was present on a given day (point prevalence). Period prevalence, on the other hand, requires only a determination that the person was mentally ill at some time during a defined period of time.

While the main use of period prevalence is in the study of mental illness, it may be used for other conditions as well. For example, for purposes of planning hospital beds, the medical administrator may be interested in the number of cancer cases, both new and old, to be anticipated during a given year.

In population surveys of mental illness Leighton and colleagues (1963) have reported morbidity in terms of *lifetime prevalence*. This may be defined as the proportion of the population who have ever been mentally ill at any time in their lives. The use of this term would seem to have little operational value since many of the individuals who would contribute to a lifetime rate currently may be well and no longer in need of psychiatric care. Furthermore, estimates of lifetime prevalence, even more than yearly prevalence, can be distorted by deaths from competing causes and migrations over the years in the population under study.

Incidence: Further Specifications

From a consideration of prevalence, we now move to a more detailed consideration of incidence rates.

Time of Onset. As stated before, determination of date of onset is necessary for studies of incidence. For some events this determination is relatively simple. The onset of illnesses such as influenza, staphylococcal gastroenteritis, acute myocardial infarction, and cerebral hemorrhage can often be pinpointed to a specific hour. However, this is not true of conditions characterized by an indefinite onset. For these, the earliest definite, objectively verifiable event that can be identified is taken as the time of onset. In cancer, the date of onset is defined by the date of definitive diagnosis, not the date when symptoms were first noted or when a physician became suspicious that the person had cancer.

In independent studies on the incidence of heroin use, de Alarcon (1969) and Hughes (1972) both found date of first heroin use to be a workable standard of onset, since addicts are better able to recall this event than to specify a date on which they became addicted. Date of first heroin use also permits a fuller examination of the sequence of drug use over time. For similar reasons, in epidemiologic studies of psychiatric outpatients, Bahn (1961) found it useful to define a "patient" in terms of date of first clinic visit rather than date of referral to the clinic or of commencement of treatment.

Period of Observation. Incidence rates must always be stated in terms of a definite period of time. Although the period of study for incidence is usually one year, it can be any length of time.

When the population is at risk for a limited period only, the study period can readily encompass the entire epidemic. When this is true, the incidence rate is generally referred to as an *attack rate*. For example, in studying an outbreak of food-borne disease, the attack rate among those who ate a certain food (i.e., population at risk) is compared with the attack rate among those who abstained from that food.

On the other hand, for a disease of low frequency, incidence may be recorded for periods of several calendar years. Under these conditions the population being studied (i.e., the denominator of the incidence rate) is likely to change over the time period so that the number at risk of developing the disease will vary. The simplest way of handling this is to let the population at the midpoint of the period represent the average population at risk. However, more elaborate adjustments may be necessary, as shown in the next section.

Use of Person-Years (Unequal Periods of Observation). Studies which require observation of individuals for long periods of time often encounter problems of attrition: patients die, move away, or become lost to follow-up. In addition, it is sometimes desirable to continue to enroll patients after a study is already underway. For all these reasons, people may be observed for varying lengths of time and therefore not contribute equally to the "population at risk." In order to utilize fully the period of observation for each individual and to weigh properly his contribution to the study, a person-time unit, *person-year*, is created for the denominator of any rates calculated. For example, in a ten-year study of the incidence of peptic ulcer, if three people were observed for three, eight, and ten years each, they would contribute a total of 21 person-years of observation to the denominator of the incidence rate.

There are several problems with regard to the use of person-years. First, it is necessary to remember that the total number of person-time units does not represent that number of independent observations. The sum of 100 person-years, for example, could represent ten persons observed for ten years each or 20 persons observed for five years each. Second, there is an implicit assumption that the risk of disease or death is constant throughout the entire period of observation. This assumption often does not hold true. For example, in a condition with a long latent period, the incidence rate may be relatively high in the latter part of the observation period. The opposite trend may also occur. The occurrence of contraceptive failures tends to decrease as the period of observation lengthens, since couples who are successful over long periods are likely to be conscientious users or low in fecundity or both (Potter, 1963). For these reasons division of the observation period into several subperiods may be necessary. Finally, if the disease under study is so rapidly fatal that individuals are observed for less than a full unit of time, the rate will be artificially high. Such persons will be counted as a new case, or "one" in the numerator, but as "less than one" person-time unit in the denominator.

Denominator. There are two points to be raised in relation to the denominator of incidence rates. First, as with period prevalence, incidence covers a period of time, so that the numbers of persons at risk are likely to change, as noted above.*

Secondly, since incidence refers to new cases of disease, theoretically only those who are at risk of developing the disease under consideration, i.e., *population at risk*, should form the denominator. The denominator should not include those who already have the disease, or have had it, or are not susceptible by virtue of previous immunizations. Usually this correction to the denominator is not made, either because the disease is of low frequency or because the needed data are not available. However, if the condition is frequent and if precision is desired, then the denominator should be corrected to include only those at risk.

For example, to test the effectiveness of measles vaccine in a

---

*For annual rates the estimated midyear population is usually taken as the average population at risk. This practical solution is deficient because the rate does not represent a true probability value. (This matter is discussed further on page 209.)

group of six-year-old children, one should include only those who are still susceptible. Thus, in the trials of measles vaccines, children with antibodies at the beginning of a trial were either excluded physically or eliminated from the analyses of results since they were not at risk of developing measles. In contrast, denominators in **prevalence** rates always include everybody in the population since the numerator contains "old" as well as "new" cases.

Numerator.   In certain circumstances more than one event can occur to the same person within a stated time period. This gives rise to two types of incidence rates from the same set of data. For example, since a person may have more than one cold in a year, the following two rates could be constructed:

$$\frac{\text{Number of people who developed a cold}}{\text{People at risk}} \text{ in one-year period}$$

$$\frac{\text{Number of colds}}{\text{People at risk}} \text{ in one-year period}$$

Each rate tells us something different. The first gives the probability that any person will develop a cold in one year. The second rate tells us the number of colds to be expected among the group of people in that year. When number of persons and number of events can differ, the numerator should be clearly specified. Without such specification it is generally assumed that the numerator refers to persons and that an incidence rate represents a statement of probability or risk per person.

Uses of Incidence and Prevalence

As mentioned earlier, incidence and prevalence rates serve different purposes. Incidence rates are the fundamental tool for etiologic studies of both acute and chronic illness since they are direct indicators of risk of disease. High incidence is synonymous with high risk of disease. In contrast, high prevalence does not necessarily signify high risk; it may merely reflect an increase in survival, perhaps due to improved medical care. Conversely, low prevalence may reflect a rapidly fatal process or rapid cure of disease as well as low incidence. A final limitation of prevalence data for studies of etiology results from the fact that in prevalence surveys both cause and effect are observed simultaneously as in an instantaneous snapshot. In order to determine antecedents of disease it is necessary to establish a time sequence and show that the presumed independent variable or variables antedated the dependent one. Such temporal relations cannot be established by "cross-sectional" data.

It is important to remember these limitations because it is often tempting to use prevalence data for causal inferences since they are more readily obtained than incidence data. This is true because prevalence can be determined from one survey while measurement of incidence, if it is to be precise, requires at least two sets of observations: first a survey to determine whether each individual has the disease or has ever had it, then a resurvey of the nondiseased persons to see how many have become ill since the initial examination.

The different impressions that can be obtained from incidence and prevalence data will be demonstrated in material excerpted from the Framingham study of heart disease. If one examines frequency of coronary heart disease by sex, the impression given by prevalence data (Table 7–1) is quite different from that conveyed by incidence (Table 7–2).

If only prevalence rates were available, it would appear that CHD existed with equal frequency in young males and young females (rate of 5 per 1000 for both sexes). However, the incidence figures indicate a risk more than 20 times as high in young males as young females. The explanation for this discrepancy lies in the different course of disease in young men and young women. In the men the disease manifests itself as myocardial infarction and sudden death. In women the disease is more likely to present as anginal attacks, i.e., attacks of chest pain of brief duration which do not generally endanger life. With the longer duration of disease in women, prevalence can actually be equal in the two sexes despite

TABLE 7–1 Prevalence of Coronary Heart Disease (CHD) at Initial Examination among 4469 Persons 30–62 Years of Age, Framingham Study

Age (years)	Males			Females			Male/Female Ratio of Prevalence Rates
	Number Examined	Number with CHD	Rate per 1000	Number Examined	Number with CHD	Rate per 1000	
30–44	1083	5	5	1317	7	5	1.0
45–62	941	43	46	1128	21	19	2.4
Total	2024	48		2445	28		

TABLE 7–2 Incidence of Coronary Heart Disease (CHD) over an Eight-year Period among 4995*Persons 30–59 Years of Age Free of Coronary Heart Disease at Initial Examination

Age (years)	Males Number Examined	Number with CHD	Rate per 1000	Females Number Examined	Number with CHD	Rate per 1000	Male/Female Ratio of Incidence Rates
30–39	825	20	24.2	1036	1	1.0	24.2
40–49	770	51	66.3	955	19	19.9	3.3
50–59	617	81	131.3	792	53	66.9	2.0
Total	2212	152		2783	73		

*It may be noted that there is a larger number of persons in Table 7–2 than in Table 7–1. Table 7–2 includes a volunteer group of 740 persons enrolled in the study before the formal sampling plan was fully developed and implemented. The addition of this group should not alter significantly the relationships being presented here.

the much greater incidence in males. One should note that the sex differential in incidence rates declines with age. The male to female incidence ratio is only 3.3 in persons 40 to 49 and 2.0 for those 50 to 59.

In spite of their limitations, prevalence figures are useful for determining the extent of a disease problem, and hence valuable for rational planning of facilities and services, e.g., number of hospital beds required, number of clinic visits anticipated, manpower needs, and so on. Furthermore, for control of disease, information is needed about factors which produce chronicity or recurrence once a disease has developed. Since prevalence reflects duration as well as incidence, it can be useful for monitoring control programs for chronic conditions such as mental illness.

CRUDE, SPECIFIC, AND ADJUSTED RATES

Any rate can be expressed in terms of a *total* population or of a *subgroup (specific rates)*. Rates expressed in terms of the total population are either crude or adjusted.

Crude rates are summary rates based on the actual number of events (e.g., births or deaths) in a total population over a given time period. *Adjusted rates* are fictitious summary rates constructed to permit fair comparison between groups differing in some important characteristic. For example, an age-adjusted rate is a total (summary) rate which has been standardized for age distribution so that it is, in effect, independent of the age structure of the particular population being studied.

Crude Rates

Two crude rates are widely used in descriptions of populations. These are crude birth rate and crude death rate. They are defined as follows:

$$\text{Crude birth rate} = \frac{\text{number of live births to residents in an area in a calendar year}}{\text{average population}^* \text{ in the area in that year}} \times 1000\dagger$$

$$\text{Crude death rate} = \frac{\text{number of deaths among residents in an area in a calendar year}}{\text{average population}^* \text{ in the area in that year}} \times 1000\dagger$$

Even brief reflection shows that the total population is really not an appropriate denominator for births since these arise only from females in child-bearing ages. Similarly, for inspection of death rates the total population is not an ideal denominator. Since people in different age groups differ in risk of death, differences between populations in age composition will create differences in crude rates even where rates specific for the various age subgroups are the same.

Despite their limitations, crude birth and death rates continue to be widely cited, in part because they are summary rates and in part because they can be constructed from a minimum of informa-

---

*Usually midyear population (July 1). As a specific example, the 3,521,000 live births in the United States in 1967 occurring in the total resident population of 197,864,000 yielded a crude birth rate of 17.5 per 1000 persons. The 1,851,000 deaths in the same year were equivalent to a crude death rate of 9.4 per 1000.

†Rates can be given in any convenient form, i.e., they may be expressed in percentage (i.e., per 100), or per 1000, or per 100,000, depending on convention and the absolute magnitude of the numbers involved. In general it is wise to avoid fractions; 4 per 100,000 is easier to deal with than 0.04 per 1000. For some rates it is customary to use a specific format (e.g., infant mortality is almost invariably given as the rate per 1000 live births, crude birth and death rates per 1000 total population). Age-specific and cause-specific death rates are generally given per 100,000.

tion. For example, crude birth rates require only knowledge of the number of births in a year and the total population of the area. A measure of births limited to females of child-bearing age would require additional information about the age and sex composition of the population. Therefore crude birth and death rates continue to be used for international and temporal comparisons of fertility and health.

Specific Rates

For understanding epidemiologic aspects of disease and population dynamics, detailed rates specific for age and other demographic components, such as sex or race, are needed. The J-shaped mortality curves presented in Figure 3–1 illustrate the great variation in death rates at different ages. The basic formula for specific rates can be seen from the following example of an age-specific rate.

$$\text{Age-specific death rate (ages 25–34)} = \frac{\text{number of deaths among residents aged 25–34 in an area in a calendar year}}{\text{average population aged 25–34 in the area in that year}} \times 100{,}000$$

Translated into actual numbers, the 37,249 deaths among the estimated population of 23,684,000 persons aged 25 to 34 years in the United States in 1968 yielded an age-specific death rate of 157.3 per 100,000. In marked contrast, the age-specific death rate for those 65 to 74 years of age was 3848.5 per 100,000.

Adjusted Rates

While specific rates can provide valuable information, there is a need for a summary type of rate which does not share the limitations of crude rates. Such a rate is the *adjusted* or *standardized rate*. Like the crude rate the *adjusted rate* presents one summary figure for a total population, but statistical procedures are carried out to "remove the effect" of differences in composition for any comparisons. Age is the variable for which adjustment is most often required because of its marked effect on morbidity and mortality. Although the following discussion will refer to adjustment for age, one should remember that at times it may be necessary to adjust for variables other than age, such as sex or race.

There are basically two methods for holding constant the age composition of a population.* In the *direct method,* age-specific rates observed in two or more study populations are applied to an arbitrarily chosen population structure known as a "standard" population. Any difference then found in these standardized rates must be due to differences in age-specific rates.

The *indirect method* is used to compare two populations in one of which the age-specific rates are not known or, if known, are excessively variable because of small numbers. In this method the more stable rates of the larger population are applied to the smaller study group. Comparison of the expected deaths thus obtained with the number actually observed in the smaller population yields a measure known as the *standardized mortality ratio,* or SMR.

$$\text{Standardized mortality ratio (SMR)} = \frac{\text{observed deaths}}{\text{expected deaths}}$$

Similarly it is possible to use a standardized morbidity ratio if the event of interest is occurrence of disease rather than death.

---

*See Appendix 7–1 for a more detailed explanation of age-adjustment.

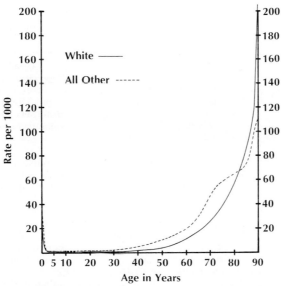

Figure 7–1 Death rates per 1000 by age and color, United States, 1968. (From National Center for Health Statistics: Vital Statistics of the United States, 1968, Vol. IIA. U.S. Govt. Printing Office, Washington, D.C., 1972.)

Many of the tables and figures in this book show standardized mortality or morbidity ratios. For example, in Table 5–4 the age-specific rates of nonsmokers are applied to the age distribution of various smoking categories to derive expected deaths for each group. The observed deaths divided by the expected deaths yields the standardized mortality ratio for that group. In the Framingham data (Figures 1–2, 13–2), the age-specific incidence rate of stroke or CHD for the total study cohort is applied to the age distribution of each subgroup (e.g., hypertension absent, hypertension present) to first obtain expected cases and then a standardized morbidity ratio.

Sometimes the direction or magnitude of differences in rates is not consistent across all age groups. Under such circumstances, an overall summary rate will mask some of the details of the comparison. For example, Figure 7–1 shows higher age-specific death rates for nonwhites than whites in the United States at all ages until 80 years. After that the picture reverses and the whites have higher rates. Because trends may differ for different age groups, one should always inspect age-specific rates before doing any age-adjustment.

Table 7–3 summarizes the advantages and disadvantages of the three kinds of rates we have been discussing — crude, specific, and adjusted.

TABLE 7–3   Advantages and Disadvantages of Crude, Specific, and Adjusted Rates

	Advantages	Disadvantages
Crude Rates	Actual summary rates Readily calculable for international comparisons (widely used despite limitations)	Since populations vary in composition (e.g., age), differences in crude rates difficult to interpret
Specific Rates	Homogeneous subgroups Detailed rates useful for epidemiologic and public health purposes	Cumbersome to compare many subgroups of two or more populations
Adjusted Rates	Summary statements Differences in composition of groups "removed," permitting unbiased comparison	Fictional rates Absolute magnitude dependent on standard population chosen Opposing trends in subgroups masked

MAJOR SOURCES OF ERROR IN MEASUREMENT OF DISEASE

In all scientific endeavors one must be concerned with the possibility of error in the measurements being made. There are two basic kinds of error, random (chance) and systematic.

Random error refers to fluctuations around a true value because of sampling variability. *Systematic error*, also known as *bias*,* may be formally defined as any difference between the true value and that actually obtained due to all causes other than sampling variability. Of the two sources of error, systematic error is generally the more important and the more insidious.

For a simple example of systematic error, consider the effects of an inadequate measuring instrument. If a ruler is incorrectly calibrated, there will always be an error in the measurement and it will always be in the same direction. The only way to detect such an error is to compare the results with those obtained by an independent standard (i.e., a correctly calibrated ruler). Several sources of bias, most more subtle than an erroneously calibrated instrument, are particularly likely to enter epidemiologic studies, and will therefore be discussed briefly.

Use of Nonrandom Samples of the Target Population

Since we are interested in inferences about populations in epidemiologic studies, it is essential to study either an entire population or a satisfactory sample thereof.

Inferences will be incorrect if the sampling procedure does not permit the development of accurate estimates of the population of interest. A classic example of this type of error is afforded by the Literary Digest poll of 1936. This now-famous poll attempted to forecast the outcome of the presidential election in which Franklin D. Roosevelt ran against Alfred Landon. The persons responsible for the poll erroneously predicted a victory for the Republican candidate; Roosevelt actually won the election by a landslide. How could the poll-takers have been so wrong? Their problem lay in the fact that they obtained a sample of people to be queried from telephone listings. The people who had telephones were typically the

---

*In statistics and epidemiology the term "bias" carries no imputation of prejudice or other subjective factor, such as the experimenter's desire for a particular outcome. This differs from conversational usage in which bias refers to a particular, partisan point of view.

more prosperous citizens who were also more likely to vote for a Republican candidate. Thus the sample was not representative of the entire universe of voters.

Similarly, in epidemiology much information about health comes from nonrandom samples of the population—from findings based on autopsy studies, from the data of insurance companies and specific occupational groups. The biases inherent in autopsy data are discussed in Chapter 8; the effects of self-selection into occupational groups on disease rates has been mentioned in Chapter 3. A major advance toward reducing this type of bias is achieved by the use of population-based samples to replace or supplement more readily obtained data from nonrandom samples of the population.

Nonparticipation of a Segment of the Target Group

Another problem in making inferences about a population stems from the fact that some of the people designated as the target group decline to participate or are not available for the study. If the nonparticipants are either more or less healthy, on the average, than the participants, or more or less likely to have had some specific exposure related to the purposes of the study, then a serious source of bias is introduced.

This is a problem which bedevils all kinds of studies. In household surveys, for example, if no one is home in a previously designated household, then it might seem convenient and harmless to substitute the family next door. This may make the sample unrepresentative since the fact of being home may be related to illness, employment status, life style, and so on. It is therefore necessary to make as many revisits as practicable to complete the study.

Nonparticipation or nonresponse is particularly troublesome in mailed surveys. Unless the survey is of particular interest to the respondents, or is sponsored by an organization of great prestige in the eyes of the persons surveyed, substantial nonresponse is the rule.

Differences between participants and nonparticipants have been demonstrated repeatedly in surveys based on clinical examination. For example, in the Framingham study of arteriosclerotic heart disease mentioned previously, the initial nonresponse rate was considerable, a little over 30 per cent. On follow-up, both male and female nonrespondents were found to have a higher death rate than respondents.

Figure 7–2 presents an intriguing illustration of systematic relations between tendency to participate and disease. The figure

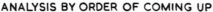

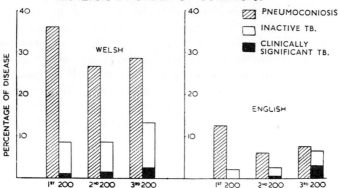

Figure 7–2 Percentage of volunteers found to have disease, analyzed by order of participation. (From Cochrane, A. L.: The application of scientific methods to industrial and social medicine. In Morris, J. N., Uses of Epidemiology. The Williams & Wilkins Company, Baltimore, 1964, p. 51.)

shows the amount of disease uncovered by a screening examination according to the order in which groups of volunteers appeared for the examination. Those who appeared later had more tuberculosis than the group which responded promptly. The opposite relationship was found for pneumoconiosis (lung disease due to occupational exposure to dust); this condition was more common among the early respondents. The fact that the same pattern was found in two groups, one English, the other Welsh, makes it more likely that this is not a chance happening.

These data suggest that the extent and direction of bias introduced by nonparticipation cannot be estimated *a priori* but must be determined empirically. However, it seems to be generally true that persons of low educational attainment tend to participate in medical surveys at a lesser rate than those with better educational background.

There are several approaches to the reduction of bias from nonparticipation. Firstly, diligent efforts should be made to keep nonparticipation at a minimum. Participation should be as convenient and painless as possible. Flexible schedules and use of mobile examination vans have been found helpful. However, even under the most favorable circumstances problems of non-response should be anticipated. The number of call-backs planned for a household interview survey, for instance, should be specified and provided for in the budget of the study. Secondly, insofar as possible the final group of nonrespondents should be evaluated to see if they differ in demographic characteristics and health status from the respondents. This might be done by search of death certificates or hospital records or by extraordinary efforts (e.g., repeated telephone calls or home visits) to gain some basic information about a subsample of the nonparticipants. Lastly, analyses can be carried out based on extreme assumptions, i.e., that **all** or **none** of the nonrespondents would have a disease or factor. The maximum and minimum possible values for the item obtained in this way establish the outer limits of variation around the true value.

Variation in Making and Recording Observations

Epidemiologic studies generally require observations of large numbers of persons. This makes it necessary to pool data from multiple observers, often working in different institutions or different countries and under differing organizational, technical, and climatic constraints. The main approaches to reducing this kind of variation lie in standardization of methods and training of personnel to carry out procedures and record observations, and in the use of duplicate or multiple observers.

Variability in findings due to variation among observers, (*observer variation*), has been of concern for several decades. A major impetus to awareness of the phenomenon was a study in the late 1940's by Yerushalmy to compare the value of different types of chest x-rays for mass screening purposes. Several kinds of miniature films had recently been developed and it was hoped that they would provide a cheaper way to x-ray larger numbers of persons than the standard (14×17) chest films. However, it was not known whether the results would be as dependable. To test this, some 1200 persons were each x-rayed with four different techniques. The resulting films were read independently by five experts. Yerushalmy concluded that the four techniques were essentially equivalent for tuberculosis case-finding in mass survey work (1947). Surprisingly, the variations in reading for each technique were so great that in effect they exceeded the variation among techniques. One conclusion from the study was the recommendation that survey films be read independently by at least two observers and that all persons whose films were read as positive or suggestive for tuberculosis by either reader be recalled for further study.

In the years since this study the phenomenon of variability among observers, as well as inconsistency for the same observer, has been documented for many kinds of medical data — history-taking, physical examination, and laboratory tests of various kinds.

These demonstrations of observer variation have heightened awareness of the need for careful training of participants in studies, for specification of criteria to be used in classifying subjects, and for the development of a standard protocol and standard equipment at the various study centers. They also provide a powerful argument for the application of double blind techniques whenever possible.

Variation in Perceptions of Illness and Illness Behavior

One factor contributing to biased morbidity statistics is *illness behavior*. This has been defined (Mechanic, 1062) as "the ways in which given symptoms may be differentially perceived, evaluated, and acted (or not acted) upon by different kinds of persons." Differences in the perception of disease and consequent action will affect all kinds of morbidity statistics, from those based on household surveys to those based on hospital records.

Severe, life-threatening symptoms almost always lead to specific action. As one moves along the spectrum from severe to mild symptoms, the proportion of situations in which aid is sought decreases and, conversely, factors in the individual and in his environmental setting assume increasing importance in determining whether or not action is taken and aid is sought. Thus the same illness, such as a moderately severe respiratory infection, might have several outcomes. The affected individual might carry on his daily activities and seek no medical advice; another might continue to work, but visit a doctor; a third might not only seek medical consultation, but take a day off from work. The first example of illness would not be known except to the person himself; the second and third would contribute to morbidity statistics, but to different extents. Only the third would contribute to days lost from work, a measure of disability. While the origins of such variability are not the issue at the moment, we might just note in passing that whether or not medical aid is sought will depend on a number of factors. Among them are the past history of the person, his cultural, ethnic, and family background, as well as situational factors, such as whether the person is a civilian or a member of the military, the nature of his arrangements for medical care, i.e., does he have to pay for care, does he have paid sick leave, is reporting of minor illnesses encouraged by his employer, is care accessible, and so on.

Measures of utilization of medical care have importance in their own right. However, based on the considerations just discussed, they have serious weaknesses as tools for the study of etiology of disease. When etiologic hypotheses are being tested, it is im-

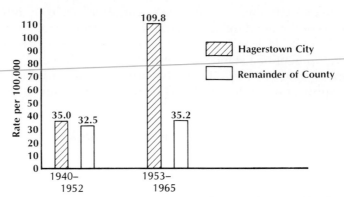

Figure 7–3 Average annual rates per 100,000 population aged 15–64 of first hospitalization for specified psychoses, Washington County, Maryland, 1940–1952 and 1953–1965. (Based on Silverman, C.: Epidemiology of Depression. Johns Hopkins University Press, Baltimore, 1968.)

portant to be aware of the potential contribution of illness behavior to statistics.

Variation in Availability of Treatment Resources

Differences between areas in the availability of treatment facilities can lead to misleading statistics. For example, a higher rate of hospitalization may reflect availability of hospital beds as well as extent of illness. This is shown clearly in Figure 7–3, which compares rates of first hospitalization for certain psychoses for Hagerstown, Maryland, and for the remainder of the county in which Hagerstown is located, in two time periods (Silverman, 1968).

It is apparent that there was a striking increase in first admissions for psychosis for Hagerstown in the second time period as compared with the rest of Washington County, whereas in the previous decade the rates had been quite similar. To interpret these rates correctly it is necessary to know that in 1959 a well-run, private mental hospital was opened in Hagerstown which attracted people from the local area.

SUMMARY

This chapter has discussed the principal methodologic tools developed to assure unbiased measurement and analysis of disease. Incidence and prevalence are the fundamental measures of morbidity. These rates, as well as mortality rates, may be expressed as total rates (crude or adjusted) or as specific rates. The need for adjustment to prevent biased comparisons of populations differing in composition is emphasized; age is the usual factor for which adjustment is carried out. Other important sources of error in measurement were also identified and discussed.

APPENDIX 7-1
ADJUSTMENT OF RATES

The purpose of this appendix is to provide more detailed background and examples of why and how rates are adjusted.

NEED FOR ADJUSTING RATES

We will start with an example which shows that differences in population structure can, by themselves, affect crude rates. In Table 7-4 we see that two populations, A and B, have the same age-specific death rates (column 4); that is, a person in a specific age group in A is at the same risk of dying as a person of the same age group in B. There is no true difference in risk of death. However, A has relatively more older people, i.e., 30 per cent over 45 years compared with only 10 per cent over 45 years in B (column 3). Because death rates are higher at older ages (Figure 3-1) and because A has more older people, this will lead to a higher crude death rate for the population in A.

The difference in crude death rates for Populations A and B can be explained mathematically as follows: The age-specific death rates (column 4) multiplied by the number in the population at each age (column 2) determines the number of deaths in each age group

TABLE 7-4 Comparison of Death Rates in Two Populations by Age

	Age (years)	Population Number	Population Proportion	Annual Age-specific Death Rate per 1000	Annual Number of Deaths	Crude Death Rate per 1000
	(1)	(2)	(3)	(4)	(5)	(6)
Population A	less than 15	1500	.30	2	3	
	15–44	2000	.40	6	12	
	45 and over	1500	.30	20	30	
	All ages	5000	1.00		45	$\frac{45}{5000} = 9.0$
Population B	less than 15	2000	.40	2	4	
	15–44	2500	.50	6	15	
	45 and over	500	.10	20	10	
	All ages	5000	1.00		29	$\frac{29}{5000} = 5.8$

and, therefore, the total deaths (column 5). The latter divided by the total population gives the crude (average) death rate. The crude rate can also be obtained by multiplying each age-specific rate (column 4) by the corresponding population proportion (column 3) and summing the resultant number of deaths. The crude death rate is, therefore, really a *weighted average* of the age-specific death rates in which the numbers (or proportions) in each age group are the weights. Since A has a higher proportion (increased weighting) of older persons for whom the age-specific death rates are higher, the crude death rate is higher in A (9.0 per 1000) than B (5.8 per 1000) even though the risk of dying for persons in each age group is the same.

DIRECT ADJUSTMENT OF RATES

Table 7–5 shows how this difference in age composition or weighting can be eliminated, thus permitting fair comparison of the two populations. This requires the selection of some population, called a *standard population*, to which the age-specific rates for each population (columns 2 and 4) can be applied. In this instance, we have arbitrarily chosen the combined populations of A and B as standard (column 1). Multiplying the standard population by the age-specific rates in A and B yields the number of *expected* deaths in A and B respectively as shown in columns 3 and 5.

Note that the expected deaths in columns 3 and 5 answer the question: What would be the number of deaths in the standard population (column 1) if people were dying at the age-specific rates observed in each population (columns 2 and 4)? The answer is, of course, fictitious. Nevertheless, we see that the number of expected deaths (74) would be the same for populations A and B. Also, the age-adjusted rates (7.4 per 1000) are the same for A and B. This must be so since A and B have the same age-specific death rates and population differences have been eliminated by use of the same (standard) population. Thus age-adjustment has demonstrated there is truly no difference between A and B in risk of death.

Let us now assume that the age-specific death rate for age 15 to 44 is *higher* in B than A, 10 vs. 6 per 1000 (columns 2 and 4), as seen in Table 7–6. Multiplying the age-specific death rates in these columns by the standard population now yields more expected deaths for B (column 5) than for A (column 3). As a result, the age-adjusted rate is now higher for B than A, as expected.

TABLE 7–5 Computation of Expected Number of Deaths by Direct Method: Example 1: Identical Age-specific Rates

Age (years)	Standard Population (A and B Combined)	Population A Age-specific Death Rates per 1000
	(1)	(2)
less than 15	3500	2
15–44	4500	6
45 and over	2000	20
All ages	10,000	

Adjusted death rates based on Table 7–6:

$$A = \frac{74}{10,000} = 7.4 \text{ per } 1000$$

$$B = \frac{92}{10,000} = 9.2 \text{ per } 1000$$

We should point out that the choice of a standard population is arbitrary. In the example above the standard was the **combined** populations of A and B, but **either** one of the two could have been chosen. For comparability among studies it is advantageous that the same standard be used by different investigators. Thus, for many years the United States population of 1940 was widely used as a standard, even when population data for subsequent years were already available. The choice of standard, while affecting the magnitudes of the age-adjusted rates, will usually not affect the relative ranking of the populations unless the standard chosen is grossly different in age distribution from the population or populations under study.

TABLE 7–6 Computation of Expected Number of Deaths by Direct Method: Example 2: Different Age-specific Rates

Age (years)	Standard Population (A and B Combined)	Population A Age-specific Death Rates per 1000
	(1)	(2)
less than 15	3500	2
15–44	4500	6
45 and over	2000	20
All ages	10,000	

TABLE 7–5 Computation of Expected Number of Deaths by Direct Method: Example 1: Identical Age-specific Rates (*Continued*)

Expected Deaths	Population B Age-specific Death Rates per 1000	Expected Deaths
$(3) = (2) \times (1)$	(4)	$(5) = (4) \times (1)$
7	2	7
27	6	27
40	20	40
74		74

INDIRECT ADJUSTMENT OF RATES

There are circumstances in which age-adjustment is required but the procedure just described cannot be applied because the small number of deaths in one group leads to unstable age-specific rates or its age-specific rates may not be known. When this is true, another method is available. This is referred to as indirect adjustment.

The indirect method of age-adjustment may be viewed as a mirror image of the direct method. In the direct method just described, an age-adjusted rate is achieved by applying age-specific rates of the population (or populations) of interest (e.g., A or B) to a population of known age structure (e.g., A and B combined) to yield an "expected" number of deaths. The group of known age structure is called the "standard" population.

In the indirect method standardization is based on age-specific *rates* rather than on age composition. Here the population whose

Table 7–6 Computation of Expected Number of Deaths by Direct Method Example 2: Different Age-specific Rates (*Continued*)

Expected Deaths	Population B Age-specific Death Rates per 1000	Expected Deaths
(3)	(4)	(5)
7	2	7
27	10	45
40	20	40
74		92

rates form the basis for comparison is referred to as the "standard" population. If two populations are to be compared by the indirect method, the larger of the two is usually chosen as standard because its rates tend to be more stable. However, if a developed and an un-derdeveloped country are being compared, the developed country would probably be taken as the standard, regardless of comparative size, since age-specific rates might be available only for this country.

The process of indirect adjustment consists of applying the age-specific rates of the standard population to a population of interest (e.g., population A) to yield a number of "expected" deaths. This process is equivalent to asking, what would be the number of deaths (i.e., expected deaths) in population A if people in that population were dying at the same (age-specific) rate as people in the standard population.

A common way of carrying out indirect age-adjustment is to relate the total expected deaths thus obtained to observed deaths through a formula known as the *standardized mortality ratio* (SMR):

$$\text{SMR} = \frac{\text{total observed deaths in a population}}{\text{total expected deaths in that population}}$$

If this mortality ratio is greater than 1, it means that more deaths are observed in the smaller population than would be expected based on rates in the larger (standard) population. If the ratio is less than 1, fewer deaths are observed than expected.*

The use of indirect age-adjustment through calculation of SMR can be illustrated by the Muscogee County, Georgia, study of tuberculosis (Comstock, 1953). In 1946, 70-mm. photofluorograms (Pf) were taken primarily for the information they would yield about tuberculosis. However, since they were also read for possible cardiovascular abnormalities, it became possible to compare the subsequent mortality experience of those whose Pf was read as negative with those whose Pf suggested possible cardiovascular disease. Data for three and one-half years of observation are shown in Table 7–7.

The crude death rate for suspects (17.9) is higher than that for the negatives (1.15). However, since the distribution of ages for the

---

*The SMR is a ratio resulting from a *relative* form of indirect age-adjustment. A more complicated method of indirect adjustment, which yields an *absolute* age-adjusted rate, involves the calculation of an *index death rate* and a *standardizing factor* for each population of interest.

TABLE 7-7 Deaths by Age and Pf Reading (Whites) for Three and a Half Year Observation Period, Muscogee County, Georgia, 1946

Age in 1946 (years)	Negative for Cardiovascular Disease			Suspect for Cardiovascular Disease	
	Population	Number of Deaths	Age-specific death rates per 100	Population	Number of Deaths
15–34	13,681	35	0.25	23	1
35–54	8838	102	1.15	24	5
55 and over	2253	149	6.61	65	14
All ages	24,772	286		112	20
Crude death rate per 100		1.15			17.9

two groups is quite dissimilar (Table 7–8), age-adjustment is necessary.

TABLE 7–8 Percentage Distribution by Age of Negatives and Suspects, Muscogee County, Georgia

Age (years)	Negative for Cardiovascular Disease		Suspect for Cardiovascular Disease	
	Number	Percentage of Population	Number	Percentage of Population
15–34	13,681	55.2	23	20.5
35–54	8838	35.7	24	21.4
55 and over	2253	9.1	65	58.0
All ages	24,772	100.0	112	99.9

Because the suspect group was small and gave rise to only 20 deaths during the three and a half year period of observation, the age-specific death rates of this group would be quite unstable. Accordingly, we use the larger group of negatives as the standard population (Table 7–9) and apply the age-specific death rates noted in this group (column 2) to the suspects (column 1) in order to determine an expected number of deaths among the suspects (column 3). The total number of expected deaths among "suspects" (4.7) is then compared with the number actually observed in this group through the standardized mortality ratio, as shown below.

$$\text{SMR} = \frac{\text{observed deaths}}{\text{expected deaths}} = \frac{20}{4.7} = 4.25$$

TABLE 7–9 Calculation of Standardized Mortality Ratio for Suspects Compared with Negatives, Muscogee County, Georgia

Age (years)	Number of "Suspects"	Death Rates per 100 for Persons Negative for Cardiovascular Disease	Expected Deaths among "Suspects" According to Rates for Negatives	Observed Deaths among "Suspects"
	(1)	(2)	(3) = (1) × (2)	(4)
15–34	23	0.25	.1	1
35–54	24	1.15	.3	5
55 and over	65	6.61	4.3	14
All ages			4.7	20

We see that the SMR is 4.25, indicating that even after age-adjustment the overall death rate is still higher for "suspects" than for "negatives." However, the much larger original ratio of the crude rates, 15.5 (i.e., 17.9 to 1.15) has been much reduced by adjustment.

SUMMARY *

In direct age-adjustment, a common age-structured *population* is used as standard. This population may actually exist (e.g., United States population, 1940) or may be fictitious (e.g., two populations may be combined to create a standard). Application of the observed age-specific rates in each area to the same standard population yields numbers of expected deaths and summary death rates which can be compared for any number of populations.

In indirect age-adjustment, a common set of age-specific *rates* is applied to the populations whose rates are to be standardized. The simplest and most useful form of indirect adjustment is the standardized mortality ratio (SMR). With this method, when more than two populations are to be compared, each may be compared to the standard population, but not directly to the others. The SMR is used in many situations, such as clinical trials and observational studies. It permits adjustment for age and other factors where age-specific rates are unavailable or are unstable because of small numbers. A typical application is comparison of death rates for a specific occupational group with those of an entire population.

STUDY QUESTIONS

7–1 Define the following terms and give an example when appropriate:
Rate (page 126)
Morbidity (page 126)
Incidence rate (page 126)
Prevalence rate (point, period, and lifetime prevalence) (page 127ff.)
Attack rate (page 130)
Person-years (page 130)

---

*For more detailed discussion of the methods and issues involved in age-adjustment, the reader is referred to Hill, A. Bradford: Principles of Medical Statistics, 9th ed. Lancet Ltd., London, 1971, pp. 201–219.

Population at risk (page 131)
Crude rate (crude birth and death rates) (page 134)
Specific rates (page 134)
Adjusted (standardized) rate (direct and indirect age-adjustment) (page 136)
Standardized mortality ratio (SMR) (page 137)
Sources of error (random vs. systematic) (page 139)
Bias (systematic error) (page 139)
Observer variation (page 142)
Illness behavior (page 143)

7–2 From Figure 7–4 calculate the following rates for a group of 300 persons.

    A. Point prevalence on July 1, 1973
    B. Incidence rate, July 1, 1973 to June 30, 1974
    C. Period prevalence, July 1, 1973 to June 30, 1974

Answer on page 347.

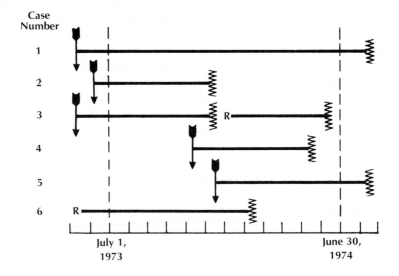

Date of onset of disease

Date of death or termination of disease

R   Date of recurrence of disease

Figure 7–4 A diagrammatic representation of cases of a disease in a group of 300 persons.

7-3 In 1970, the crude death rate (all causes) for Guyana was 6.8 per 1000; for the United States it was 9.4 per 1000.

> A. Can the lower crude death rate in Guyana be explained by the fact that the United States has a larger population? Explain your answer.
> B. Cite two other possible explanations for the lower rate in Guyana.
> C. Additional information about these countries for the same year is as follows:

	Guyana	United States
Crude birth rate (per 1000 population)	38.1	18.2
Infant mortality rate (per 1000 live births)	38.3 (provisional, 1968)	19.8

> How does this additional information assist you in interpreting the difference in crude death rates?

> Answer on page 348.

7-4 Crude and age-adjusted death rates from "arteriosclerotic and degenerative heart disease" are shown for Chile and the United States for 1967:

	Rates per 100,000 Persons	
	Crude Rates	Age-adjusted Rates
Chile	67.4	58.2
United States	316.3	131.4
Ratio United States/Chile	4.7	2.3

> Which of the two summary rates is preferable for comparing the death rate from heart disease in the two countries? Why? Why do the ratios of the crude and age-adjusted rates for the two countries differ?

> Answer on page 348.

7-5* Three successive surveys of the prevalence of pulmonary tuberculosis were carried out by the National Tuberculosis Institute, Bangalore, India. A complete population census (household survey) was taken of 119 villages randomly selected from a total of 734 villages in three administrative units (taluks). The study group included the entire population of these 119 villages except for children under the age of five years, persons previously vaccinated with BCG,†

---

*Study questions 7–5, 7–6, and 7–7 are based on Narain, R., Naganna, K., et al.: *Incidence of pulmonary tuberculosis.* Am. Rev. Respir. Dis., *107*:992, 1973.

†BCG is a vaccine prepared from an attenuated bovine strain of tubercle bacillus (see page 296).

TABLE 7–10 Incidence of Pulmonary Tuberculosis (Culture-positive Cases)

Age (years)	Number of Persons Examined at Survey 2 and/or 3	Males Number of New Cases	Rate per 1000 Person-years
0–4	2325	—	—
5–14	6354	8	1.3
15–24	3009	4	1.3
25–44	4868	7	1.4
45 and over	2375	9	3.8
All ages	18,931	28	1.5

and persons with an abnormal chest x-ray on initial survey. The study population was tuberculin tested and offered a 70 mm. chest photofluorogram. Specimens of sputum were also examined for persons with abnormal chest x-rays. The average interval between surveys was approximately 18 months. Some persons were examined at all three surveys, some only at surveys one and two, or one and three.

Incidence rates of pulmonary tuberculosis calculated on the basis of the three surveys are shown in Table 7–10.

A. Was it necessary to conduct two or more surveys in order to obtain incidence rates? Explain your answer.

B. The authors present incidence rates as "rates per 1000 person-years." Why did they express the rates in this way?

Answer on page 348.

7–6 Table 7–11 shows tuberculosis incidence for households with and without a case of tuberculosis at survey one.

Comment on the difference in new case rate by type of household. What are the implications of Table 7–11 for a tuberculosis control program?

Answer on page 349.

7–7 A. Study Figure 7–5. What factors might account for the higher incidence, but lower prevalence, for females than males at ages 15 to 44? Which factor is the most likely explanation? Why?

B. In light of Figure 7–5, comment on the dangers of prevalence surveys for estimating the relative risk of ac-

among Persons with Normal Photofluorograms at Survey One, by Age and Sex

Number of Persons Examined at Survey 2 and/or 3	Females	
	Number of New Cases	Rate per 1000 Person-years
2163	—	—
6210	8	1.3
2526	7	2.8
4989	9	1.8
2366	2	0.8
18,254	26	1.4

quiring a disease for different subgroups (e.g., males vs. females)?

Answer on page 349.

7–8 The usefulness of age-adjustment of rates is illustrated in Figure 7–6. Curves (1) and (2) represent two ways of showing the secular trend in overall mortality in the United States between 1900 and 1960. One curve represents crude death rates, the other age-adjusted death rates.

    A. The United States population of what year was used as the standard for age-adjustment? Explain your answer.

    B. Looking at the rates in 1900, which is the crude rate and which the age-adjusted rate? Explain your answer.

TABLE 7–11 Incidence of Pulmonary Tuberculosis (Culture-positive Cases) among Members of Three Different Categories of Households

Category of Household at Survey 1	Number of Persons Reexamined at Survey 2 and/or 3	Number of New Cases	New Case Rate per 1000 Person-years
Household with a culture-positive case	491	8	5.9
Household with a culture-negative case of radiographic category 1 or 2*	11,124	17	0.6
Household with no case	19,301	27	0.5
Total	30,916	52	0.6

*Category 1, active or possibly active pulmonary tuberculosis; category 2, inactive tuberculosis or nontuberculous pulmonary disease.

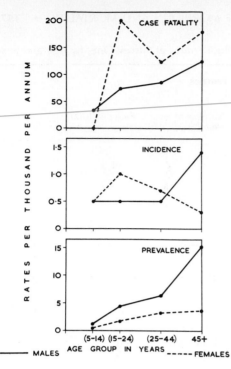

Figure 7–5 Prevalence, incidence, and case fatality rates for the culture-positive cases, shown separately for males and females in four age groups. (From Narain, R., Naganna, K., et al.: Incidence of pulmonary tuberculosis. Am. Rev. Respir. Dis., *107*:992, 1973.)

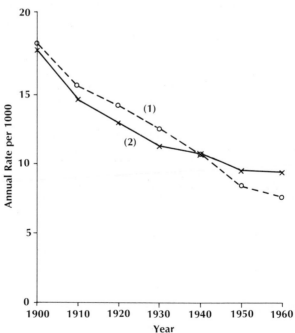

Figure 7–6 Crude and age-adjusted death rates, United States (1900–1930, death registration states; 1940–1960, total United States).

158

C. Why has one curve levelled off after 1940, while the other has continued to decline?

Answer on page 349.

REFERENCES

Bahn, A. K.: Methodologic Study of Population of Outpatient Psychiatric Clinics, Maryland 1958–1959. USPHS Pub. No. 821 (Public Health Monograph No. 65), U.S. Govt. Printing Office, Washington, D.C., 1961.

Comstock, G. W.: Mortality of persons with photofluorograms suggestive of cardiovascular disease. N. Engl. J. Med., 248:1045, 1953.

de Alarcon, R.: The spread of heroin abuse in a community. Bull. Narc., 21, 3:17, 1969.

Hughes, P. H., Barker, N. W., et al.: The natural history of a heroin epidemic. Am. J. Public Health, 62:995, 1972.

Leighton, D. C., Harding, J. S., et al.: The Character of Danger. Basic Books, New York, 1963.

Mechanic, D.: The concept of illness behavior. J. Chronic Dis., 15:189, 1962.

Potter, R. G., Jr.: Additional measures of use-effectiveness of contraception. Milbank Mem. Fund Q., 41:400, 1963.

Silverman, C.: The Epidemiology of Depression. Johns Hopkins University Press, Baltimore, 1968.

Yerushalmy, J.: Statistical problems in assessing methods of medical diagnosis, with special reference to X-ray techniques. Public Health Rep., 62:1432, 1947.

SOURCES OF DATA ON COMMUNITY HEALTH

8

Earlier chapters emphasized the importance of epidemiology in furnishing a conceptual framework and tools for studying the etiology of disease. Epidemiology is also of value to administrators and health planners for identifying health problems and needs, allocating resources, and measuring the effectiveness of new programs. For these purposes data are required in three areas: (1) the population and its demographic components; (2) health status, illness, and deaths; and (3) health resources, i.e., physician and allied manpower and facilities. Discussion of health resources is outside the scope of this text, but the first two subjects will be covered in the next three chapters. Sources of data will be discussed in this chapter. Chapter 9 will outline the specific indices used for measuring the health of population groups. Chapter 10 will focus on the population itself, the dynamics of population change, and their implications for health.

THE CENSUS

Planning and programming in all fields, including health, is predicated on knowledge of the size and composition of a population, the forces which determine present size and composition, and projected trends. The importance of accurate information on population is recognized by governments everywhere. In the United States, the Congress allocates large sums for periodic enumerations of the population.

160

The term *census*, which comes from the Latin word meaning "to estimate or assess," refers to periodic counts or enumerations of a population. Records of population enumerations go back over 5000 years to the Babylonians, Chinese, and Egyptians. Following the disintegration of the Roman Empire, there were relatively few attempts to maintain accurate population records in Europe until the late eighteenth century, when a number of Western European countries instituted a formal census.

In this country, a census has been taken every ten years since 1790. The original purpose of the census was to count heads in order to apportion the number of logislators each state would send to the House of Representatives. Since its beginnings the census has gradually been expanded to encompass data on many characteristics of the population. Name, address, age, sex, color, marital status, and relation to the head of the household, as well as some characteristics of housing, are obtained from all persons. Information on nativity, migration, education, parity, employment status, income, and so on are obtained from a sample. Information from the census is vitally important to each jurisdiction because it forms the basis for the allocation of federal and state funds under a variety of programs. This has recently become particularly important owing to the decentralization of federal activities and the introduction of revenue-sharing.

There are two principal methods for enumeration of a population: *de facto*, which allocates persons according to their location at the time of enumeration, and *de jure*, which assigns them according to their usual place of residence. For example, a salesman living in Cincinnati but working in Boston on the day of the census would be assigned to Boston on a *de facto* census, to Cincinnati if the *de jure* method were employed. The United States Census uses *de jure* enumeration because it provides a better indication of the permanent population and household composition of an area.

The Bureau of the Census has attempted to compensate for the cost and complexity of enumerating an ever increasing population by utilizing technological advances, such as punched cards (1890) and optical scanning of forms (1960). Through 1950 the census was taken primarily by trained enumerators who visited each household to collect data. The 1960 census introduced self-enumeration by households, the 1970 census reliance on the mails for distribution and return of census forms. In the latter year enumerators were used in urban areas only to obtain missing information and to verify questionable items.

Census information is analyzed and presented for the country as a whole and for progressively smaller subdivisions — four regions

(Northeast, North Central, South, and West), nine divisions (e.g., New England, Middle Atlantic), states, counties, cities or munici-palities, census tracts, blocks, and, where requirements for ano-nymity permit, block faces. In addition, areas are classified as urban or rural. The definitions of urban and rural have changed from time to time. The term "urban" is now normally used for places with at least 2500 inhabitants, but the complete definition specifies a number of exceptions.

Since 1950 emphasis has been placed on classification of areas as metropolitan or nonmetropolitan as well as rural or urban. The political boundaries of cities in the United States no longer de-scribe meaningful units. The proliferation of a network of highways in and around cities has been followed by the establishment of not only dormitory suburbs and shopping centers but also industrial parks and commercial complexes. Because of the extensive interac-tions between a city and its surrounding areas, a unit encompassing both is needed as a base for statistical description.

The concept of a *Standard Metropolitan Statistical Area* (SMSA) was introduced to furnish such a unit. To qualify as an SMSA an area has to meet criteria related to size (at least one city of 50,000 residents), social and economic integration of the city and sur-rounding county or counties, minimum population density, and minimum proportion of the labor force engaged in nonagricultural work. In the 1970 census there were 228 SMSA's in the United States. Over two-thirds of the population (69 per cent) lived within an SMSA; of this number more than half (37.6 per cent) lived out-side the central city, the remainder (31.4) within it. The actual level of integration among the political entities within an SMSA varies greatly. The degree to which the metropolitan area functions as a unit has profound import for the planning and delivery of health services.

Within cities there is often a need for statistical analysis of smaller geographic areas. To meet this need, units called census tracts were established. These are relatively permanent subdivi-sions of large cities and adjacent areas. The boundaries of tracts were originally set so that each tract would contain 3000 to 6000 persons and would be relatively homogeneous in ethnic and so-cioeconomic composition. However, with the passage of time many tracts have become quite heterogeneous. Population growth has necessitated subdivision of some tracts.

The Bureau of the Census makes detailed studies to check on the completeness and accuracy of the census. The 1970 census has been estimated to err by a net undercount of about 2.5 per cent, but the percentage is much higher for certain groups — young children, especially infants, young males, and Blacks. The underenumeration of Blacks was estimated to be 7.7 per cent.

A serious current limitation of the census is that a decennial count cannot provide the accurate and up-to-date information needed by a growing, highly mobile population. This limitation is partially overcome by monthly sample surveys of approximately 50,000 households known as the Current Population Survey (or CPS). However, these surveys cannot provide information in sufficient detail to meet all intercensal needs. There is continued interest in reducing the interval between total population censuses to five years.

The information furnished by individuals to the census is confidential and is not available to private or other government agencies except in the form of summary statistical compilations. Tabulations for small areas are suppressed if they would permit identification of individuals. Despite this, in the past there have been complaints about invasion of privacy. Indignation has been expressed at questions such as whether the toilet and bathroom in a house are shared with another household. The consensus of reactions among public health workers to these objections was expressed in an editorial in the American Journal of Public Health (1969).

[While] this controversy may appear to have its humorous aspects, it is potentially serious in its implications. . . . Valuable statistical information is provided by the census and it is necessary, in fact essential, to have it so as to know where we are and to plan for the future.

VITAL STATISTICS

Probably the major source of information about the health of a population is its vital statistics. By *vital statistics* we mean the data collected from ongoing recording, or registration, of all "vital events"—births and adoptions; deaths and fetal deaths; marriages, divorces, legal separations, and annulments. We will discuss only those aspects of registration with which physicians are mainly concerned—certification of death, birth, and fetal death.

Although certificates are filed locally, legal responsibility for registration of vital events is centralized in the governments of individual states and territories and several large cities. Figure 8–1 outlines the flow of information through the Vital Statistics Registration System in the United States. Although each state determines the format and content of its own certificates, the federal government through its National Center for Health Statistics recommends standard forms which the states tend to adopt. The standard certifi-

RESPONSIBLE PERSON OR AGENCY	BIRTH CERTIFICATE	DEATH CERTIFICATE	FETAL DEATH CERTIFICATE (Stillbirth)
Physician, Other Professional Attendant, or Hospital Authority	1. Completes entire certificate in consultation with parent(s). Physician's signature required. 2. Files certificate with local office of district in which birth occurred.	1. Completes medical certification and signs certificate. 2. Returns certificate to funeral director.	1. Completes or reviews medical items on certificate. 2. Certifies to the cause of fetal death and signs certificate. 3. Returns certificate to funeral director. 4. In absence of funeral director, files certificate.
Funeral Director		1. Obtains personal facts about deceased. 2. Takes certificate to physician for medical certification. 3. Delivers completed certificate to local office of district where death occurred and obtains burial permit.	1. Obtains the facts about fetal death. 2. Takes certificate to physician for entry of causes of fetal death. 3. Delivers completed certificate to local office of district where delivery occurred and obtains burial permit.
Local Office (may be Local Registrar or City or County Health Department)	1. Verifies completeness and accuracy of certificate. 2. Makes copy, ledger entry, or index for local use. 3. Sends certificates to State Registrar.	1. Verifies completeness and accuracy of certificate. 2. Makes copy, ledger entry, or index for local use. 3. Issues burial permit to funeral director and verifies return of permit from cemetery attendant. 4. Sends certificates to State Registrar.	

City and county health departments use certificates in allocating medical and nursing services, followups on infectious diseases, planning programs, measuring effectiveness of services, and conducting research studies.

State Registrar, Bureau of Vital Statistics	1. Queries incomplete or inconsistent information. 2. Maintains files for permanent reference and as the source of certified copies. 3. Develops vital statistics for use in planning, evaluating, and administering State and local health activities and for research studies. 4. Compiles health related statistics for State and civil divisions of State for use of the health department and other agencies and groups interested in the fields of medical science, public health, demography, and social welfare. 5. Prepares copies of birth, death, and fetal death certificates or records for transmission to the National Center for Health Statistics.
Public Health Service National Center for Health Statistics	1. Prepares and publishes national statistics of births, deaths, and fetal deaths; and constructs the official U.S. life tables and related actuarial tables. 2. Conducts health and social-research studies based on vital records and on sampling surveys linked to records. 3. Conducts research and methodological studies in vital statistics methods including the technical, administrative, and legal aspects of vital records registration and administration. 4. Maintains a continuing technical assistance program to improve the quality and usefulness of vital statistics.

Figure 8–1   The Vital Statistics Registration System in the United States. (From Physicians' Handbook on Medical Certification: Death, Fetal Death, Birth. USPHS Pub. No. 593–B, U.S. Govt. Printing Office, Washington, D.C., 1967.)

cates were last revised in 1968. This revision produced little change in the standard death certificate, but several important changes in the certificates of birth and fetal death.

Historically, registration of vital events goes back a variable length of time for the different states. In Virginia and Massachusetts, the pioneer states, registration of births, marriages, and deaths had been instituted by the middle of the seventeenth century. The federal government began to compile national statistics on deaths in 1880 and on births in 1915 on the basis of copies of certificates submitted by the states. Over the years, the minimum standards for reporting established by the federal government have been met by an increasing number of states. By 1933 the quality of reporting births and deaths had improved to the extent that all states were included in what is known as the *Birth and Death Registration Area.* Since then, registration of births and deaths has continued to improve, partly because an increased proportion of these events take place in hospitals, partly because registration is advantageous to each individual and his family. Proof of birth is required for obtaining a passport and for school entrance. Death certificates are needed for establishing insurance claims, for receipt of veterans' or Social Security benefits, and so on.

Death Certificate

The death certificate is so important for epidemiologic study that it deserves further comment. Death certificates provide information not only on the number of deaths and the decedent's characteristics (e.g., age, sex, color, usual occupation) but also on the conditions which led to death. (Figure 8-2 presents a copy of the recommended standard form.)

It is important to be aware of some problems inherent in obtaining and interpreting information on cause of death. The amount of information available about decedents varies; it depends on the extent to which the person had been studied medically before death, on the familiarity of the certifying physician with the deceased, and on whether or not an autopsy was done. Problems of particular importance for comparative purposes are variation from one area to another in medical practices and diagnostic labelling.

In this connection we might consider the value of autopsy data. The pathologic information obtained from the autopsy is often the basis for a final judgment about the individual patient and is, therefore, of great value in the continuing education of physicians. However, autopsy results can be misleading for epidemiologic pur-

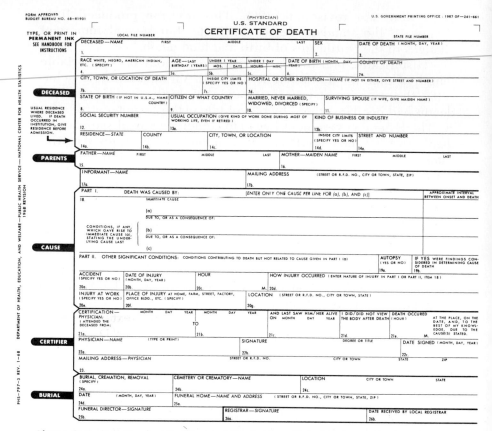

Figure 8–2 U.S. Standard Certificate of Death. (From United States Standard Certificates, 1968 Revision. U.S. Dept. of Health, Education, and Welfare, USPHS.)

poses because autopsies are done on a nonrandom sample of all deaths. The difficulty in obtaining permission for some autopsies owing to religious and other factors adds a further selective process to those which determine admission to hospital.

Nevertheless, autopsy data have contributed significantly to an understanding of the natural history of disease and knowledge of trends in frequency. For example, a cornerstone in modern thinking about atherosclerotic heart disease was the finding of a high prevalence (77 per cent) of atherosclerotic lesions in the coronary arteries of young soldiers killed in action in the Korean war (Enos et al., 1951). Among the earliest indications of a rise in the incidence of lung cancer were reports that this condition was being found with increasing frequency on autopsy.

Medical Examiners' and Coroners' Cases.   If death is due to an accident, if there is any suspicion of "foul play" (i.e., either homicide or suicide), or if a physician has not been in attendance, the private physician cannot complete the certificate but, instead, must notify the local authority, i.e., the medical examiner or the coroner. These terms are not identical. The *medical examiner* is a public officer who must be a physician and who is usually trained in forensic pathology. It is his function to investigate the cause of death in the circumstances outlined above. A *coroner* is also a public official, but he need not be a pathologist or even a physician. In fact, his qualifications often are more political than scientific. Most jurisdictions still have a coroner's system. For example, in Pennsylvania, Philadelphia is the only one of the 67 counties which has a medical examiner's office. Even the adoption of a medical examiner's system does not guarantee adequate information on all cases of sudden death. Investigation of an unexplained death is not mandatory; rather, the medical examiner decides on the need for an autopsy on the basis of a preliminary investigation. For persons previously under medical care but not attended by a physician immediately prior to death, the medical examiner may defer to the judgment of the decedent's physician.

Assignment of Cause of Death.   The physician's major contribution to the death certificate is his certification of cause of death. The decisions he must make can best be understood by examining the standard certificate of death in Figure 8–2. For each death, one condition must be assigned as the underlying cause of death (Part I, item 18c). There is also provision for reporting the immediate cause or causes of death (items 18a and 18b), as well as other significant conditions which contributed to the death (Part II).

The diagnostic terms used on the certificate must follow an internationally accepted classification, International Statistical Classification of Diseases, Injuries and Causes of Death (ICD). This is revised every ten years. In 1949 a major change was introduced in the method of assigning cause of death. Before that date, if more than one cause was recorded on a certificate, the cause was assigned according to a system of fixed priorities. Since 1949 the cause of death which is incorporated into all statistics is the one recorded on the death certificate by the individual physician as *the underlying cause*. Practicing physicians thus participate directly in the official vital statistics system. This, of course, makes it essential for physicians to understand the certificate and to complete it so that it reflects the best current medical thinking.

The above change in the system for assigning cause of death

had a pronounced effect on the recording of some diseases. Figure 8–3 shows an apparent sudden drop in mortality from diabetes. Deaths attributed to this cause were reduced by almost 50 per cent. About half of the deficit was accounted for by assignment to arteriosclerotic heart disease, the other half to several other conditions. In contrast, rates for malignant neoplasms showed an abrupt upward shift.

In completing a death certificate, the physician must choose one condition as the underlying cause of death. In earlier days when the major causes of death were infectious diseases it was relatively easy to assign a death to cholera, typhoid fever, tuberculosis,

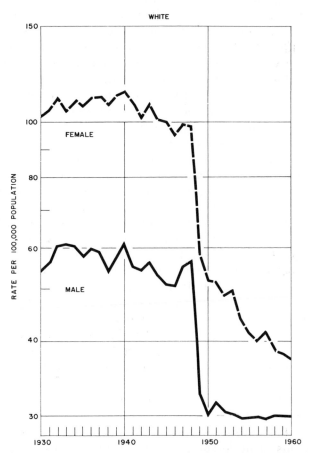

Figure 8–3 Death rates for diabetes, 55–64 year old white males and females, United States, 1930–1960. (From The Change in Mortality Trend in the United States. USPHS Pub. No. 1000, Series 3, No. 1, U.S. Govt. Printing Office, Washington, D.C., 1964.)

or similar cause. Today, with increased life expectancy, people are more likely to die with multiple afflictions (e.g., diabetes and a malignant neoplasm) or conditions which affect multiple organ systems (cardiovascular-renal disease). As a result, assignment of **one** cause of death is increasingly difficult and unsatisfactory as an indication of the major disease processes present in an individual.

The impact on mortality statistics of coding only one cause of death was studied by Dorn and Moriyama (1964). Their analysis of United States death certificates for 1955 revealed that, overall, limiting the tabulations to a single cause resulted in the loss of about half of the diagnostic information on the death certificate. This was more of a problem for some diseases than others. For cancer the loss of information was relatively small, since about 95 per cent of the certificates which mentioned cancer cited it as the underlying cause of death. On the other hand, generalized arteriosclerosis and hypertension without indication of heart disease were listed as contributing to death about eight times as often as they were cited as the underlying cause of death. Statistics based on one cause of death would miss such information. To extend the amount of medical information available from the death certificate, the National Center for Health Statistics is developing a computer based system (called Automated Classification of Medical Entities for Selection of Causes of Death, or ACME), which will not only record the underlying cause of death but also prepare tabulations which reflect multiple causes of death.

Certificate of Live Birth

As noted before, registration of live births is one of the cornerstones in the system of vital statistics. In addition, it provides identification essential to individuals as citizens.

The standard certificate of live birth is shown in Figure 8–4. Note that the certificate contains two parts. The first, which is an open public record, primarily identifies the child and his parents. A separate section, marked confidential for medical and health use only, contains information useful for epidemiologic study. This section calls for information on the race and education of the parents, previous pregnancies, amount of prenatal care, birth weight, complications of pregnancy and delivery, and congenital abnormalities. Most of this information, although gathered previously by some states, was added to the standard certificate only recently. The changes resulting from the 1968 revision are indicated by dark areas in Figure 8–4.

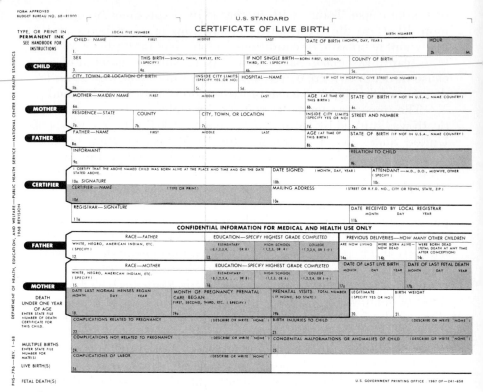

Figure 8-4 U.S. Standard Certificate of Live Birth. (From United States Standard Certificates, 1968 Revision. U.S. Dept. of Health, Education, and Welfare, USPHS.)

There has been some controversy over whether sensitive items, such as race and legitimacy status, should be included in the certificate. As a partial answer to such concerns, race, which has always been on the standard certificate, was moved to the confidential portion, where illegitimacy is also recorded. Inclusion of both these items is recommended because they help in the evaluation of social and health problems. Not all states require, or even permit, reporting on illegitimacy. Since there is undoubtedly underreporting even in the states where the information is requested, estimates of the extent of illegitimacy from birth certificates are certainly below the actual level.

The data on birth weight, birth injuries, and congenital malformations are potentially useful for identifying children likely to need special health, educational, and social services. In addition, they provide information for epidemiologic studies of prematurity and congenital defect. However, there are limitations to the use of birth certificates for such purposes. Whether a given birth defect is entered on the certificate depends on its severity and manifestion at birth, the thoroughness with which the child is examined, and the care with which the certificate is completed. Milham (1963) found, for example, that in a series of 143 cases of cleft lip and palate, one-fourth were not noted on the birth certificates. Hospital records may also yield an underestimate. One-fifth of these defects were not noted on the hospital records of these infants.

Certificate of Fetal Death

Statistics on fetal death provide some information on fetal wastage. These data are undoubtedly inferior to those on births and deaths in completeness and in comparability of different areas. There are minor differences from one jurisdiction to another in the criteria specified for determining the presence or absence of life at birth (live birth vs. fetal death), but the major problems result from incomplete registration and from differences among states in the stage of gestation at which registration is required. The definition of fetal death adopted by the World Health Assembly includes all fetal deaths, regardless of age of gestation. Although this definition has been recommended for use in the United States, in practice most states require registration only after 20 completed weeks of gestation.

MORBIDITY DATA

The earliest attempts by governmental authorities to investigate disease occurrence were related to the urgent need to contain serious infectious diseases, such as smallpox, diphtheria, yellow fever, typhoid fever, and cholera. To this pragmatic goal was added that of studying the occurrence of these diseases to plot their distribution in time and place. More recently, attempts have been made to extend systematic collection of data to a broader range of conditions than the catastrophic infectious diseases. This section of the chapter will outline major sources of morbidity data and comment on the utility, as well as the limitations, of each source.

Reports of Notifiable Disease

In their focus on patients as individuals, practicing physicians are likely to be concerned relatively little with their role in contributing to a community-wide network of information about disease. We will try to give a picture of that network, and also, if possible, stimulate awareness of the important role physicians can and should play in transmitting information about cases of *reportable disease.*

The control of communicable disease has long been accepted as a critically important health department function. Effective control of communicable disease requires that responsible officials know the nature and extent of the health problems within their jurisdictions so that they can take appropriate action. For example, when a case of typhoid fever is reported, an investigative team must be dispatched to determine the source of the infection so that control measures can be instituted. Prompt reports on foodborne illness are of importance in preventing future common vehicle epidemics.

Today, with immunization against measles available, health departments are most anxious to learn about its occurrence. They can then search out unimmunized segments of the population and set up immunization campaigns. Cases of venereal disease provide an entry into a chain of infection which includes the source on the one hand and persons possibly infected by the reported case on the other. Thus, control activities not only serve the immediate need for containment of a disease but also generate additional information about its distribution and transmission.

As with the collection and recording of vital statistics, the responsibility and authority for control of disease is legally vested in the individual states. The list of diseases which must be reported varies somewhat from state to state. Diseases reportable in all states are shown in Table 8–1. Note that four—cholera, plague, smallpox, and yellow fever—are covered by international regulations. Some states also require reporting for epidemics of any kind and for occupationally acquired disease; in a few areas cancer is reportable.

Unfortunately, the reporting of disease is often neglected. The more serious and rare infectious diseases, such as plague and rabies, are probably reported quite consistently because physicians can see the need for notifications of such illnesses. The value of reporting the more common diseases is less obvious. In addition, physicians are often reluctant to report diseases which carry a social stigma, such as syphilis and gonorrhea. Nonetheless, the dangers to the community as a whole from uncontrolled communicable disease are such that legally and ethically a physician is bound to report these diseases to the proper authorities.

TABLE 8-1   Diseases Reportable in All States

Amebiasis	Plague*
Anthrax	Poliomyelitis, total and paralytic
Aseptic meningitis	Psittacosis-Ornithosis
Botulism	Rabies in man and animals
Brucellosis	Rubella
Chickenpox	Rubella congenital syndrome
Cholera*	Salmonellosis, excluding typhoid fever
Diphtheria	Shigellosis
Encephalitis, primary infectious	Smallpox*
Encephalitis, postinfectious	Tetanus
Food poisoning (outbreaks)	Trichinosis
Hepatitis A	Tuberculosis (new active cases)
Hepatitis B	Tularemia
Hepatitis, viral, type unspecified	Typhoid fever
Leprosy	Typhus, fleaborne (murine)
Leptospirosis	Typhus, tickborne (Rocky Mountain
Malaria	spotted fever)
Measles	Venereal diseases
Meningococcal infections	Syphilis (primary and secondary)
Mumps	Gonorrhea
Pertussis	Yellow fever*

*Diseases covered by International Quarantine Agreement.

Recognition of the incompleteness of reporting has led health departments to streamline and simplify the reporting process, to establish multiple sources for reporting (i.e., physicians, hospitals, and laboratories), and, at times, to solicit reports from a sample of interested physicians rather than the total group. For example, in a three-year trial (1966 to 1969) in Rhode Island, 40 physicians, mostly general practitioners and pediatricians, were paid a token honorarium to report each week the communicable illnesses in their own practices. During this trial period the 40 consultants reported more cases of three common conditions—chickenpox, mumps, and streptococcal infections—than did the 400 general practitioners and pediatricians in the entire state in the period prior to the trial (Schaffner et al., 1971).

The exact procedures for reporting vary for the different states; in general, the attending physician is responsible for reporting cases to the local health authority. Hospital and laboratory directors may also be required to report. The information is channelled to the state health department, from there to the Center for Disease Control (CDC) in Atlanta, and eventually to the World Health Organization for inclusion in international statistics. CDC prepares a weekly report (Morbidity and Mortality Weekly Report, or MMWR) which summarizes the current incidence of some 20 notifiable diseases, as well as the week's deaths in 122 cities throughout the country. Other items in MMWR consist of reports of current epidemiologic investigations, recommendations from official committees on immunization policy, and reviews of disease surveillance. Because of a system of weekly telegraphic reports from state and territorial health officers to CDC, only a few days elapse between transmittal of information to Atlanta and its publication and dissemination. CDC also publishes yearly summaries of morbidity and mortality from notifiable diseases. Additional information about certain infectious diseases is derived from a series of national surveillance programs (see Chapter 12).

The fact that most infectious diseases are underreported does not mean that data from official notifications have no epidemiologic value. It is possible, at least for some diseases, to estimate the level of underreporting; data on reported illness can be used to study trends over time and place. Thus, such data, albeit incomplete, can lead to hypotheses about the etiology and mode of transmission of disease. (See section on viral hepatitis, page 292.)

Other Routine Statistics on Morbidity

Information about illness is available from a number of sources other than compulsory notifications, as a by-product of the ongoing activities of various organizations. Among these sources are hospital records, records of private physicians, data from insurance programs, industrial health plans, school records, and federal agencies, such as the armed forces and Veterans Administration. A few of these will be discussed briefly. For further detail, Murnaghan (1974) may be consulted.

Hospital Records. On first thought it might seem that records from general hospitals would be a good source of morbidity data. Unfortunately this is not true in the United States for most types of illness. Data based on hospital admissions or discharges provide a biassed picture of the illnesses in a community. Acute minor illnesses treated in a physician's office and cases which do not come to medical attention will be missed. In addition, serious chronic diseases, such as cancer and rheumatoid arthritis, followed on an outpatient basis will not appear in prevalence data based on hospital inpatients. Further, admission to a given hospital results from many selective factors, such as access to the hospital, availability of beds, desire for care by a specific physician, and insurance policies which promote inpatient care. Thus, there is usually no defined population base associated with any one hospital or even, in many instances, with all the hospitals in an area.

Further, hospital statistics even on primary diagnosis are generally difficult to collect, at least in part because of the lack of automated systems. In the United States, at the present time there is no centralized and uniform mechanism for collecting epidemiologic and utilization data from general hospitals. However, a nonprofit system, the Professional Activity Study (PAS) system, was formed in 1953 in response to the need for such information. This organization, which is sponsored by several professional groups, currently collects and compiles reports on discharges from almost 2000 short-stay hospitals. The information, which is collected on a standard abstract form, includes demographic characteristics, length of stay, diagnosis, treatment, complications, status at discharge, and details of diagnostic work-up and management.

Additional impetus to the reporting of hospital data now comes from the statistical requirements of various government programs. Examples are the utilization review mandated by Medicare and the data required by the Children's Bureau for those cared for under the Children and Youth Programs. These should serve to increase the value of hospital records for the study of morbidity.

Despite their many deficiencies, data on morbidity from hospitals lend themselves to surveillance of certain conditions. The defined populations of inpatients provide denominators for rates of events occurring during hospitalization. Two problems which are being studied in this manner are hospital-acquired (nosocomial) infections and, more recently, adverse drug reactions. Careful studies have indicated that both problems are substantively important in terms of frequency and severity. It has been estimated (National Academy of Sciences, 1971) that as many as 15 per cent of hospitalized patients suffer an adverse drug reaction during their hospital stay. This reflects in part the extensive use of potent drugs in hospitalized patients. Hospital-acquired infections will be discussed in Chapter 12.

Data on mental illness and retardation form a major exception to the limited usefulness of routine hospital statistics on admissions and discharges. Most public and private mental hospitals and psychiatric outpatient clinics routinely report uniform data on characteristics and diagnoses of patients to the state mental health agency and the National Institute of Mental Health. Of course, with chronic or remitting disease, such as mental illness, there is a great likelihood that individuals will have multiple admissions to one or more facilities during a time period. The use of case registers (see below) obviates the problem of multiple counts of the same individual.

Prepaid Group Practice Insurance Programs. Increasing use is being made of illness data available from large prepaid group practice services, such as the Health Insurance Plan (HIP) of Greater New York and the Kaiser Permanente Group which started on the West Coast. Although the membership of these groups does not form a "representative" sample of the population, their large size and excellent computerized records of illnesses and services rendered have made it possible to obtain morbidity data not available from other sources. An example of the usefulness of such records can be found in a study of outcome of pregnancy initiated by HIP in 1958 (Shapiro and Abramowicz, 1969). Using primarily routinely recorded information, they were able to study the outcome of approximately 12,000 pregnancies and to identify factors related to an unfavorable result. They found that about one-quarter of the pregnancies ended unfavorably (i.e., in fetal or neonatal death, a low-birth-weight infant, or a significant congenital anomaly) and that the history of the outcome of previous pregnancies was a useful predictor of risk for subsequent pregnancies.

Private Physicians. The records of private physicians have been rarely used in this country. In contrast, in England approximately 95 per cent of the population is covered by the National Health Service, and each individual is on the list of one general practitioner who is paid on a per capita basis. This defined relationship has made it possible to use general practitioners' records for morbidity studies which could not be duplicated in this country.

However, the National Center for Health Statistics is embarking on a sample survey of office-based physicians, the National Ambulatory Medical Care Survey (NAMCS). Participating physicians will be asked to report on demographic characteristics and medical problems of patients seen in office visits during one week of practice. This survey, which will provide the first national statistics on the use of ambulatory services in this country, is a part of the National Health Survey (page 178).

Disease Registers

In some areas *registers*, or rosters, have been established for diseases of major public health concern — tuberculosis, cancer, rheumatic fever, and mental illness. All newly diagnosed cases meeting specified criteria are identified through routine reporting (see above) to a central repository (e.g., state or local health department). Incoming case reports are matched against the current roster, and new cases are added to the existing enrollment. The roster is kept up-to-date through periodic follow-up.

For diseases such as tuberculosis and cancer a register helps in the care of patients by facilitating regular follow-up. A well-designed and conducted case register can also provide information on the natural history of a disease which is not readily obtainable from any other source. In addition, if the register is population-based, it can yield information on incidence and prevalence as well as survival. Some notable population-based registers have been the Psychiatric Case Registers in Maryland and in Monroe County, New York, and the Connecticut Cancer Registry. The latter has been in operation continuously since 1935. (Figure 13–6 shows data from this source relating to survival in cancer of the breast and cervix.)

Cancer registers which are not population-based are included in the End Results Group (1972). This organization, composed of three state and ten hospital registries, has provided valuable information on the treatment and survival experience of patients treated in over 100 hospitals throughout the country since 1940. It is now being replaced by a program of cancer Surveillance, Epidemiology and End Results Reporting (SEER), which will be population-based and will provide information on incidence as well as treatment and survival.

In view of the substantial work and expense entailed in establishing and maintaining a population-based register, the decision to set up a new register should not be made lightly. A register should be attempted only in situations where there are good prospects for exploiting the information to be collected. This necessitates cooperation from the local medical community and stable financial support for a competent professional staff.

Morbidity Surveys

It can be seen that routinely collected data on illness from physicians, hospitals, and other sources of medical care do not yield a complete picture of the illness and disability experience of the total population of a defined region. To provide more comprehensive data for monitoring the health status of a population, sample surveys, known as *morbidity surveys,* have been undertaken.

Large-scale surveys of illness in selected geographic areas of the country were first carried out in the early years of this century. Some were single-visit surveys (e.g., the National Health Survey conducted by the United States Public Health Service in 1935 and 1936). In others, the same households were revisited periodically over months or years (e.g., Hagerstown, Maryland, 1921 to 1924). The most extensive and ambitious survey undertaken to date is the current National Health Survey, which has been in operation for over a decade.

The National Health Survey. The National Health Survey was established by an Act of Congress in 1956 to provide a continuing source of information about the health status and needs of the entire country. Conducted by the National Center for Health Statistics, it includes several major survey programs.

HEALTH INTERVIEW SURVEY. Each week, interviews are conducted with approximately 800 households, a sample of all households throughout the country. The methods of sampling are such that the results of weekly samples can be combined to represent data for longer periods of time, a month or a year. The interview includes a basic core of health-related questions* plus more specialized topics which are included for limited periods of time.

HEALTH EXAMINATION SURVEY (HES). To augment the information which may be obtained appropriately by household interview, additional population samples are studied through physical examinations supplemented by laboratory tests (e.g., serum cholesterol and blood glucose). The examinations are conducted in specially designed mobile units. These examinations have been carried out in cycles, each requiring approximately two years for completion. The first cycle was designed to study the prevalence of certain chronic conditions in adults 18 to 79 years of age. The second cycle included children 6 to 11 years of age; the third, adolescents 12 to 17.

In 1971 a new cycle was launched, the Health and Nutrition Examination Survey (HANES). In this survey persons 1 to 74 years of age will be examined, with particular attention to the detection of nutritional deficiency.

HEALTH RECORDS SURVEY. The National Health Survey also collects information from a sample of the many institutions (general and long-term hospitals, nursing homes, clinics, and so on) which provide medical and residential care. The purpose of these surveys is to describe the health services provided by the various facilities, to develop statistics about the facilities themselves, and to delineate the characteristics of people being served, discharge diagnoses, and surgical procedures.

NATIONAL FAMILY GROWTH SURVEY. This is a biennial household survey on fertility patterns and trends and family planning practices.

---

*Examples of questions from the National Health Survey: During the past two weeks, did anyone in the family go to a dentist? Has anyone in the family been a patient in a hospital during the past two weeks? (During the past two weeks) has anyone in the family been to a doctor's office or clinic for shots, x-rays, tests, or examinations?

SURVEYS LINKED TO VITAL RECORDS. In these "follow back surveys" information supplementary to death or birth certificates is obtained from the family, physician, or hospital. For deaths this includes data on morbidity and hospitalization in the last year of life; for births information is sought on prenatal care and fertility history.

AMBULATORY MEDICAL CARE SURVEY. This new survey has been described on page 176.

To improve the quality of the data from these surveys, the National Center for Health Statistics carries out many pilot tests of procedures and conducts various types of checks to detect sources of error and bias. For example, hospital records have been reviewed to validate self-reports of hospitalization obtained through household interviews. Such studies have shown that certain chronic illnesses (e.g., mental illness and cancer) are greatly underreported on interview. Among the probable reasons are the social stigma associated with certain diseases and people's lack of knowledge of the specific diagnoses made by physicians.

Other limitations to the National Survey are that it represents primarily prevalence rather than incidence data, and that sample sizes are such that analyses can be presented only for major geographic regions and for relatively common conditions. Nevertheless, despite these limitations, the National Health Survey is the only source of nationwide data on minor illnesses, disabilities, functional deficits, physiologic measurements, and patterns of utilization of medical care. To provide data of greater value to state and local areas, the National Center for Health Statistics is developing cooperative arrangements among the various levels of government (the Cooperative Health Statistics System).

Surveys for Specific Diseases. The National Health Survey attempts to collect comprehensive data on illness. In contrast are surveys which focus on a specific disease or group of diseases, e.g., cancer, mental illness, and diabetes. Examples of this approach are the cancer surveys conducted by the National Cancer Institute (1937, 1947, and 1969 to 1971) for selected urban and rural areas. These surveys have yielded basic data on the incidence of cancer by primary site, histologic type, and stage of disease at diagnosis.

LINKED HEALTH RECORDS

The various sources of data cited so far lead to fragmented records for many individuals. A person's birth certificate may be on file in one jurisdiction, his marriage certificate in another, his children's birth certificates in a third. In addition, he may be entered in the records of a number of hospitals and individual physicians. The possibility of integrating all of this information into one record system is attractive. The term *record linkage* was first used by Dunn in 1946 to denote a comprehensive approach to linking events of significance for health. In the words of a speech by Dunn:

> Each person in the world creates a book of life. This book starts with birth and ends with death. Its pages are made up of the records of the principal events in life. Record linkage is the name given to the process of assembling the pages of this book into a volume.

Two aspects of contemporary life in particular make such linkage highly desirable: the increase in life expectancy, with its concomitant burden of chronic disease, and widespread population mobility. With the advent of computer technology it became reasonable to consider the feasibility of linking records on vital statistics and health events for entire populations or subpopulations. The initial concept of linkage of events for individuals (personal record linkage) has since been broadened to encompass family record linkage; as the name implies, this means that the records of individuals are assembled in family units.

In the past quarter-century several projects have been developed to evaluate the feasibility of record linkage and to demonstrate its usefulness. The Oxford Record Linkage Project was established in 1962 (Acheson, 1967). In that project files are built up through entries on all births and deaths within the defined area, all episodes of in-hospital treatment, and all deliveries in hospital and at home. The files have provided material useful for planning and administration of health services, as well as findings of epidemiologic significance. Newcombe's work in British Columbia with family linkage has yielded knowledge about such matters as familial aggregation of disease and maternal fertility following stillbirth and birth of children with various diseases (Newcombe, 1966; Newcombe and Tavendale, 1965).

Data banks of computer-linked vital and health records theoretically have great potential for studies in demography, fertility, genetics, and natural history of disease. However, the high cost of initiating and maintaining such files and the need for sophisticated technical and analytical skills to exploit the data, as well as questions of confidentiality, suggest that linked records will find limited application in the near future.

There would be many advantages to having an individual's health and other records united through a unique identifying number; the Social Security number has been proposed to serve this purpose. However, many people have expressed fear that, despite official safeguards, the information on file might improperly become available to potential employers, to sources of credit, and to a variety of government agencies. No really satisfactory solution to this problem has yet been devised.

In this chapter we have presented a variety of sources of data for determination of the frequency of disease. It is important to realize that a number of factors determine the choice of source and methods for the study of a given disease problem.

Of primary importance is the nature of the disease, i.e., whether it is frequent or rare, acute or chronic, typically mild or severe, and whether it regularly serves to bring people to medical attention. For example, we might contrast lung cancer with arthritis and rheumatism. Death certificates would be a good source of information about the former, the National Health Survey about the latter.

We should also point out that in rapidly fatal conditions (e.g., acute myelogenous leukemia), mortality data are practically equivalent to data on incidence. However, in most instances, mortality and morbidity are not synonymous, and the problems of collecting information about these two aspects of a disease must be considered separately.

Other factors relevant to choice of study method include current state of knowledge about the condition, the relative costs of different methods of study, and the specific purposes of the investigation.

It is often the case that definitive answers about the etiology of disease cannot be reached through any of the sources of data discussed so far. Instead, a special study may have to be initiated to test a specific hypothesis. A number of illustrations of such studies are cited throughout the book. The Framingham study, the various studies of the effects of cigarette smoking, and the fluoridation trials are but a few examples of researches in which new data had to be generated to answer specific questions.

SUMMARY

This chapter has outlined the major sources of data about the population, for monitoring of health status and for epidemiologic investigation. The decennial census provides the basic information on the numbers of persons and their demographic, socioeconomic, and household characteristics. It thus provides the denominator of morbidity and mortality rates.

The numerators of these rates are derived from a variety of other sources. Chief among them is the reporting of vital events, principally births and deaths. The accurate information furnished on documents by the physician, particularly with respect to the cause of death, was highlighted as our main source of intelligence about the causes of death and trends in these causes.

Especially for nonfatal diseases and conditions, mortality data must be supplemented by data on illness. The uses and limitations of various types of morbidity data were enumerated. The reporting of notifiable diseases, principally communicable diseases, although incomplete, provides useful information on trends in disease.

Other routinely collected morbidity statistics are derived (or potentially derived) from the ongoing records of hospitals, private practitioners, and large prepaid group practices. A more modern source of information is the morbidity survey. This rubric includes not only surveys of specific diseases but also the more comprehensive ongoing National Health Survey, in which random samples of the population are studied through such means as household interviews, physical examinations, and analysis of vital records and utilization of health care facilities.

In the final section of the chapter the concept, potentialities, and problems of linking records of vital and health events were presented.

STUDY QUESTIONS

8-1 Define the following terms and give an example when appropriate:
Census (page 161)
Standard Metropolitan Statistical Area (SMSA) (page 162)
Vital statistics (page 163)
Registration area (page 165)
Medical examiner vs. coroner (page 167)
Underlying cause of death (page 167)
Reportable (notifiable) disease (page 172)
Disease (case) register (page 176)
Morbidity survey (page 177)
National Health Survey (page 178)
Record linkage (page 180)

8–2 What would be the single best source of available informa-mation for the following conditions? Explain your answer.

    A. Incidence of cancer of the pancreas
    B. Prevalence of arthritis
    C. Incidence of skin cancer
    D. Incidence of acute leukemia
    E. Incidence of chronic lymphocytic leukemia
    F. Incidence of meningococcal meningitis
    G. Survival rates for different cancers
    H. Current status of known tuberculous cases
    I. Number of mentally retarded children in a community

Answer on page 350.

8–3 Consider a community that you know well. List any political, social, or industrial changes that have occurred there since the 1970 census. Indicate which of these factors would create changes in the population of the area causing the 1970 census data to be inadequate as a denominator for morbidity and mortality rates for that area.

8–4 List potential uses of a record linkage system, which brought together for each person in one computer file information from the following: birth certificate, death certificate, hospitalizations, and immunization history. Indicate one possible disadvantage of such a system.

REFERENCES

Acheson, E. D.: Medical Record Linkage. Oxford University Press, London, 1967.

Dorn, H. F., and Moriyama, I. M.: Uses and significance of multiple cause tabulations for mortality statistics. Am. J. Public Health, 54:400, 1964.

Editorial: Support the 1970 census now. Am. J. Public Health, 59:897, 1969.

End Results Group, National Cancer Institute: End Results in Cancer. Report No. 4. Dept. of Health, Education, and Welfare Pub. No. (NIH) 73–272, U.S. Govt. Printing Office, 1972.

Enos, W. F., Holmes, R. H., et al.: Coronary disease among United States soldiers killed in action in Korea. J.A.M.A., 152:1090, 1951.

Milham, S., Jr.: Underreporting of incidence of cleft lip and palate. Am. J. Dis. Child., 106:185, 1963.

Murnaghan, J. H.: Health-services information systems in the United States today. N. Engl. J. Med., 290:603, 1974.

National Academy of Sciences: Report of the International Conference on Adverse Reactions Reporting Systems. Washington, D.C., 1971.

Newcombe, H. B.: Familial tendencies in diseases in children. Br. J. Prev. Soc. Med., 20:49, 1966.

Newcombe, H. B., and Tavendale, O. G.: Effects of father's age on the risk of child handicap and death. Am. J. Hum. Genet., 17:163, 1965.

Schaffner, W., Scott, H. D., et al.: Innovative communicable disease reporting. HSMHA Health Rep., 86:431, 1971.

Shapiro, S., and Abramowicz, M.: Pregnancy outcome correlates identified through medical record-based information. Am. J. Public Health, 59:1629, 1969.

SELECTED
INDICES
OF
COMMUNITY
HEALTH

=== 9

The major sources of data for epidemiologic study and for monitoring the health status of a community have been discussed in the previous chapter. To recapitulate briefly, these include data about the population, derived largely from the census, and data about births, illnesses, and deaths derived from vital statistics, routine morbidity reporting, and morbidity surveys. This chapter will be concerned with some of the more important applications of these data, the specific indices used to maintain surveillance over the health status of the population and to plan and evaluate programs for disease control.

Before discussing specific indices, however, we will elaborate on the distinction between two terms, rate and ratio. A *ratio* is a relative number expressing the magnitude of one occurrence or condition in relation to another. It is a more general term than *rate*. That is, all rates are ratios, but the converse is not true. A true rate exists only if the numerator is included as part of the denominator and if the denominator represents the entire population at risk. Only when these conditions exist can probability statements be derived. Strictly speaking, death rates as conventionally computed are not exact probability statements of the risk of death (see Appendix 9–1).

Table 9–1 lists the rates most commonly used to depict the "well-being" of a community. The United States values for a recent year are also given. Note that the rates have been grouped according to the base to which they refer: total population, live births, and live births plus fetal deaths. As you consider each rate, try to iden-

184

tify the source of information for the numerator and the denominator (census, vital registration, and so on). For example, in the crude birth rate, the numerator is derived from vital registration and the denominator from census data. We will now define those indices in Table 9–1 which have not been discussed previously.

CAUSE-SPECIFIC INDICES

The *cause-specific death rate*, which approximates the risk of death from a specific condition, is probably the most important epidemiologic index available. As pointed out in earlier chapters, differences in the magnitude of this measure in subgroups and by time and place suggest etiologic hypotheses and document the need for control measures. Cause-specific death rates are, of course, subject to the various errors and limitations previously discussed, such as difficulties in assigning cause of death (inaccurate numerator) and underenumeration of certain segments of the population (inaccurate denominator). Illustrations of the usefulness of cause-specific death rates for analyzing epidemiologic problems will not be given here since a number of examples have already been cited.

As we have noted, mortality rates are inadequate for study of the dynamics of diseases which either are not fatal or produce death only after a protracted course. For such conditions, data on morbidity are required. In examining morbidity data, it is always necessary to consider whether a specific Index represents incidence or prevalence. Infectious diseases are generally reported as annual incidence rates (i.e., new cases of hepatitis per 100,000). Reports on chronic disease may represent incidence (e.g., new cases of cancer in the population of Connecticut each year) or prevalence (chronic conditions such as diabetes reported in the National Health Survey).

Proportionate Mortality Ratio

A measure which is often confused with cause-specific death rate is the *proportionate mortality ratio*, or PMR. This measure tells us the relative importance of a specific cause of death in relation to all deaths in a population group.

Proportionate mortality ratio (PMR) =

$$\frac{\text{number of deaths from a given cause in a specified period of time}}{\text{total deaths in the same time period}} \text{ per 100 (i.e., percentage)}$$

TABLE 9–1 Major Public Health Rates*

Rates	Usual Factor	Rate for United States, 1971
Rates Whose Denominators Are the Total Population		
Crude birth rate = $\dfrac{\text{number of live births during the year}}{\text{average (midyear) population}}$	per 1,000 population	17.2 15.7‡ (1973, preliminary)
Crude death rate = $\dfrac{\text{number of deaths during the year}}{\text{average (midyear) population}}$	per 1,000 population	9.3 9.4‡ (1973, preliminary)
Age-specific death rate = $\dfrac{\text{number of deaths among persons of a given age group in a year}}{\text{average (midyear) population in specified age group}}$	per 1,000 population	5–14 years – 0.4 65–74 years – 35.9
Cause-specific death rate = $\dfrac{\text{number of deaths from a stated cause in a year}}{\text{average (midyear) population}}$	per 100,000 population	Diseases of the heart – 359.5 Malignant neoplasms – 163.2
Rates and Ratios Whose Denominators Are Live Births		
Infant mortality rate = $\dfrac{\text{number of deaths in a year of children less than 1 year of age}}{\text{number of live births in same year}}$	per 1,000 live births	19.1 17.6‡ (1973, preliminary)

$$\text{Neonatal mortality rate} = \frac{\text{number of deaths in a year of children} < 28 \text{ days of age}}{\text{number of live births in same year}}$$ per 1,000 live births — 14.2

$$\text{Fetal death } ratio = \frac{\text{number of fetal deaths}^{**} \text{ during year}}{\text{number of live births in same year}}$$ per 1,000 live births — 13.4

$$\text{Maternal (puerperal) mortality rate} = \frac{\text{number of deaths from puerperal causes in a year}}{\text{number of live births in same year}}$$ per 100,000 (or 10,000) live births — 18.8 per 100,000

Rates Whose Denominators Are Live Births and Fetal Deaths

$$\text{Fetal death rate} = \frac{\text{number of fetal deaths}^{\dagger} \text{ during year}}{\text{number of live births and fetal deaths during same year}}$$ per 1,000 live births and fetal deaths — 13.3

$$\text{Perinatal mortality rate}^{\dagger} = \frac{\text{number of fetal deaths 28 weeks or more and infant deaths under 7 days of age}}{\text{number of live births and fetal deaths 28 weeks or more during the same year}}$$ per 1,000 live births and fetal deaths — 27.6

*From National Center for Health Statistics: Vital Statistics of the United States. Vol. I and II. U.S. Govt. Printing Office, Washington D.C., 1974.
**Includes only fetal deaths for which period of gestation was 20 weeks or more or was not stated.
†This rate is for Perinatal Period I (page 194 and Figure 9–1).
‡Monthly Vital Statistics Report 22:12, U.S. Govt. Printing Office, Washington, D.C., 1974.

TABLE 9–2   Death Rates per 100,000 Population, All Causes and Accidents, and Proportionate Mortality Ratio for Persons aged 1–4 and 65–74 Years, United States, 1969*

Age	Death Rate per 100,000		Proportionate Mortality Ratio
	All Causes	*Accidents*	**For Accidents**
1–4	85	31	36.5 per cent
65–74	3739	89	2.4 per cent

*From National Center for Health Statistics: Vital Statistics of the United States, Vol. IIA. U.S. Govt. Printing Office, Washington, D.C., 1973.

Note that the proportionate mortality ratio is not a rate since it refers to total deaths and not to the population at risk. This measure answers the question, what proportion of deaths are attributable to disease X? In contrast, a cause-specific death rate answers the question, what is the **risk** of death from disease X for members of a population?

From the viewpoint of public health, the proportionate mortality ratio is useful because it permits estimation of the proportion of lives to be saved by eradication or reduction of a given cause of death. On the other hand, proportionate mortality ratios can be misleading. Because the denominator refers to total deaths, its magnitude depends on the number of deaths from other causes besides the condition under consideration. For example, Table 9–2 shows that, although the *proportion* of deaths due to accidents is greater for young children than for elderly persons, death *rates* from accidents are actually higher among the elderly. The explanation of this seeming paradox is, of course, that the total number of deaths from all other causes is also considerably higher in the elderly.

INFANT AND NEONATAL MORTALITY

Losses early in life (i.e., fetal wastage and deaths shortly after birth) present important challenges to those concerned with community health. Several measures (Table 9–1) are used to indicate the stages of development at which these losses occur. These terms are clarified in Figure 9–1, which presents schematically the relation of the various time periods.

The infant mortality rate traditionally has been considered of great significance in public health. A high rate has been taken to indicate unmet health needs and unfavorable environmental factors—economic conditions, nutrition, education, sanitation, and

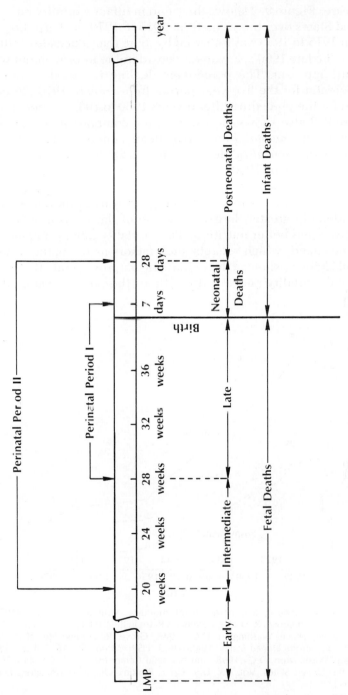

Figure 9–1 Measures of mortality in early life. Fetal death registration varies in different jurisdictions. (LMP, First day of last menstrual period.)

medical care. Figure 9–2 shows the trend in infant mortality rates in the United States over the years from 1915 to 1970. A sharp drop in rates from 1915 to 1950 was followed by more than a decade of little change. In the late 1960's, however, considerable improvement was once again apparent. The percentage decline in infant mortality rate was greater for the five-year period from 1965 to 1970 (20 per cent) than for the preceding fifteen years 1950 to 1965 (15 per cent).

Figure 9–2 also shows the trend in the components of the infant mortality rate: *neonatal mortality* (deaths under 28 days of age) and *postneonatal mortality* (deaths between 28 days and one year). It can be seen that in 1930 the neonatal mortality was somewhat higher than the postneonatal. Although both rates declined over the next 40 years, the improvement in the postneonatal mortality rate was considerably greater, largely because of the control of infectious diseases and better nutrition. The mortality rate for neonates, on the other hand, which reflects such factors as prematurity and congenital defects, showed less dramatic improvement. By 1970, the neonatal mortality rate was three times the post-neonatal rate.

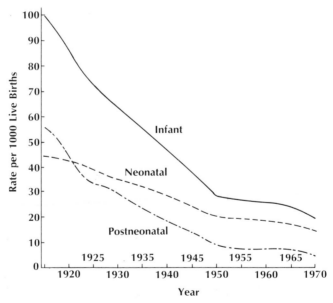

Figure 9–2 Infant, neonatal, and postneonatal mortality, United States, 1915–1970* (From Linder, F. E., and Grove, R. D.: Vital Statistics Rates in the United States, 1900–1940. U.S. Govt. Printing Office, Washington, D.C., 1943; Grove, R. D., and Hetzel, A. M.: Vital statistics rates in the United States, 1940–1960. USPHS Pub. No. 1677, U.S. Govt. Printing Office, Washington, D.C., 1968; and National Center for Health Statistics. Vital Statistics of the United States, Vol. IIA. U.S. Govt. Printing Office, Washington, D.C., selected years.)

*Prior to 1933, data are for birth-registration states only.

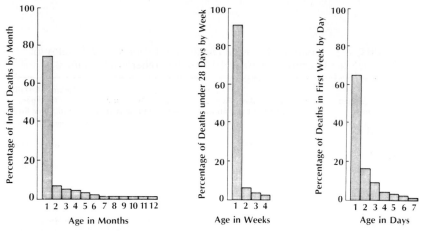

Figure 9–3   Infant deaths by age, United States, 1968. (From National Center for Health Statistics; Vital Statistics of the United States, 1968, Vol. IIA. U.S. Govt. Printing Office, Washington, D.C., 1972.)

A further breakdown of deaths within the first year is shown in Figure 9–3. It is clear that the deaths are not distributed randomly over time, not even within the first month. They are concentrated in the first week of life, and within that time period, in the first day. Accordingly, there has been an increasing focus on the hazards of the early days of life. Evidence of this can be found in the emergence of neonatology as a recognized subspecialty within pediatrics.

International Comparisons

The variations in infant mortality rates along with crude birth and death rates, are shown for selected countries in Table 9–3. In general, infant mortality rate is highly correlated with crude birth rate and, to a lesser extent, with crude death rate. The extraordinarily high infant mortality rates of the colored population of South Africa and of countries such as Guatemala, Chile, and Albania are in striking contrast to the rate of 11.7 per 1000 live births in Sweden.

The relatively poor international ranking of the United States with respect to infant mortality (i.e., thirteenth in 1971) is a matter of great concern and considerable controversy. Much of the debate has centered on the extent to which infant mortality can be directly affected by the quality and extent of medical care. Medical care is so inextricably bound to other social and economic factors that, as

TABLE 9–3 Crude Birth, Crude Death, and Infant Mortality Rates for Selected Countries (1970 or 1971 unless otherwise specified)°

Continent and Country	Crude Birth Rate per 1000 Population	Crude Death Rate per 1000 Population	Infant Mortality Rate per 1000 Live Births
Africa			
Ghana	46.6°°	17.8°°	66.9‡ (1969)
Morocco	49.5°°	16.5°°	–
Sierra Leone	44.8°°	22.7°°	*136.3* (1968)
North America			
Canada	17.0	7.3 (1969)	18.8
Costa Rica	45.1°°	7.6°°	67.1 (1969)
Guatemala	39.0	15.0	88.4†
Mexico	43.4	9.9	68.5
United States	17.3	9.3	19.8
South America			
Argentina	21.7 (1968)	9.5 (1968)	*58.3*‡ (1966)
Bolivia	44.0°°	19.1°°	–
Chile	26.6 (1968)	9.0 (1969)	87.5 (1969)
Venezuela	40.9°°	7.8°°	*48.7*
Asia			
India	42.8°°	16.7°°	72.8 (1964)
Indonesia	48.3°°	19.4°°	–
Israel	26.8	7.0	22.9
Japan	19.2	6.6	13.1†
Philippines	44.7°°	12.0°°	*67.3* (1969)
Syrian Arab Republic	47.5°°	15.3°°	*23.5*
Europe			
Albania	35.3 (1969)	7.5 (1969)	81.5 (1964)
Belgium	14.5	12.2	20.5†
Denmark	15.2	9.9	14.2
England and Wales	16.0	11.6	18.1
France	17.1	10.7	19.6 (1969)
Italy	16.8	9.6	29.2
Sweden	14.1	10.2	11.7 (1969)
Oceania			
Australia	21.7	8.7	17.9
New Zealand	22.1	8.8	16.7
Union of Soviet Socialist Republics			
U.S.S.R.	17.8	8.2	24.4

°From Demographic Yearbook, 1971, United Nations, New York, 1972.
°°Estimates prepared by the United Nations Population Division for 1965–1970.
†Provisional.
‡Italics indicate civil registers which are incomplete or of unknown reliability.

Chase has said (1972), "any attempt to attribute all of the variation in infant mortality rates to a single antecedent is an oversimplification and can lead to erroneous conclusions and misdirected action."

However, there is no doubt that, in terms of current standards, a sizable proportion of pregnant women in the United States do not receive adequate prenatal care. This is of particular significance for women who are in a high-risk category because of medical, obstetric, or sociodemographic problems (Chase, 1973; Kessner, 1973). The fact that infant mortality rate has dropped recently in the United States and that other countries have achieved even lower levels suggests that further advances should be possible in the United States. For example, one biological variable that is at least partially subject to control is infant birth weight. Of the infants born alive in the United States in 1968, 8.2 per cent weighed 2500 grams or less. At current rates, almost one-fifth of these infants can be expected to die in the first year of life (Chase, 1972). Possible primary interventions to decrease the number of low-birth-weight infants would be control over smoking during pregnancy and correction of poor nutrition due to either poor eating habits, economic factors, or overrestrictive diets prescribed by physicians. In addition, greater availability of intensive care services for low-birth-weight infants (secondary prevention) might improve salvage rates.

FETAL AND PERINATAL MORTALITY

Deaths *in utero* constitute a major public health concern. For intrauterine deaths, the term fetal death is now used in place of the older terms "abortion" and "stillbirth." While in most instances the product of gestation can readily be classified as a "live birth" or a "fetal death," there are instances in which it is difficult to make this distinction. For these reasons the following definitions have been adopted by the World Health Assembly and recommended for use in the United States by the National Center for Health Statistics:

Live Birth—Live birth is the complete expulsion or extraction from its mother of a product of conception, irrespective of the duration of pregnancy, which, after such separation, breathes or shows any other evidence of life, such as beating of the heart, pulsation of the umbilical cord, or definite movement of voluntary muscles, whether or not the umbilical cord has been cut or the placenta is attached; each product of such a birth is considered liveborn.

Important: If a child breathes or shows any other evidence of life after complete birth, even though it be only momentary, the birth should be registered as a live birth and a death certificate should be filed also.

Fetal Death—Fetal death is death prior to the complete expulsion or extraction from its mother of a product of conception, irrespective of the duration of pregnancy; the death is indicated by the fact that after such separation the fetus does not breathe or show any other evidence of life, such as beating of the heart, pulsation of the umbilical cord, or definite movement of voluntary muscles.*

The definition of fetal death given above includes all fetal deaths "irrespective of the duration of pregnancy." However, in the United States, most of the states require registration only at or after 20 weeks of gestation. National statistics for the United States are based on all deaths in gestations 20 weeks or longer plus those for which length of gestation is unspecified.

Let us now consider two indices used for measuring fetal wastage, *fetal death ratio* and *fetal death rate*. These terms are defined in Table 9–1. In the fetal death ratio, fetal deaths are related only to the number of live births $\frac{\text{fetal deaths}}{\text{live births}} \times 1000$. In the fetal death rate, the numerator is included within the denominator $\frac{\text{fetal deaths}}{\text{fetal deaths + live births}} \times 1000$. Therefore, in contrast to the fetal death ratio, the fetal death rate can provide an indication of the probability that a pregnancy will end in a fetal death. However, the fetal death ratio is more commonly used because, in comparison with live births, the registration of fetal deaths is relatively incomplete.

Perinatal mortality rate, a relatively recent rate, combines losses of late fetal life and early infancy. In contrast to fetal deaths, statistics on perinatal mortality are usually based on fetal deaths occurring 28 weeks or later rather than 20 weeks or later in gestation (i.e., Perinatal Period I rather than II). This choice excludes products of conception which are unlikely to be viable. In addition, it usually includes only the deaths during the first week following birth rather than the full four weeks included in the neonatal mortality rate. In practice this latter distinction is not of great importance since most of the neonatal deaths occur during the first week of life (Figure 9–3). There are several advantages to use of the perinatal death rate rather than the fetal death rate (or ratio) or the neonatal mortality rate. For one, it facilitates comparison for different areas because it eliminates the need to distinguish between a

---

*From Physicians' Handbook on Medical Certification: Death, Fetal Death, Birth. Dept. of Health, Education, and Welfare Pub. No. 73–1108, U. S. Govt. Printing Office, Washington, D. C., 1973.

fetal death and a live birth. Further, concern with perinatal mortality fosters collaborative efforts between obstetricians and pediatricians.

MATERNAL MORTALITY

Maternal mortality rate is a measure which reflects not only the adequacy of obstetric care but also the general level of socioeconomic development. Maternal deaths represent particularly tragic losses because they affect young adults, often at the peak period of family responsibility.

The definition of maternal mortality rate is given in Table 9–1. It can be seen that this rate is approximately 1 per cent of the infant mortality rate. Note that the denominator consists only of live births. If this were a true rate, the denominator should include all pregnancies, since each pregnancy puts the woman at risk regardless of the outcome for the fetus. However, since registration is more complete for live births than for fetal deaths, it has been customary to express this rate in terms of live births only.

There have been dramatic decreases in maternal mortality rates in many parts of the world in recent years. Figure 9–4 shows on a semi-logarithmic scale the decline in the rates for white and nonwhite women in the United States between 1935 and 1971. Although the rates have declined for both groups, the ratio of the rates for nonwhite to those for white women has increased from about 2 in 1935 to 3.5 in 1971. The higher maternal losses among nonwhites reflects a variety of social and economic handicaps, including inadequate medical care antepartum and at delivery. As these unfavorable conditions improve, the rate for nonwhite women can be expected to approach that for whites. The high maternal mortality rate for nonwhites is probably a major component in the relatively low international ranking of the United States in maternal mortality (tenth in 1970).

Age appears to be a key factor in risk of death for the mother. Figure 9–5 shows a J-shaped curve for maternal mortality, with high rates at both extremes of age. Specific medical problems associated with these high rates are toxemia in very young mothers, and a greater tendency to hypertension and uterine hemorrhage in older women. However, it is difficult to say how much of the risk can be attributed to maternal age *per se.* For one thing, maternal age and parity are inevitably intertwined. Further, a woman's social class position influences the likelihood that she will bear children at the extremes of her reproductive period.

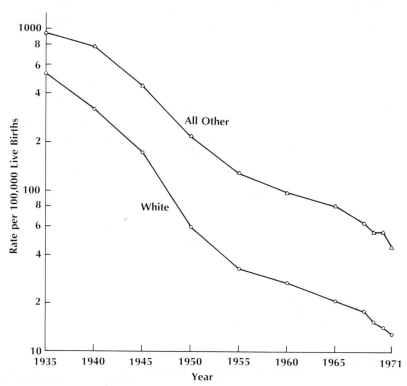

Figure 9–4 Maternal mortality rate per 100,000 live births, by color, United States, 1935–1971 (semi-logarithmic scale). (From National Center for Health Statistics: Vital Statistics of the United States. U.S. Govt. Printing Office, Washington, D.C., annual.)

Figure 9–5 Maternal mortality rate per 100,000 live births, by maternal age,* United States, 1968. (From National Center for Health Statistics: Vital Statistics of the United States, 1968, Vol. IIA. U.S. Govt. Printing Office, Washington, D.C., 1972; rates for those under 20 years of age were supplied in unpublished form through the courtesy of Mr. R. Israel of the National Center for Health Statistics.)

*The rate for the group under 15 years is based on only 5 deaths, for women 45 and over, 9 deaths. However, for the period 1960–1968, the death rate for those under 15, based on a much larger number of deaths, 51, was also high, 71.8 per 100,000 live births.

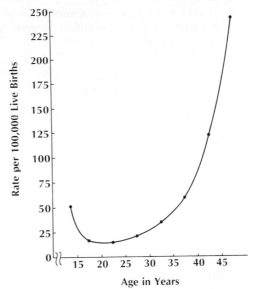

Until recently in this country sophisticated methods of contraception have been utilized largely by those favored in educational opportunity and social position. More widespread availability and use of effective contraception should decrease maternal mortality, since it would probably increase the proportion of births occurring to mothers in the relatively favorable third decade of life and would also decrease grand parity (Hellman, 1973).

It is likely that a significant portion of the maternal mortality in this country has been related to the indeterminate but large number of illegal abortions performed yearly. Indirect evidence can be found in the sharp drop in maternal mortality (from 53 to 29 per 100,000 live births) in New York City between 1969 and 1971 after the laws of that state were changed to permit abortion on demand.

In 1972 the Supreme Court struck down laws banning abortion. The implementation of this decision in the various states has been uneven. In time, however, the increased availability of abortions under medically controlled conditions should have a favorable effect on maternal mortality.

We have referred to the beneficial effects of contraception and therapeutic abortion on maternal mortality. However, we should also note that even the best available methods of contraception are not without some risk. The increased risk of thromboembolism

TABLE 9–4 Illustrative Annual Rates of Pregnancies and of Deaths Associated with Contraception, Pregnancy, and Induced Abortion per 100,000 Women of Reproductive Age in Fertile Unions[*]

Condition	Pregnancies	Maternal Deaths
1. No contraception, no induced abortion	40,000–60,000	8–12
2. No contraception, all pregnancies aborted out of hospital	100,000	100
3. Ditto, aborted in hospital	100,000	3
4. Highly effective contraception	100	3
5. Moderately effective contraception, no induced abortion	11,800–13,000	2.5
6. Ditto, all pregnancies aborted out of hospital	14,300	14.3
7. Ditto, aborted in hospital	14,300	0.4

[*]From Tietze, C.: Mortality and Contraception and Induced Abortion, Studies in Family Planning, No. 45. The Population Council, New York, 1969.

among users of oral contraceptives is well established (Sartwell et al., 1969; Vessey and Doll, 1968). There is concern that these agents may have a carcinogenic potential as well, especially for cervix or breast, but at present there is no evidence that any increased risk exists (Thomas, 1972; Sartwell et al., 1973). Hazards associated with the use of intrauterine devices are also under study.

Several attempts have been made to compare the dangers of effective contraception with the complications of the pregnancies and deliveries that would inevitably occur in the absence of contraception. Table 9–4 projects the number of pregnancies and deaths to be anticipated over a one-year period among 100,000 sexually active women of reproductive age under a variety of assumptions. It provides a cogent argument for a combination of contraception with availability of early legal abortion. Of course, the hope is that effective contraception will largely eliminate the need for abortion.

LIFE EXPECTANCY

Life expectancy, the average number of years an individual is expected to live, is a very important summary measure for comparing death rates within and between countries and over time. One practical application of this measure is its use for life insurance purposes.

The term "life expectancy" is generally used to refer to expectation of life at birth, the average number of years of life that a newborn infant is expected to live. However, expectation of life can be calculated for any age. Expectation at age 20, for example, indicates the average number of remaining years of life for those who have attained the age of 20.

There has been an impressive change in life expectancy in the United States since the turn of the century. On the average, white males born in 1900 could expect to live only 48 years. By 1971, life expectancy for this group had increased to 68.3 years. While similar increases have occurred for all race-sex groups, life expectancy has consistently been highest for white females and lowest for nonwhite males. For 1971, these rates were 75.6 and 61.2 years, respectively.

The biggest advance has come from the salvage of life in infancy and early childhood. Both the expectation of life and the percentage of survivors at different ages (Figure 9–6) for children born in 1971 are higher than for those born in 1901. This advance is reflected also in the change over time in the median length of life, the age at which half of a cohort remains alive and half have died. This measure of survival increased from 58.4 years in the 1901 life table to 74.9 years in 1971.*

---

*Note that the median length of life is greater than the mean (life expectancy) because the distribution of deaths by age is skewed.

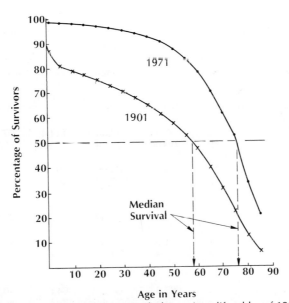

Figure 9–6 Percentage of survivors at specified ages from life tables of 1901 and 1971, United States. (From Bureau of the Census, Dept. of Commerce: U.S. Life Tables 1890, 1901, 1910, and 1901 through 1910. U.S. Govt. Printing Office, Washington, D.C., 1921; National Center for Health Statistics: Vital Statistics of the United States, 1971, Vol. II, Sect. 5. Dept. of Health, Education, and Welfare Pub. No. (HRA) 74–1147, U.S. Govt. Printing Office, Washington, D.C., 1974.)

There has been proportionately less change in the expectation of life for those who survive to middle age. Figure 9–6 suggests that there has been relatively little progress in extending the life span, a reflection primarily of the toll of cardiovascular disease and cancer (see Chapter 13, page 308).

As might be expected, the populations of different countries vary greatly in life expectancy. Table 9–5 shows the extent of international variation in life expectancy for a few selected countries at about the same period of time. The range of values is seen to vary from approximately 30 to more than 70 years. In comparison with other countries, the United States ranked twenty-second in life expectancy for males and eighth for females in 1971.

Life expectancy is calculated from tables known as *demographic life tables*. These tables are constructed from current age-specific death rates as if these rates will remain unchanged for the lifetime of the cohort, about 85 or more years. That is, life expectancy for infants born in 1970 is calculated from 1970 age-specific death rates even though the 1970 birth cohort will, as it ages, be subject to the age-specific death rates existing in 1980, 1990, 2000, and so on. The demographic life table is explained further in Appendix 9–1.

TABLE 9–5   Expectation of Life at Specified Ages by Sex for Selected Countries*

Area and Period	Sex	Expectation of Life in Years at Age				
		0	1	5	30	60
Belgian Congo						
African population	M	37.64	42.45	44.04	27.69	10.63
1950–52	F	40.00	44.14	45.87	29.78	12.27
India	M	32.45	39.00	40.86	26.58	10.13
1941–50	F	31.66	37.30	40.91	26.18	11.33
England and Wales	M	67.46	68.46	64.77	40.81	15.04
1953–55	F	72.86	73.52	69.80	45.52	18.67
Netherlands	M	71.0	71.8	68.2	44.2	17.8
1953–55	F	73.9	74.3	70.6	46.2	18.9
United States						
white population	M	67.3	68.2	64.5	40.9	16.0
1955	F	73.6	74.2	70.4	46.2	19.3

*From Swaroop, S.: Introduction to Health Statistics. E. & S. Livingstone, Ltd., London, 1960, p. 207.

MEASUREMENT OF DISABILITY

Most of this chapter has focussed on measures of mortality. While these measures tell us much about a society, they convey little information about the quality of life. Information that life expectancy is high in a given population does not tell us whether the population is predominantly well or is heavily burdened with chronically ill or disabled individuals.

It is only recently that life expectancy has increased to the point where concern has become focussed on functional measures of ill-health. For many years statistics have been available from public agencies on persons with severe impairments (e.g., blindness, severe physical disability). More recently information is becoming available on more subtle deviations from optimal function, and on the extent and causes of such problems.

Disability can be defined in a variety of ways. For insurance purposes disability is usually defined as inability to engage in gainful employment. The National Health Survey (1972) defines *disability* more broadly as "any temporary or long-term reduction of a person's activity as a result of an acute or chronic condition." It specifies three measures of disability. The most general is the "restricted-activity day," defined as follows:

Restricted-activity day—one on which a person cuts down on his usual activity for the whole of that day on account of an illness or injury.

Within this general definition more severe restrictions of activity are specified by the work-loss day and the bed-disability day.

Work-loss day—one on which a person would have worked but instead lost an entire work day because of an illness or injury.
Bed-disability day—one on which a person stays in bed for all or most of the day (i.e., more than half the daylight hours). Hospital days are classed as bed-disability days even if the person is ambulatory within the hospital.

The National Health Survey has produced much information on extent of disability for the population as a whole and for subgroups according to age, sex, geographic region, color, and family income. In 1968, for example, the overall yearly average per person was 15.3 days of restricted activity; of these, 5.4 were work-loss days and 6.3 were bed-disability days. Disability rates are higher for nonwhites than whites, and within color groups, for low-income compared with high-income families.

The average number of restricted-activity and bed-disability days per person per quarter-year over a six-year period is shown in

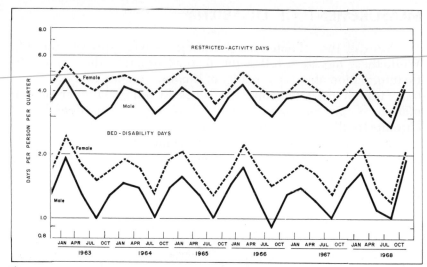

Figure 9–7 Disability days per person per quarter, by type of disability and sex. (From Bauer, M. L.: Current estimates from the Health Interview Survey, United States – 1968. USPHS Pub. No. 1000, Series 10, No. 60, U.S. Govt. Printing Office, Washington, D.C., 1970.)

Figure 9–7. The marked seasonality can be attributed mainly to seasonal fluctuations in acute diseases, especially respiratory conditions.

OTHER HEALTH-RELATED INFORMATION

Additional types of information relevant to the general mental, physical, and socioeconomic health of a community are available from a variety of sources – vital statistics; the United States census; data routinely collected by health and mental health departments and law enforcement agencies; and surveys of the labor force. Among these indices are:

1. Marriage and divorce rates
2. Illegitimacy rate
3. Proportion of babies without prenatal care
4. Unemployment rate
5. Rates of drug and alcohol abuse
6. Rates of adult crime and juvenile delinquency
7. Utilization rates of mental hospitals and psychiatric outpatient clinics
8. Proportion of the population in substandard housing

9. Proportion of the population living at the poverty level

While many of these are not direct measures of health and the supporting data are often incomplete, they are important indices of the quality of life in a community and indicate deviations from "complete physical, mental and social well-being" (WHO, 1948).

Of particular concern is the "nesting" of health and social problems in certain areas, both urban and rural, and in certain "hard core" families. This was demonstrated in a classic study which showed that 6 per cent of the families in St. Paul, Minnesota, absorbed 25 per cent of the total social and health service efforts (Buell et al., 1952). An ecological analysis of Baltimore by Klee et al. (1967) combined data from the Maryland Psychiatric Case Register and the 1960 census with information supplied by a variety of agencies. This analysis showed that census tracts which ranked high on various indices of poverty, social disorganization, and public health problems tended also to have high total psychiatric admission rates. In one tract (1960 population of 1400, mainly white) there were 48 arrests per 100 adults yearly, a three-year tuberculosis morbidity rate of 1 per 100, and a three-year psychiatric admission rate of 11 per 100.

The difficulties of elucidating the etiologic relationships in such a complex of medical and social pathology were noted previously in relation to schizophrenia (page 53). To what extent does living in this tract cause a high arrest, tuberculosis, or psychiatric admission rate? To what extent do the high rates represent the drift or migration to this area of persons already incapacitated mentally and physically? Whatever the contribution of each factor, the findings certainly underscore the need for comprehensive approaches to the measurement of health.

SUMMARY INDEX OF HEALTH*

Many health workers feel that a summary index of health in a community would be valuable. Among the suggested approaches to this concept (Sullivan, 1971; Fanshel and Bush, 1970) is a scale which treats the health of each individual as a continuous variable from zero to one. The numeric value is obtained by summing various dimensions of physical and psychosocial health, each weighted according to the importance or "desirability" of that

---

*Adapted from a personal communication from G. W. Torrance (1974).

particular aspect of health. With such a health scale for individuals, a health index for an entire population may be derived which also falls between zero and one. For example, it would be zero if everyone in a community had died prematurely, and one if everyone were in complete health and there had been no premature deaths.

Although there are many conceptual and practical difficulties in developing such an index, the notion that a single number could represent the overall level of health for a community has great appeal because of its simplicity. Such an index could assist, for example, in evaluating the effect of changes in the system of health care delivery. Further research in this area is needed.

SUMMARY

In this chapter we continued the presentation of the major measures of morbidity and mortality needed for epidemiologic study and for monitoring the health status of a community. Cause-specific death rates were highlighted as fundamental to epidemiologic knowledge and control programs, particularly for diseases with high case fatality rates. Proportionate mortality ratio (i.e., proportion of all deaths due to a disease) was contrasted with the death rate from a disease; only the latter indicates risk of death.

Indices related to early life include the infant mortality rate as an indicator not only of the adequacy of medical care but also of general conditions of health, nutrition, and education. A study of the neonatal period reveals that, in the first week of life and, more specifically, in the first day, the infant is at greatest risk; it is this early period of life as well as the prenatal period to which preventive measures should be directed. Other indices of fetal wastage include the fetal death rate, the fetal death ratio, and, more recently, the perinatal mortality rate.

Although there has been a marked decline in the maternal mortality rate, further improvement is needed, particularly for non-whites. The factors related to maternal risk include age of the mother and parity, as well as medical care. The widespread use of contraceptives and liberalization of the restrictions against abortion will have a significant impact on this rate.

Finally, life expectancy, a measure which summarizes current levels of mortality, was described. While life expectancy has changed markedly largely owing to reduction of death in infancy and early life, it is apparent that there has been no significant exten-sion of the life span of man during this century. The ranking of the United States internationally on several measures indicates that ad-vances being achieved elsewhere are yet to be made here.

The chapter concluded with a discussion of measures of the quality of life, such as disability rates and indices of social deviance and other health-related problems. The nesting of problems in cer-tain families and areas was noted, as was the need for a summary index of the health status of a community.

APPENDIX 9–1

CALCULATION OF LIFE EXPECTANCY (THE DEMOGRAPHIC LIFE TABLE)

Life expectancy is determined from *demographic life tables.* Such tables are used by actuaries as the basis for setting insurance rates, for comparing survival of special study groups, and for making awards in legal suits relating to injury or death.

To see how a demographic life table is constructed, let us assume a hypothetical stationary* population into which 100,000 babies are born alive, evenly distributed over the calendar year. (Table 9–6, column 3). We estimate how many of these 100,000 babies will die during the first year of life (column 4) and therefore how many will be alive at the beginning of the next age-interval (column 3). These data are obtained by estimating the probability of death in the first year of life, (column 2), an estimate based on the observed infant mortality rate for 1969. Similarly, we estimate the number of one-year-olds who die before age two based on the one- to two-year-old death rate for the same year. We continue to estimate the decrement for successive ages, with 1969 age-specific death rates applied to each year's survivors, until the last person of this hypothetical population has died.

A detailed life table presents data by single years of age. For compactness, ages can be grouped in what is called the abridged life table (Table 9–6). Column 5 represents a census (or count) of the number of persons in each age interval at any time (i.e., person-years) which would result from a stationary population. Because of the five year age grouping, there are almost five times as many persons present in the age interval 5 to 10 years as are alive at the beginning of that age interval (column 3).

Column 6, obtained by cumulating column 5 upwards, shows the total number of persons (or person-years) in that age interval and in all subsequent age intervals. This figure is equivalent to the total

---

*In a stationary population, the number of persons living in any age interval remains constant. The demographic life-table population, an example of a stationary population, assumes a constant number of births, constant age-specific death rates, and absence of migration.

Age Interval	Proportion Dying	Of 100 000 Born Alive		Stationary Population		Average Remaining Lifetime
Period of life between two exact ages stated in years (1)	Proportion of persons alive at beginning of age interval dying during interval (2)	Number living at beginning of age interval (3)	Number dying during age interval (4)	In the age interval (5)	In this and all subsequent age intervals (6)	Average number of years of life remaining at beginning of age interval (7)
x to $x+n$	$_nq_x$	l_x	$_nd_x$	$_nL_x$	T_x	$\overset{\circ}{e}_x$
0–1	0.0211	100,000	2,108	98,117	7,044,699	70.4
1–5	.0034	97,892	332	390,773	6,946,582	71.0
5–10	.0021	97,560	203	487,238	6,555,809	67.2
10–15	.0021	97,352	202	486,304	6,068,571	62.3
15–20	.0057	97,150	556	484,474	5,582,267	57.5
20–25	.0074	96,594	710	481,227	5,097,793	52.8
25–30	.0072	95,884	691	477,717	4,616,566	48.1
30–35	.0087	95,193	832	473,981	4,138,849	43.5
35–40	.0126	94,361	1,192	469,023	3,664,868	38.8
40–45	.0191	93,169	1,779	461,715	3,195,845	34.3
45–50	.0287	91,390	2,621	450,875	2,734,130	29.9
50–55	.0437	88,769	3,877	434,725	2,283,255	25.7
55–60	.0661	84,892	5,610	411,209	1,848,530	21.8
60–65	.0978	79,282	7,755	377,955	1,437,321	18.1
65–70	.1424	71,527	10,183	333,143	1,059,366	14.8
70–75	.2084	61,344	12,786	275,678	726,223	11.8
75–80	.2842	48,558	13,802	208,872	450,545	9.3
80–85	.4010	34,756	13,939	138,226	241,673	7.0
85 and over	1.0000	20,817	20,817	103,447	103,447	5.0

*From National Center for Health Statistics: Vital Statistics of the United States, 1969, Vol. IIA, Section 5. US. Govt. Printing Office, Washington, D.C., 1973.

number of person-years of life remaining for all those who reach that age or birthday (column 3). Therefore, to obtain an average number of years of life remaining (column 7) we must divide column 6 by column 3. Column 7 gives us the life expectancy at birth, as well as at all other ages.

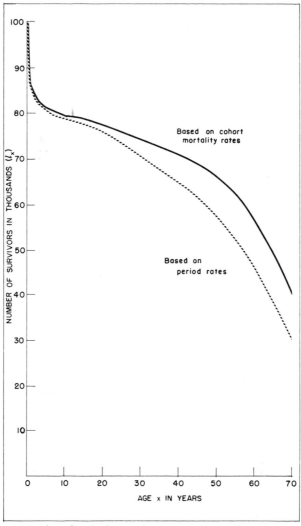

Figure 9–8 Survivorship (l_x) of white males in birth cohort of 1901 as compared with corresponding period survivorship, by single years of age, death-registration states, 1900–1968. (From Moriyama, I. M. and Gustavus, S. O.: Cohort mortality and survivorship: United States death-registration states, 1900–1968. USPHS Pub. No. 1000, Series 3, No. 16, U.S. Govt. Printing Office, Washington, D.C., 1972.)

Demographic life tables actually project a fictitious picture, since they are based on age-specific death rates existing in one calendar year (e.g., 1969) and not on the age-specific death rates of a birth cohort followed throughout their lifetime. This model assumes that these period age-specific death rates for any calendar year will remain unchanged for a life span. When age-specific death rates improve over time, as has occurred in the United States during this century, survivorship based on period death rates understates the actual survivorship, as shown in Figure 9–8.

Note that the demographic life table requires the use of probabilities of death by year of age. Conventional death rates are not exact probability statements of the risk of death. They actually overstate the risk slightly, for the following reason. A true probability of death, between ages 25 and 26, for example, would have as the denominator all persons who reach their twenty-fifth birthday. The numerator would consist of those from this group who die before their twenty-sixth birthday.

In conventional death rates, the denominator is derived from census data and is a count of the population at a point in time. Since the persons aged 25 (i.e., between 25 and 26 years of age) present in the population at any time include only those in the age interval who have survived to that point, this number is smaller than the original cohort.

Expressing this concept in mathematical terms, if we let m_x denote the conventional death rate, then:

$$m_x = \frac{\text{deaths during calendar year of}}{\text{person age x at census count}} = \frac{d_x}{P_x}$$

The probability of death during the year, q_x, is then obtained from m_x by the following formula:

$$q_x = \frac{2m_x}{2 + m_x} = \frac{2\,\dfrac{d_x}{P_x}}{2 + \dfrac{d_x}{P_x}} = \frac{d_x}{P_x + \dfrac{d_x}{2}}$$

This formula shows why conventional death rates overstate the probability of death — they are based on denominators which are actually too small $\left(P_x \text{ instead of } P_x + \dfrac{d_x}{2}\right)$.

Because the force of mortality is so much greater near the time of birth than near the end of the first year of life (Figure 9–3), special procedures are followed for estimating the probability of death in the first year of life.

A further discussion of the estimation of probability of death from vital statistics rates, including adjustment for changes in succeeding calendar years, may be found in Spiegelman (1968).

STUDY QUESTIONS

9–1 Define the following terms and give an example when appropriate:
Ratio (page 184)
Rate (page 184)
Cause-specific death rate (page 185)
Proportionate mortality rate (PMR) (page 185)
Infant mortality rate (page 188)
Neonatal and postneonatal mortality rates (page 190)
Live birth (page 193)
Fetal death (page 194)
Fetal death rate and ratio (page 187, 194)
Perinatal mortality rate (page 187, 194)
Maternal mortality rate (page 187, 195)
Life expectancy (page 198)
Demographic life table (page 200, 206 ff.)
Disability (restricted activity, work-loss, and bed-disability days) (page 201)

9–2 Following are imaginary population and vital statistics for a U.S. county for 1970.

Total midyear population	80,000
Population 45 years of age and over	20,000
Number of infants born alive	2000
Fetal deaths (reported)	32
Maternal deaths	1
Total deaths	648
Death under 1 year of age	42
Deaths of persons 45 and over	300
From heart disease	98
From cancer	60
From stroke	48
From all other causes	94

From the above data, calculate the following indices of health for the community, applying the usual constant (e.g., × 1000, or × 100,000).

    A. Crude birth rate
    B. Crude death rate
    C. Infant mortality rate
    D. Fetal death ratio
    E. Maternal mortality rate
    F. Age-specific death rate for persons 45 and over
    G. Age-cause-specific death rates for those 45 and over for: (1) heart disease, and (2) cancer
    H. Proportionate mortality ratios for those 45 and over for: (1) cancer, and (2) stroke

Answer on page 351.

9-3 Approximately 12 per cent of the deaths in children, aged five through nine, in the United States in 1967 were due to cancer. In contrast, approximately one-fourth of the deaths at ages 60 to 64 were due to this condition. Is it correct to say that the risk of death from cancer was approximately twice as great in the older age group? If not, why not?

Answer on page 352.

9-4 Except for the first year of life, the census count is used for the denominator of age-specific death rates. Explain why the number of live births rather than the census count of infants under one year of age is taken for the denominator of the infant mortality rate.

Answer on page 352.

9-5 In several areas of the United States in the past few years, there has been a sharp increase in the number of legally performed abortions. Reports to the abortion surveillance program maintained by the Center for Disease Control indicates that in 1972 there were 315 abortions for every 1000 live births in 27 states plus the District of Columbia.

    Which of the following public health indices might be affected by an increase in legal abortions: (1) crude birth rate, (2) crude death rate, (3) infant mortality rate, (4) maternal mortality rate, (5) ratio of illegitimate to legitimate births. Comment on the anticipated direction of change.

Answer on page 352.

9–6   Inspect Table 9–5. From the data there, which sex has the less favorable life expectancy? In the United States, which diseases would account for the higher death rate in this sex?

Answer on page 353.

9–7   One might expect that life expectancy (average remaining years of life) would decrease steadily with each year of life. Explain the **increase** in life expectancy at age one as compared with life expectancy at birth for almost every country shown in Table 9–5.

Answer on page 353.

REFERENCES

Buell, B., and associates: Community Planning for Human Services. Columbia University Press, New York, 1952.

Chase, H. C.: The position of the United States in international comparisons of health status. Am. J. Public Health, 62:581, 1972.

Chase, H. C. (ed.): A study of risks, medical care and infant mortality. Am. J. Public Health, 63(supp.), 1973.

Constitution of the World Health Organization, 1948. In Basic Documents, 15th ed. WHO, Geneva, 1964.

Fanshel, S., and Bush, J. W.: A health-status index and its application to health-services outcomes. Operations Research, 18:1021, 1970.

Hellman, L. M.: Conception control as a health practice: An emerging concept in government and medicine. Perspec. Biol. Med., 16:357, 1973.

Kessner, D. M., Singer, J., et al.: Contrasts in Health Status, Vol. 1. Infant Death: An Analysis by Maternal Risk and Health Care. Institute of Medicine, National Academy of Sciences, Washington, D.C., 1973.

Klee, G. D., Spiro, E., et al.: An Ecological Analysis of Diagnosed Mental Illness in Baltimore in Psychiatric Epidemiology and Mental Health Planning. Monroe, R. R., Klee, G. D., et al. (eds.), American Psychiatric Association (Psychiatric Research Report No. 22), 1967.

National Health Survey: Health Household–Interview Survey. USPHS Pub. No. 584–A3, U.S. Govt. Printing Office, Washington, D.C., 1972.

Sartwell, P. E., Arthes, F. G., et al.: Epidemiology of benign breast lesions: Lack of Association with oral contraceptive use N. Engl. J. Med., 288:551, 1973.

Sartwell, P. E., Masi, A. T., et al.: Thromboembolism and oral contraceptives: An epidemiologic case-control study. Am. J. Epidemiol., 90:365, 1969.

Spiegelman, M.: Introduction to Demography (rev. ed.), Harvard University Press, Cambridge, Mass., 1968.

Sullivan, D. F.: A single index of mortality and morbidity. HSHMA Health Rep., 86:347, 1971.

Thomas, D. B.: Relationship of oral contraceptives to cervical carcinogenesis. Obstet. Gynecol., 40:508, 1972.

Tietze, C.: Mortality and Contraception and Induced Abortion, Studies in Family Planning, No. 45. The Population Council, New York City, 1969.

Vessey, M. P., and Doll, R.: Investigation of relation between use of oral contraceptives and thromboembolic disease. Br. Med. J., 2:199, 1968.

POPULATION
DYNAMICS
AND
HEALTH
10

Knowledge of the complex interdependence between the demographic* characteristics of a population and its health status and health needs is essential to those responsible for providing health services. We have already discussed the measurement of population through the census (Chapter 8). In this chapter, we will outline the factors which influence size and composition of populations, and then present the current status of world population, with emphasis on the great disparities in population dynamics, economic levels, and health problems in different countries. Finally, we will indicate the major current trends in United States population.

FACTORS IN POPULATION DYNAMICS

Three variables determine the population of any defined area: births (fertility), deaths (mortality), and migration. The balance among these three factors determines whether a population decreases, remains stationary, or increases in number. The relation between births and deaths is referred to as *natural increase*. When the net effect of migration is added to natural increase, this is referred to as *total increase*. Demographers have evolved a number of specific measures of these dynamic factors. Since mortality rates have already been discussed, only fertility and migration will be outlined here.

---

*The study of population is known as *demography*. Demography has been defined as the statistical study of the characteristics of human populations, especially with reference to size and density, growth, distribution, migration and vital statistics, and the effect of all these on social and economic conditions (Webster's Third New International Dictionary).

213

Fertility

Many factors influence the fertility of individuals and populations. It is now widely accepted that control of fertility, like the prevention of avoidable deaths, is a public health responsibility. Both lay people and public health professionals have become increasingly concerned about the recent unprecedented growth of population. The societal consequences of uncontrolled fertility have been summarized in a formula which states that level of living is directly related to resources of all kinds and inversely related to population.

$$\text{Level of living} = \frac{\text{resources of the earth}}{\text{number of people}}$$

That is, the greater a country's resources, the higher its possible standard of living. These resources include the creative potential of the population. However, since each person is also a consumer and since only a fraction of the population is economically productive, the number of people who must be supported by the country's resources is, in general, inversely related to the level of living. Uncontrolled fertility influences adversely the economic, physical, and psychologic health of populations and family units, especially those existing at marginal and poverty levels.

For these reasons, measurement of fertility is extremely important. One measure of fertility, the crude birth rate, has already been discussed in Chapter 7. This is a very rough indicator of fertility, since everyone in the population — male, female, old, young — contributes equally to the denominator of this rate despite the fact that only females of childbearing age are actually at risk of giving birth. The percentage of the population in this category varies with past events and trends. Thus, the crude birth rate can be high either because of a currently high rate of childbearing among women of reproductive age or because women in this age group constitute a high proportion of the population.

A more refined measure of fertility is the *general fertility rate,* whose denominator is restricted to the number of women of childbearing age (i.e., 15 to 44 or 15 to 49).

$$\text{General fertility rate} = \frac{\substack{\text{number of live births in an area} \\ \text{during a year}}}{\substack{\text{midyear female population aged} \\ \text{15–44 in same area in same year}}} \times 1000$$

Other, more specific measures are *age-specific, parity-specific,* and *age–parity-specific birth rates.*

Age-specific birth rate:

$$\text{Birth rate for 15–19 year old females annual} = \frac{\begin{array}{c}\text{number of live births to females} \\ \text{aged 15–19 in an area} \\ \text{during a year}\end{array}}{\begin{array}{c}\text{midyear female population aged} \\ \text{15–19 years in same area in} \\ \text{same year}\end{array}} \times 1000$$

Parity-specific birth rate:

$$\text{Parity-specific birth rate (annual)} = \frac{\begin{array}{c}\text{number of live births of a given} \\ \text{birth order occurring in an} \\ \text{area during a year}\end{array}}{\begin{array}{c}\text{midyear female population of} \\ \text{appropriate parity group in same} \\ \text{area in same year}\end{array}} \times 1000$$

The above rates are called *period* measures of fertility since they refer to births in a population over a specified period of calendar time, usually a year. Another way of looking at fertility describes the fertility of a cohort (i.e., *cohort fertility*) of women up to a certain age or over their total reproductive life. A commonly used cohort measure of fertility is the *completed birth rate* (also called the final birth rate or completed fertility rate). This is defined as the number of children ever born per 1000 women (or married women) by the end of the childbearing period (i.e., age 44 or 49).

The relation between period and cohort measures of fertility is complex. For example, economic recession or war, which can create short-term decline in period fertility, usually does not affect final cohort fertility. Poor economic conditions in one year may cause a couple not to have a child in that year but may not affect their ultimate number of children. Lowering of the average age at which childbearing begins will create a temporary rise in period fertility, which may or may not result in an increase in cohort fertility.

Migration

Migration is defined as a change in residence in which a recognized boundary of some type is crossed. Migration does not affect world population. However, international and internal (intranational) migration can be important sources of change within a particular area. For example, in this country the proportion of whites who were foreign-born reached a peak around the turn of the century; the census of 1910 indicates that almost one of every five whites in the country was foreign-born (Table 10–3). This vast influx not only contributed a cheap source of labor and increased the total size of the population but also, as implied by the concept of the "melting pot," enriched and diversified the cultural heritage of the country. There were also less desirable consequences, such as crowded, unwholesome living conditions which gave rise to disease and crime.

More recently, changes in the technology of agriculture and expanded opportunities for employment in urban areas during World War II led to a mass migration of Blacks from rural areas in the South to the northeastern cities. At the same time new patterns of housing and transportation increased the movement of middle-class whites from inner cities to suburbs. Current trends in internal migration are continued shifts from rural to urban areas, from central cities to suburbs, and from inland to coastal areas. These changes have had a massive impact on the relative requirements of different areas for facilities and personnel to meet health needs. Adequate social response to such changing needs is immeasurably aided by the use of census data, in conjunction with other kinds of social statistics, to register current population distribution and forecast trends.

Different kinds of population movement within the country compound the problem of satisfactory enumeration. Groups of people without a single, fixed residence include migratory workers, who are mainly but not exclusively engaged in agriculture, and military families; college students essentially have two residences; skid row inhabitants and street people essentially have none. The Bureau of the Census makes a limited attempt to register internal migration, but it does not request information on all moves made during the ten-year intercensal period. The lack of good information from these migratory groups can be a serious handicap to health planners and other public officials.

Population Pyramids: The Age-Sex Composition of Populations

The effects of the three factors which influence population — births, deaths, and migration — can be shown pictorially by a population pyramid. *Population pyramids* present the population of an area or country in terms of its composition by age and sex at a point in time. By convention, males are shown on the left of the pyramid, females on the right, young persons at the bottom, and the elderly at the top. The pyramid consists of a series of bars, each drawn proportionately to represent the percentage contribution of each age-sex group (often in five-year groupings) to the total population; that is, the total area of the bars represents 100 per cent of the population. The shape of the pyramid reflects the major influences on births and deaths, plus any changes due to migration, over the three or four generations preceding the date of the pyramid. The following pyramids (Figure 10 1) contrast the differences in composition in 1959 of Mauritius, with high birth and death rates, and the United Kingdom, in which birth and death rates have been low over a period of years.

The essentially triangular, broad-based pattern of Mauritius reflects high birth and death rates over a long period of time. Only a small proportion of persons have survived into the older age groups; as a result, the median age is relatively young. In contrast, the pyramid for the United Kingdom has a narrow base and steep

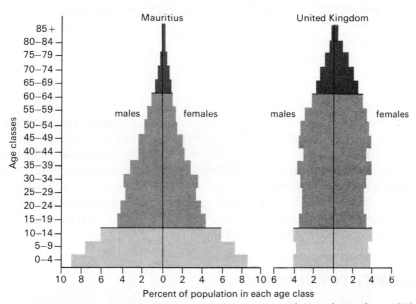

Figure 10–1 Age structure of populations of Mauritius and United Kingdom, 1959. Self-supporting portion of population is shown in medium gray, young dependent in pale gray, and elderly dependent in dark gray. (From Ehrlich, P. R., and Ehrlich, A. H.: Population, Resources and Environment. Issues in Human Ecology. W. H. Freeman and Company, San Francisco, Copyright © 1972, after Desmond, A., and Morris, J. K.: The story of Mauritus—From the dodo to the stork) Population Bulletin (Population Reference Bureau, Washington, D.C.), *18*(5):106, 1962.)

sides. Life expectancy is higher and, therefore, a higher proportion of the population survives into old age, leading to a higher median age. In other words, Mauritius is a "young" country, the United Kingdom an "old" one. The differences in population dynamics of the two countries will be discussed further. Here we will just note that the triangular pyramid shown for Mauritius is typical of "developing" countries, the straighter sides of the pyramid for the United Kingdom typical of economically developed areas.

Irregularities in the shape of a pyramid mirror prior events in the history of a country. Severe famines affect age distribution by taking a disproportionately high toll of infants, young children, and the aged. Wars not only reduce the number of young males but also affect patterns of conception by delaying or reducing births. In Figure 10–1, for example, the slight bulge for ages 10 to 14 for the United Kingdom suggests that the number of births was higher during 1945 to 1949 (post–World War II baby boom) than it was during 1950 to 1954.

Dependency Ratio. Figure 10–1 also illustrates another important concept, the *dependency ratio*. The dependency ratio describes the relation between the potentially self-supporting portion of the population and the dependent portions at the extremes of age.

Dependency ratio =
$$\frac{\text{population under 20 + population 65 and over}}{\text{population 20–64}} \times 100$$

The period of economic self-sufficiency is defined variously as starting at age 15, 18, or 20. The upper limit of the working population is usually set at 64, but is sometimes defined as 59. In Figure 10–1, we see that the dependency ratios for Mauritius and the United Kingdom are very different. (In this figure, economic self-sufficiency is considered to start at age 15.) The dependency ratio is much greater in Mauritius than in the United Kingdom owing to the higher proportion of young dependents (i.e., 44 per cent vs. 23 per cent under the age of 15).

WORLD POPULATION

Concern about the size of world population goes back at least to Thomas Malthus (1766-1834), the English clergyman who warned of the dire effects of uncontrolled population growth. Malthus proposed that production of food can only increase arithmetically, whereas population increases geometrically. Malthus' concern with the harmful effects of unchecked fertility is echoed by many modern scientists with more accurate insights into the mathematical aspects of demography.

Data about the past numbers of people on the planet are fragmentary, but available evidence indicates an exponentially increasing rate of population growth (Dorn, 1962). Figure 10–2, which is based on United Nations projections prepared in the 1950's, has been widely reproduced as an estimate of past, current, and future population figures. In considering the figures, it is well to note that no accurate information is available on the current population of many countries, and that the projections for the future are based on a number of assumptions, such as the assumption that food supply will be adequate to permit continued rapid growth of population.

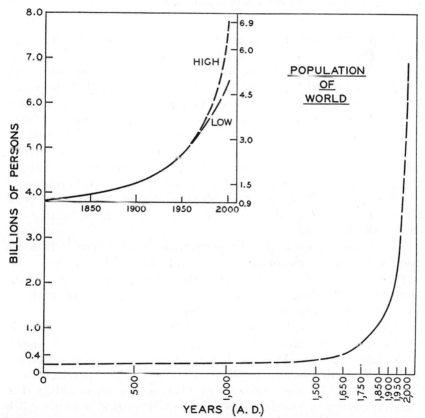

Figure 10–2 Estimated population of the world, A.D. 1 to A.D. 2000. (From Dorn, H. F.: World population growth: An international dilemma. Science, 135:283, 1962.)

TABLE 10–1   Estimated World Population and
Doubling Time in Different Eras*

Year (A.D.)	Population in Billions	Number of Years to Double
1	0.25	1650
1650	0.5	200
1850	1.1	80
1930	2.0	45
1975	4.0	35
2010	8.0†	?

*From Dorn, H. F.: World population growth: An international dilemma. Science, 135:283, 1962. Copyright 1962 by the American Association for the Advancement of Science.
†Projection based on United Nations estimates.

It is estimated that there are about four billion people on earth today. This number is greater than it has ever been. Estimates of the length of time that man has been on the earth vary widely. Nevertheless, there is general agreement that the numbers of people on earth increased very slowly in the early millennia; by the start of the Christian era there were perhaps one-quarter of a billion people on earth. It took approximately 1650 years for this number to double, but the rate of growth has continued to accelerate so that the next doubling, i.e., to one billion, took about 200 years, the next 80, and the next only 45 years. It is projected that the next doubling will take 35 years, so that by the year 2010 there will be eight billion people on earth. These figures are summarized in Table 10–1.

The major factor in the recent increase in world population has been a decline in death rates, especially in childhood. As a consequence, more people live into the reproductive ages. Local increases in fertility have not been of sufficient magnitude to account for the rapid rise in population.

The rapidity with which change in death rates can occur is demonstrated in Figure 10–3. Age-specific death rates are shown for Sweden and the Moslems in Algeria, each at two different time periods. Note that between 1946 to 1947 and 1954, the decrease in the death rate for the Moslems in Algeria was greater than that which occurred in Sweden over the 100-year period between 1771 to 1780 and 1871 to 1880.

In 1966, the United Nations prepared a second set of world pop-

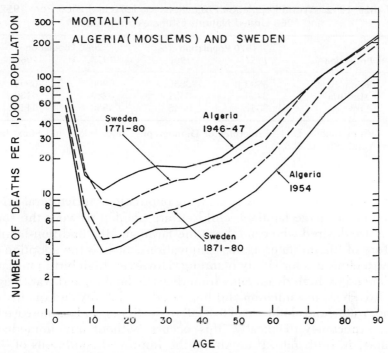

Figure 10–3 Age-specific death rates per 1000 per year, Sweden and the Moslem population of Algeria, various time periods from 1771–1954 (semi-logarithmic scale). (From Dorn, H. F.: World population growth. An international dilemma. Science, *135*:283, 1962.)

ulation projections (Table 10–2). Comparison of the earlier (1957) and later (1966) figures shows that, on the whole, the two sets agree, with the disturbing exception that the 1957 "low" projections for the year 2000 were revised upwards in the later estimate.

THE STAGES IN DEMOGRAPHIC DEVELOPMENT

The explosive increase in the number of people in the world in the recent past has resulted from the complex series of developments accompanying the industrial revolution and the worldwide spread of advanced technology. It is possible to characterize trends in population by describing several stages in the transition from agrarian, preindustrial cultures to technologically advanced societies. These stages are summarized in Figure 10–4. The overall change is referred to as the *demographic transition*.

TABLE 10–2 World Population Projections for 1970 and 2000 from 1957 and 1966 United Nations Estimates (in Millions)*

| | 1970 Population | | 2000 Population | |
Projection	1957	1966	1957	1966
High	3500	3659	6900	6994
Medium	3480	3592	6280	6130
Low	3350	3545	4880	5449

*From Bogue, D. J.: Principles of Demography. John Wiley and Sons, Inc., New York, 1969, p. 878.

From a demographic viewpoint, agrarian civilizations are characterized by stable or slowly growing population. Agricultural existence favors large families; children are needed to work the soil; sons are desired who can inherit the farm; and the tradition-bound nature of life militates against innovations, such as the adoption of new techniques for family planning. However, high birth rates are balanced by high death rates from disease, famine, and war (Stage 1). Advances in sanitation and improved availability and quality of food, water, and shelter lead to a fall in death rate and an increase in life expectancy. Typically, this occurs without any immediate change in birth rate. If anything, the improved conditions of life may favor an increase in fertility. During this stage (Stage 2) a marked excess of births over deaths develops, leading to rapid expansion in population.

After a time, birth rates tend to fall as a reflection of industrialization and consequent urbanization. With industrialization, people tend to migrate from rural areas to cities. Urban living not only breaks the traditional patterns, but also creates positive incentives for small families. Living quarters are cramped. Children come to represent a financial liability rather than an asset. There is a greater

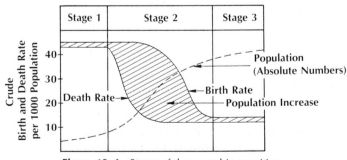

Figure 10–4 Stages of demographic transition.

need for cash since food and clothing cannot be produced at home. For these reasons, wives are impelled to seek work outside the home for wages. There is a greater geographic proximity to health care, including sources of information about family planning. These various factors increase the likelihood that contraceptive practices will be adopted. In some places abortion has also been included in the measures available for the control of fertility. Post–World War II Japan is an example of a country in which all of the mechanisms outlined above have contributed to a dramatic drop in fertility.

The end-stage (Stage 3) of this demographic transition is a situation in which birth and death rates are again essentially in balance, but at a much lower level (e.g., around 10 to 15 per 1000 population) than in the primitive stage, where both were in the vicinity of 35 to 45 per 1000. The extent to which the demographic transition has been completed varies for different parts of the world. Many countries in Europe and North America are well into Stage 3, although few, if any, are at a point of zero population growth. Since 1945 the introduction of public health and medical advances (e.g., sanitation, DDT, and antibiotics) has led to a precipitous drop in death rates in many South American, Asian, and African countries, whereas their birth rates have not declined commensurately.

Figure 10–5, which gives birth and death rates for England and Wales from 1700 to 1930, shows the stages of demographic transition. Until 1740 birth and death rates were similar in magnitude. Thereafter they diverged. The birth rate remained elevated, dropping only slightly toward the end of the nineteenth century,

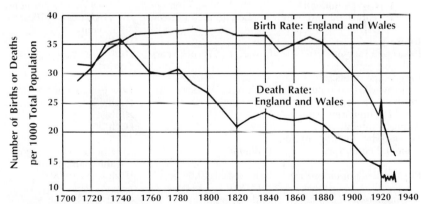

Figure 10–5 Birth rate and death rate, England and Wales, 1700–1930. (Adapted from Carr-Saunders, A. M.: World Population. Past Growth and Present Trends. Frank Cass & Co., Ltd., London, 1965.)

whereas, for reasons which are not fully understood, the death rate dropped quite precipitously during the second half of the eighteenth century. The final figures (1930) show that birth and death rates have both reached low levels, although the birth rate still exceeds the death rate.

To sharpen our understanding of the profound differences between countries at different stages in the demographic transition, it might be useful (Table 10–3) to compare the developed countries (industrialized, Stage 3) with those which are essentially agrarian (Stage 1) or only partly through the process of demographic change ("developing," Stage 2).

As we look at the features of the developing countries we can see a constellation of forces which operate to maintain a static level of economic development and create a cycle of poverty and ill health. Solutions to the total complex of problems presented by developing countries cannot be simple, nor can "health" problems be resolved solely through provision for health needs alone, since these are woven so firmly into the total fabric of life.

TABLE 10–3 Comparison of Some Major Demographic and Economic Characteristics of Developing and Developed Countries

Characteristic	Developing	Developed
Birth rate	High (e.g., 35 per 1000)	Low (e.g., 15 per 1000)
Infant mortality rate	High (e.g., 50 per 1000 live births)	Low (e.g., 18 per 1000 live births)
Crude death rate°	High°(e.g., 25 per 1000)	Low (e.g., 10 per 1000)
Life expectancy	Low (e.g., 40 years)	High (e.g., 65–70 years)
Average age of population	Young	Old
Percentage under 15	High (35–40 per cent)	Low (20–25 per cent)
Percentage 65 and over	Low (e.g., 3 per cent)	High (e.g., 9–10 per cent)
Literacy	Low	High
Per capita income	Low (e.g., $70 per year)	High (e.g., $2500 per year)
Percentage of males engaged in agriculture	High (e.g., 80 per cent)	Low (e.g., 15 per cent)
Productivity of land	Low	High
Food to population ratio	Low	High
Animal protein in diet	Low	High
Disease due to poor environmental conditions	Common	Rare but increasing with industrialization
Physician to population ratio	Low (e.g., 1:10,000–15,000)	High (e.g., 1:800)
Accumulation of capital	Little or none	Great

°Crude death rate may be low because of young age of population even with high age-specific death rates.

Whatever the optimal combination or sequence of interventions, it is clear that decreased fertility is an essential component in economic advance. In a number of countries herculean efforts at economic development have been negated by an ever increasing number of people to be fed, housed, clothed, educated, and given medical care. The problem of population in technically developed nations is somewhat less acute but nonetheless real.

Even today various countries (e.g., U.S.S.R., Canada, France) are concerned about underpopulation and oppressed by the fear that their population might decline in numbers, making the country unable to resist military encroachments. This has been particularly true, for example, of France since 1870. On a worldwide basis, it is generally agreed that the potential threat lies in over-, not underpopulation, and efforts should be directed toward the control of fertility, not its encouragement.

TRENDS IN UNITED STATES POPULATION

In the final section of this chapter we would like to point out the major, current trends in population in this country (Figure 10–6,

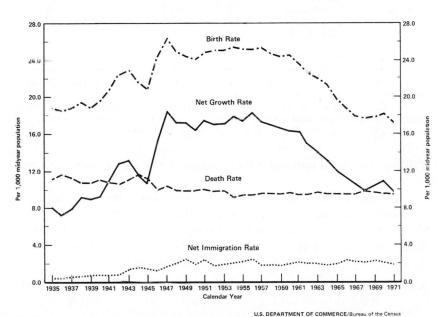

U.S. DEPARTMENT OF COMMERCE/Bureau of the Census

Figure 10–6 Annual rates of net growth, birth, death, and net immigration, 1935–1971. (From Current Population Reports. Population Estimates and Projections. Series P–25, No. 481. U.S. Dept. of Commerce, U.S. Govt. Printing Office, Washington, D.C., 1972.)

TABLE 10–4 Summary of United States Population Growth and Change, 1770–1970*

Census Year	Total Population	Percentage Increase in Previous Decade	Percentage Nonwhite	Percentage White Foreign-born	Percentage Urban-C†
1770-A†	2,205,000	37.0	D†	D†	D†
1780-A	2,781,000	26.1	D	D	D
1790	3,929,214	41.3	19.3	D	5.1
1800	5,308,483	35.1	18.9	D	6.1
1810	7,239,881	36.4	19.0	D	7.3
1820	9,638,453	33.1	18.4	D	7.2
1830	12,866,020	33.5	18.1	D	8.7
1840	17,069,453	32.7	16.8	D	10.8
1850	23,191,876	35.9	15.7	11.6	15.3
1860	31,443,321	35.6	14.4	15.2	19.8
1870	39,818,449	26.6	12.9	16.4	25.7
1880	50,155,783	26.0	13.5	15.1	28.2
1890	62,947,714	25.5	12.5	16.6	35.1
1900	75,994,575	20.7	12.1	15.3	40.0
1910	91,972,266	21.0	11.1	19.5	45.7
1920	105,710,620	14.9	10.3	16.9	51.2
1930	122,775,046	16.1	10.2	14.5	56.2
1940	131,669,275	7.2	10.2	9.7	56.5
1950	150,216,110	14.1	10.5	7.5	64.2
1960-B†	179,323,175	19.4	11.4	5.9	69.9
1970-E†	203,211,926	13.3	12.6	4.9	73.5

*From U.S. Decennial Censuses. Bureau of the Census, U.S. Govt. Printing Office, Washington, D.C., selected years.

†A, Estimated; B, includes Alaska and Hawaii; C, definitions of "urban" have changed many times, and generally reflect contemporary political, social, and economic developments; D, data not available; E, preliminary.

Table 10–4), with particular focus on their relevance for health and social needs.

The *net growth rate* of a population reflects the net difference between additions to the population through births and immigration and losses from deaths and emigration. Thus, for the United States the net growth rate in 1971 was 9.7 per 1000 population, or approximately 1 per cent. Its components were:

Net growth rate* = birth rate − death rate + net immigration rate
9.7   =   17.2   −   9.3   +   1.8

*Rates can only be added or subtracted directly if they are based on the same population denominator.

Figure 10–6 shows yearly rates of net growth of population and its components over a 35-year period. The outstanding feature evident is the abrupt rise in net growth rate in the late 1940's followed by a decline after the peak period (1947 to 1956). Crude death rates and net immigration have been relatively constant during the entire 35-year interval; the major influence on growth rate has been fluctuation in births. The birth rate has been declining since 1957.

The striking increase in the size of the United States population from 1790 to 1970 is evident in Table 10–4. Other features of population change are also indicated:

Variation in the Rate of Increase. In general, the rate of increase has declined. Until 1860 the population increased by more than 30 per cent each decade (i.e., 3 per cent per year). Then between 1860 and 1910 the rate of increase each decade was between 20 and 30 per cent. Since 1910 it has consistently been below 20 per cent. The lowest rate, 7.2 per cent, was recorded in 1940 as an aftermath of the depression.

Changes in Proportion of Nonwhites. Until 1920 there was a constant decline in the proportion of nonwhites (from 19 per cent to 10 per cent, explained in part by the large immigration of whites. Since 1940 the proportion of nonwhites has increased slightly, from 10.2 per cent to 12.6 per cent, because of higher birth rates and greater proportionate gains in life expectancy among nonwhites. However, in interpreting these figures it is well to remember, as we noted previously, that the census has tended to miss more Blacks than whites. The extent of undercounting of Blacks may have varied from one census to the next.

Changes in the Proportion of Foreign-born. The variations in the proportion of the white population born abroad was discussed earlier in the chapter (Migration, page 216).

Steady Increase in Urbanization. Whereas in 1790 only one out of 20 were city dwellers, now three of four people live in urban areas. The small apartments and homes characteristic of urban areas tend to reduce the size of households. Three-generation households have become less common. The difficulty in absorbing persons other than members of the nuclear family has led to a need for nursing homes and similar facilities for elderly and chronically ill persons.

There have been other trends in population which are not apparent from the figure or table.

Move from the Cities to the Suburbs. The implications for health of this shift in population have been outlined in Chapter 4.

Increase in the Proportion of Women. The male to female ratio, which was 104 in 1920, dropped to 99.2 in 1950, and to 97.1 in 1960. This decrease has been due primarily to proportionately greater increase in life expectancy for females than males, and also to changes in patterns of migration.

Industrialization. Closely tied to the urbanization noted previously is industrialization. Over the years there has been a progressive decrease in the proportion of people engaged in farming and an increase in those working in industry and service occupations. The 1970 census indicated that less than 4 per cent of the working population was engaged in agriculture, forestry, and fisheries. This was an all-time low. Within industry, automation and changes in the relative importance of capital-intensive and labor-intensive industrial processes have led to a massive shift away from production toward service and white-collar activities. The change from the relative self-sufficiency characteristic of farm life to specialization and dependence on monetary earnings has resulted in a greater need for old age, unemployment, and disability benefits.

Increase in Literacy and Level of Education. The increased level of education in the population over the past decades, along with advances in medical science, has generated a rising level of expectation for medical services. The concept of medical care as a right rather than privilege has increasingly permeated social thinking.

Increase in the Proportion of Women in the Labor Force. This is one of the more important trends of our times. For instance, whereas women comprised 28 per cent of the labor force in 1950, this had risen to 37 per cent by 1970. This is only partly due to a decrease in the proportion of older men who work. In 1970 one of four women with a husband and a child under the age of six worked either full- or part-time.

Current Economic Status. The majority of Americans are more prosperous than any people in the history of the human race. Nevertheless, segments of the population suffer from extremes of poverty. This may in part explain the country's low ranking in international comparisons on some indices of heath. Overall, 13 per cent of the population in 1970 was living below the "poverty" line as defined by federal standards. The proportion was higher among nonwhites (34 per cent), the elderly (25 per cent), and rural residents (18 per cent).

Implications for Health

Each of the trends and population features just outlined has important consequences for health and needs for health services. For example, the high proportion of working mothers requires that there be adequate arrangements for child care and for health supervision to accommodate the working mothers' schedules. This is particularly true in view of the current high rate of divorce and separation. In 1970 one-sixth of all children under the age of 18 were living with either no or only one parent. An attempt is being made to meet these needs through the development of day care centers.

Our high rates of utilization of resources create, and urbanization and associated industrialization intensify, environmental problems of all kinds, such as water and air pollution, solid waste disposal, and noise "pollution." In addition, shifts in population have left the inner cities with a concentration of problems at the interface of medical and social pathology: alcoholism, delinquency, drug abuse, suicide, venereal disease, tuberculosis, and mental illness. These problems are compounded by the loss of revenue-producing industries and the flight of middle-class householders from the cities.

The convergence of several forces has led to a consensus that the time is ripe for some form of National Health Insurance. Pertinent factors include the aging of the population, advances in medical care technology, the increasing costs of medical care (especially in hospitals), and the relative shortage of primary physicians, as well as concepts of egalitarianism and medical care as a right. There is also interest in the development of new health care delivery systems (especially the so-called Health Maintenance Organizations) which, it is hoped, would emphasize preventive and ambulatory services and continuity of care.

United States Population Projections

In 1972 a Presidential Commission on Population Growth and the American Future published an important document entitled *Population and the American Future.* Following a comprehensive exploration of the implications of current population trends, the commission presented such cogent arguments for slowing the rate of growth and achieving population stabilization as the expanding demand for government services and the impact of a growing population upon finite resources of water, arable land, and areas for outdoor recreation.

An analysis by the commission (Figure 10–7) demonstrates the enormous impact on population made by a difference of even one child in average family size. By 2070, under the same conditions of

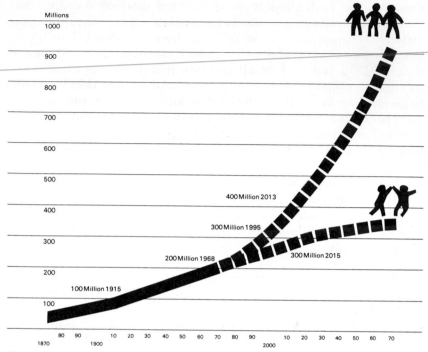

Figure 10–7 United States population projections through 2070: 2- vs. 3-child family. (From Population and the American Future, Final Report, Commission on Population Growth and the American Future. U.S. Govt. Printing Office, Washington, D.C., 1972.)

migration and mortality, the two-child average would result in a population of 350 million, while the three-child family would lead to a population of almost a billion people.

The difference in average family size would affect the composition of the population as well as its total numbers. Table 10–5 presents the same two projections (i.e., two-child vs. three-child average family) for the year 2000. It shows that the difference in total population would be 50 million and that most of the difference would be due to an increase in young people. Thus, the overall effect would be not only an increase in total numbers, but also a markedly higher dependency ratio.

The population problems facing the United States are well expressed in the following quotation from the Presidential Commission:

Demographic events have the quality of persisting over time, for example, the baby boom generation born after World War II is still working

TABLE 10–5   United States Population in Millions, 1970 and 2000,
under Two Assumptions about Family Size*

Age	1970	2000	
		2-child Average	3-child Average
All ages	205	271	322
Under 5	17	20	34
5–17	53	55	80
18–21	15	17	24
Under 18	70	75	114
18–64	115	167	179
65 and over	20	29	29
Dependency ratio†	78	62	80

*From Census Bureau: Projections of the Population of the United States by
Age and Sex, 1970–2000. Current Population Reports, Series P-25, No. 470, U.S.
Govt. Printing Office, Washington, D.C., 1971.
†Number of persons 65 and over plus persons under 18, per 100 persons aged
18–64.

its way through the age structure, with many repercussions. . . . Because
the lead time is decades in length, it is necessary to face the issue now and
come to deliberate and informed decisions about population problems. . . .
The major contribution to growth now comes from the advantaged majority
in our society. Because of their smaller number, our "have-not"
groups — our racial and ethnic minorities — do not bear the primary responsibility for population growth, and inducing them to limit the number of
children they have would not in itself stabilize our population. However,
there are strong connections between high fertility and the economic and
social problems that affect the 13 per cent of our people who are poor.
Therefore, we recognize that unless we address our racism and poverty we
will not be able to resolve the question of population growth for our racial
and ethnic minorities. As deprived groups are brought into the educational,
occupational, and residential mainstream, their fertility will probably
decline to the level of the people already there.

SUMMARY

Births, deaths, and migration are the three variables which determine the size and composition of the population of any defined
area. The operation of these factors over several decades is mir-
rored in population pyramids which depict percentage distribution
of the population by age and sex at a point in time. Developing
countries with high birth and death rates have a triangularly shaped
pyramid, whereas countries with low birth and death rates have

pyramids of a more rectangular shape. Past levels of fertility and mortality determine the dependency ratio, a measure of the relative proportions of economically productive and unproductive persons (i.e., those at the extremes of life) in the population.

In this chapter, an historical account of trends in world population was followed by a discussion of projections for the future. The demographic transition was identified by the changes in birth and death rates which have typically accompanied the shift from agrarian to industrialized societies. The rapid population growth characteristic of countries in the process of transition was noted. The economic status and health needs of developed and developing countries were contrasted.

Lastly, we focussed on trends in United States population and the implications of different projected levels of fertility. Excerpts of the report of the Presidential Commission on Population Growth and the American Future were cited in support of the need for stabilization of the United States population.

STUDY QUESTIONS

10–1 Define the following terms and give an example when appropriate:
Demography (page 213)
Natural increase in population (page 213)
Total increase in population (page 213)
General fertility rate (page 214)
Period vs. cohort measures of fertility (page 215)
Completed birth rate (page 215)
Migration (page 215)
Population pyramid (page 216)
Dependency ratio (page 218)
Demographic transition (page 221)
Net growth rate (page 226)

10–2 In Figure 10–8 it can be seen that population pyramids reflect the major events in a country's history and that the record of these events persists throughout the lifespan of birth cohorts. Study these four pyramids and comment on their major features.

Answer on page 353.

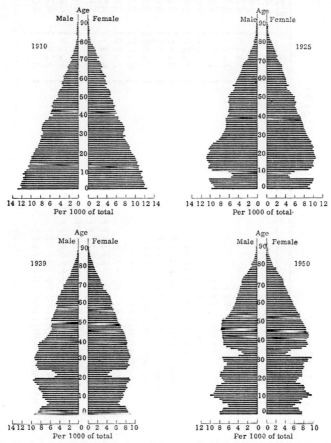

Figure 10–8 Age and sex distribution of the population of Germany, 1910, 1925, 1939, and 1950. (From The Federal Minister for the Interior (ed.): Leben und Sterben in der Bundesrepublik Deutschland. Department of Health, Bonn, 1953 [Der Bundesminister des Intern. Abteilung Gesundheitswesen].)

10–3 Figure 10–9 represents computer print-outs derived from census data for one section of Montgomery County, Maryland, for 1970. (Figure 10–9A is for whites, Figure 10–9B for nonwhites.) The figure shows population pyramids, i.e., the numbers and percentage distribution of the population by five-year age groups and by sex. Each symbol (M or F) represents 0.33 per cent of the total population in the pyramid.

A. Calculate dependency ratios for whites and nonwhites separately for (1) youths (ages 0 to 19 years), and (2) the aged (ages 65 years and over). How do the white and non-white groups differ in the contributions of young people and the aged to their dependent populations?

WHITE POPULATION OF CATCHMNT
TAK.PARK-SS AREA II, MD.
TOTAL POP 109208 MALES (51819) FEMALES (57389)

NUMBER	%	AGE	9 8 7 6 5 4 3 2 1	1 2 3 4 5 6 7 8 9	%	NUMBER
184	0.17	85+		F	0.45	490
313	0.29	80-4		FF	0.69	749
646	0.59	75-9	M	FFF	1.13	1238
1123	1.03	70-4	MMM	FFFF	1.63	1777
1526	1.40	65-9	MMMM	FFFFF	1.95	2133
2469	2.26	60-4	MMMMMM	FFFFFFF	2.64	2884
2955	2.71	55-9	MMMMMMMM	FFFFFFFFF	3.20	3499
3291	3.01	50-4	MMMMMMMMM	FFFFFFFFFF	3.48	3800
3291	3.01	45-9	MMMMMMMMM	FFFFFFFFFF	3.55	3876
3119	2.86	40-4	MMMMMMMM	FFFFFFFFF	3.05	3329
2756	2.52	35-9	MMMMMMM	FFFFFFF	2.62	2859
3278	3.00	30-4	MMMMMMMMM	FFFFFFFF	2.88	3144
4423	4.05	25-9	MMMMMMMMMMMM	FFFFFFFFFFFF	4.17	4551
4794	4.39	20-4	MMMMMMMMMMMMM	FFFFFFFFFFFFFFF	5.12	5595
4377	4.01	15-9	MMMMMMMMMMMM	FFFFFFFFFFFFF	4.35	4746
4509	4.13	10-4	MMMMMMMMMMMM	FFFFFFFFFFFF	4.09	4468
4558	4.17	5-9	MMMMMMMMMMMM	FFFFFFFFFFF	3.88	4238
4207	3.85	0-4	MMMMMMMMMMM	FFFFFFFFFFF	3.67	4013

Figure 10–9 Mental Health Demographic Profile System, Takoma Park-Silver Spring, Catchment Area II, Montgomery County, Maryland. *A*, White population; *B*, nonwhite population.

```
NEGRO  POPULATION OF CATCHMNT
TAK.PARK-SS AREA II, MD.
TOTAL POP    7874                   MALES (  3755)                 FEMALES (  4119)

NUMBER|  %  |AGE 9  8  7  6  5  4  3  2  1 | 1  2  3  4  5  6  7  8  9 |  %  |NUMBER
     8| 0.10|85+                            |                           | 0.05|     4|
     6| 0.08|80-4                           |                           | 0.24|    19|
     9| 0.11|75-9                           |                           | 0.27|    21|
    25| 0.32|70-4                           |F                          | 0.38|    30|
    32| 0.41|65-9                          M|F                          | 0.56|    44|
    66| 0.84|60-4                         MM|FF                         | 0.75|    59|
    98| 1.24|55-9                        MMM|FFF                        | 1.32|   104|
   114| 1.45|50-4                       MMMM|FFFF                       | 1.65|   130|
   163| 2.07|45-9                     MMMMMM|FFFFFFF                    | 2.49|   196|
   220| 2.79|40-4                   MMMMMMMM|FFFFFFFF                   | 2.86|   225|
   287| 3.64|35-9                 MMMMMMMMMM|FFFFFFFFFFF                | 3.99|   314|
   339| 4.31|30-4               MMMMMMMMMMMM|FFFFFFFFFFFFF              | 4.58|   361|
   448| 5.69|25-9          MMMMMMMMMMMMMMMMM|FFFFFFFFFFFFFFFFFFF        | 6.46|   509|
   319| 4.05|20-4               MMMMMMMMMMMM|FFFFFFFFFFFFFFFFFFF        | 6.41|   505|
   336| 4.27|15-9               MMMMMMMMMMMM|FFFFFFFFFFFFFFF            | 5.12|   403|
   384| 4.88|10-4             MMMMMMMMMMMMMM|FFFFFFFFFFFFFF             | 4.70|   370|
   427| 5.42| 5-9           MMMMMMMMMMMMMMMM|FFFFFFFFFFFFFF             | 4.99|   393|
   471| 5.98| 0-4          MMMMMMMMMMMMMMMMM|FFFFFFFFFFFFFFFF           | 5.47|   431|
```

Figure 10–9 *Continued.*

B. How would you use the information from the figure for planning health services for the county?

C. What other kinds of demographic information about the population would be desirable for planning purposes?

Answer on page 354.

10–4 Which set of annual vital statistics rates* shown below would be typical of: A. a developing country? B. a developed country?

	Crude Birth Rate	Infant Mortality Rate	Crude Death Rate
(1)	15	18	35
(2)	35	18	25
(3)	15	18	10
(4)	15	60	10
(5)	35	60	25
(6)	15	60	25

Answer on page 355.

*Rates per 1000.

REFERENCES

Bogne, D. J.: Principles of Demography. John Wiley & Sons, Inc., New York, 1969.

Dorn, H. F.: World population growth: An international dilemma. Science, *135*: 283, 1962.

Ehrlich, P. R., and Ehrlich, A. H.: Population, Resources and Environment. Issues in Human Ecology. W. H. Freeman and Company, San Francisco, 1970.

Population and the American Future. Final Report, Commission on Population Growth and the American Future. U.S. Govt. Printing Office, Washington, D.C., 1972.

SCREENING
IN THE
DETECTION
OF
DISEASE
AND
MAINTENANCE
OF
HEALTH

11

In the previous chapter we discussed aspects of population, such as size and composition by age, sex, and other characteristics, which determine need for health care. Here we examine one approach to control of disease in population groups, early detection.

If early detection and treatment can affect favorably the ultimate course of a disease, then these measures can serve as a secondary line of defense against ailments which are not currently susceptible to primary prevention. There are two possible avenues to early diagnosis. One depends upon prompt attention to the earliest *symptoms* of disease, the other attempts to detect disease in *asymptomatic* individuals.

Achievement of early investigation of incipient symptoms of disease requires education of the public and physicians so that they learn to respond promptly to cues which may be indicative of disease. The efforts of the American Cancer Society to publicize "the seven signs of cancer" (e.g., unusual bleeding or discharge, a sore that does not heal, and so on) are an example of this approach.

Delays in response occur all too frequently; studies of the sequence of events in the diagnosis of cancer have repeatedly shown that, in a substantial proportion of patients, there is delay before appropriate action is taken after the patient becomes aware of the problem. Most of this delay has been found to be attributable to patients, particularly those of lower social class (Hackett et al., 1973), but physicians also contribute to delay. In this chapter we will not be concerned with early response to signs or symptoms, even though this is an important problem. Rather, we will focus on active detection of disease in *asymptomatic, apparently healthy individuals,* i.e., screening.

Theoretically, at least, detection of disease in asymptomatic individuals should be superior to reliance on response to symptoms.

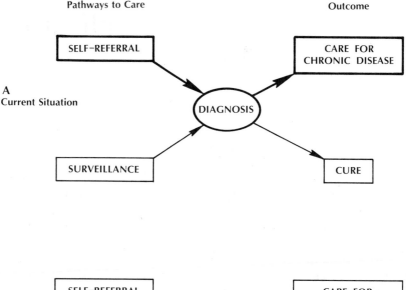

Figure 11–1 Schema relating path of detection to outcome. (Based on a presentation by Dr. M. Henderson.)

If a disease has not yet reached the threshold of clinical visibility, the chances that it is curable should be better. This assumption, however, must be tested for each disease. With respect to cancer, for example, it must be ascertained whether tumors detected by screening are not those that grow slowly and would therefore have a relatively good prognosis even without screening. But, at least in the abstract, detection of disease before symptoms develop should improve the chances for preventing death and disability.

The importance of the path by which disease is brought to diagnosis is illustrated by Figure 11–1. Currently (Figure 11–1A), disease is diagnosed primarily because people refer themselves to medical care for the investigation of specific symptoms. Only a few cases of disease are detected in the asymptomatic state because of participation in an ongoing surveillance program. Since many of the cases come to attention relatively late, the proportion cured is small compared with the proportion that require protracted care.

In contrast, our goal for the future could be a situation more like that depicted in Figure 11–1B. If this utopian condition were reached, most disease would be detected in the course of regular surveillance rather than through self-referral for symptoms. Since this should facilitate detection early in the course of disease, the percentage of cures should be increased and the load of care for chronic illness decreased. The principles underlying surveillance, or screening programs, will be discussed later in the chapter. First we have to understand more about screening tests and the criteria used to evaluate them.

DEFINITION OF SCREENING

Screening was defined some years ago as:

the *presumptive* identification of *unrecognized* disease or defect by the application of tests, examinations, or other procedures which can be applied *rapidly* to sort out apparently well persons who *probably* have a disease from those who *probably do not*. A screening test is *not* intended to be diagnostic. Persons with positive or suspicious findings must be referred to their physicians for diagnosis and necessary treatment. (Commission on Chronic Illness, 1957. Italics added for emphasis.)

Figure 11–2 presents this definition of screening in the form of a flow diagram. Note that essentially two groups are formed by the screening procedure. One is presumed to be well (negative on screening), the other to require further diagnostic tests. In addition, there may be some individuals whose results are so clearly abnormal that the screening test may be virtually diagnostic.

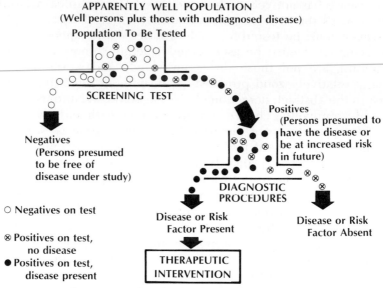

APPARENTLY WELL POPULATION
(Well persons plus those with undiagnosed disease)

Population To Be Tested

SCREENING TEST

Positives
(Persons presumed to
have the disease or
be at increased risk
in future)

Negatives
(Persons presumed
to be free of
disease under study)

DIAGNOSTIC
PROCEDURES

○ Negatives on test

⊗ Positives on test,
no disease

● Positives on test,
disease present

Disease or Risk
Factor Present

Disease or Risk
Factor Absent

THERAPEUTIC
INTERVENTION

Figure 11–2   Flow diagram for a mass screening test.

Identification of Normal Values

The concept of "normal" and the specifications for separating "positives" from "negatives" deserve some discussion. The term "normal" can refer to the usual, or typical, value of a characteristic for a population group (e.g., average height or weight). It can also be used to describe *functional* status, either present or future. In this sense, any value can be considered normal if no increased risk has been found to be associated with it. In addition, the term "normal" has a technical, *statistical* meaning, i.e., the normal or Gaussian distribution.

Since the goal of screening is to identify persons who have a disease or are at increased risk for the future, screening is concerned ultimately with a functional definition of normality. However, we must also consider how the statistical use of the term "normal" relates to the goal of screening.

The normal curve refers to a continuous, symmetrical distribution which has certain properties. A major property is that two units of variation (standard deviation units*) above and below the mean

---

*See Bahn, A. K.: Basic Medical Statistics. Grune & Stratton, Inc., New York, 1972 or other standard statistics text for definition of standard deviation and other technical terms.

correspond to the central 95 per cent of the area under the curve. That is, the central 95 per cent of the cases will be included in the values identified by the mean value ±2 S.D. (Figure 11–3 depicts a normal curve.) By extension, the normal range in laboratory tests or physiologic measures is often defined in terms of the central 95 per cent (or 68 per cent) of values derived from a series of presumably healthy individuals.

This statistical approach to normality is often unsatisfactory for purposes of classification of disease. For one thing, some biochemical measures are not normally distributed (Elveback et al., 1970) and, therefore, items corresponding to the mean ± 2 S.D. do not represent the middle 95 per cent of the values. But beyond this, a dichotomous classification of people as "normal" or "abnormal" with respect to a certain value often oversimplifies a complex situation. We know, for example, that even within the central 95 per cent of the total range of blood pressures, there is a gradient such that persons at the upper end are at greater risk of coronary heart disease or stroke than those at the lower end.

In response to problems of this nature, Elveback (1972) has suggested that laboratory data on individuals be presented in terms of a *percentile level*, and, furthermore, that this be specific for age and sex. Such specificity is needed because the same level of cholesterol might represent one percentile value for a 60-year-old female, another for a 30-year-old male. The use of age-sex-specific percentiles rather than the 95 per cent central range would emphasize that (1) no assumptions are made that the distribution is normal; (2) the same biochemical value, e.g., 300 mg. per 100 ml. of cholesterol, could represent a common value for an older woman,

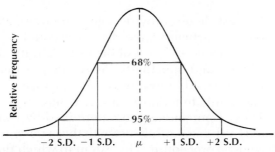

Figure 11–3 Diagram of the areas under a normal curve in standard deviation units.

but a distinctly unusual one for a young man; and (3) health and disease lie along a continuum and that separation of the two on the basis of a single "cut-off" point may be arbitrary.

The study group from which the values are derived also deserves consideration. Ideally, norms should be based on random samples of defined, healthy populations. With few exceptions, notably the population samples examined in the National Health Survey, random samples have not been used in setting norms for physical measurements (i.e., height, weight, and blood pressure) or laboratory determinations (e.g., serum cholesterol, blood glucose, and serum uric acid). The "normal" ranges for many tests currently used in screening programs have been derived from small numbers of highly selected groups both in and out of hospitals. The development of screening programs for large numbers of healthy persons and the increasing automation of laboratory procedures should make it feasible to retrieve normative data on better samples.

CRITERIA FOR EVALUATION OF SCREENING TESTS

Several criteria are needed for the evaluation of a screening test. These include its *validity*, determined by measures of sensitivity and specificity; its *reliability* (that is, repeatability); and its *yield*, or amount of disease detected in the population. It is perhaps superfluous to note that since screening is designed to be applied to large groups of people, screening tests should be innocuous, rapid, and inexpensive; they should also be able to be carried out largely by technicians rather than professionals.

Validity

A screening test should provide a good preliminary indication of which individuals actually have the disease and which do not. This is referred to as the *validity* of the test. Validity has two components: sensitivity and specificity. *Sensitivity* is defined as the ability to identify correctly those who have the disease. *Specificity* is defined as the ability to identify correctly those who do **not** have the disease. These components are determined by comparing the results obtained by the screening test with those derived from some definitive diagnostic procedure. The extent to which the screening results agree with those derived by the more definitive tests provides a measure of sensitivity and specificity. For simplicity, we will assume that there is no error in the final diagnosis reached by the more definitive procedure.

An ideal screening test would be 100 per cent sensitive and 100 per cent specific. In practice this does not occur; sensitivity and specificity are usually inversely related. That is, one usually achieves high sensitivity at the expense of low specificity, and vice versa. This can be demonstrated readily with tests which measure a continuously distributed variable (e.g., hemoglobin, blood pressure, serum cholesterol, and intraocular pressure). For such tests, it is possible to vary the sensitivity and specificity by changing the level at which the test is considered positive. The determination of intraocular pressure as a screening test for glaucoma will be used as an example.

Determination of Sensitivity and Specificity: An Example. Glaucoma is an abnormality of the eyes in which increased intraocular pressure causes organic changes in the optic nerve and defects in the visual fields. In general, for the unequivocal diagnosis of glaucoma, three factors must be present: increased intraocular pressure, optic nerve atrophy, and typical defects in the visual fields.

The level of intraocular pressure on any one examination is not an infallible indication of glaucoma. Intraocular pressure varies during the day, and the variability is greater in persons with glaucoma than in others. In addition, people vary in the extent to which pathologic changes occur at a given level of pressure. Therefore, although persons with elevated intraocular pressure on casual examination are more likely to have glaucoma than those with lower pressure, further studies are needed for a definitive diagnosis. In addition to examining for changes in the optic nerve and defects in the visual field, the ophthalmologist may also conduct provocative tests (e.g., have the person drink a large quantity of water within a few minutes), which create a significant rise in intraocular pressure in persons with glaucoma.

How do the results of screening by determination of intraocular pressure relate to the presence or absence of glaucoma? The following discussion derives largely from a monograph by Thorner and Remein (1961). These authors suggest that screening tests may be understood in terms of overlapping distributions of an attribute for a diseased and a nondiseased group.* For some values of the test the distributions overlap, and it is not possible to assign per-

---

*Wilson and Jungner (1968) cite studies which do not support the existence of two overlapping distributions of intraocular pressure. Nevertheless, the model is presented because it is helpful for understanding of sensitivity and specificity.

sons with these values to the normal or diseased group on the basis of the screening test alone. When the screening value is clearly outside the normal range its interpretation poses less of a problem.

This situation is illustrated in Figure 11–4. Note that there are two groups, those without the disease (A) and those with the disease (B). The nonglaucomatous group (A) is much larger than Group B and has a lower average intraocular pressure, with values ranging from approximately 14 to 26 mm. Hg. Intraocular pressure in Group B partially overlaps that in Group A, lying between 22 and 42 mm. Hg. The range from approximately 22 to 26 mm. Hg thus includes both glaucomatous and nonglaucomatous eyes.

Now let us consider screening for glaucoma carried out by determination of intraocular pressure. If the screening level is set at 26 mm. Hg, all of the nonglaucomatous eyes will be called negative. In other words, the test will be 100 per cent specific. However, since all of the glaucomatous eyes which lie between 22 and 26 mm. Hg will also be called negative, the sensitivity of the test will be low. When diseased persons are labelled negative, the test results are referred to as *false negatives.*

On the other hand, if the screening level were set at 22 mm. Hg, all eyes which are truly glaucomatous will be positive on the test. That is, the test will now be 100 per cent sensitive. However, since the nonglaucomatous eyes with pressures between 22 and 26

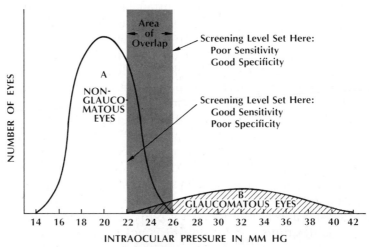

Figure 11–4 Hypothetical distribution of intraocular pressures in glaucomatous and nonglaucomatous eyes, measured by tonometer. (Adapted from Thorner, R. M., and Remein, Q. R.: Principles and procedures in the evaluation of screening for disease. USPHS Pub. No. 846, U.S. Govt. Printing Office, Washington, D.C., 1961.)

Result of Screening Test	Disease State	
	Disease	No Disease
Positive	*true positive* TP	false positive FP
Negative	false negative FN	*true negative* TN

$$\text{Sensitivity} = \frac{\text{TP}}{\text{TP} + \text{FN}} \quad \text{Specificity} = \frac{\text{TN}}{\text{TN} + \text{FP}}$$

Figure 11–5 Results of screening test illustrating sensitivity and specificity.

mm. Hg will also be called positive, the test will have poor specificity. Such test results are referred to as *false positives.*[*]

Of course, the level may be set anywhere between 22 and 26 mm. Hg. The decision about where to set this level will be determined by a number of considerations — the cost of diagnostic testing of false positives, the importance of not missing a possible "case," the likelihood that the population will be rescreened at a reasonable interval, and the prevalence of the disease.

From what has been said so far, it can be seen that each person falls into one of four groups (Figure 11–5), depending upon whether or not he has the disease and whether or not he is classified as positive on the screening test.

From Figure 11–5 formal definitions are obtained,

Percentage sensitivity = percentage of people with the disease who are detected by the test $= \frac{\text{TP}}{\text{TP}+\text{FN}} \times 100$

Percentage false negatives = percentage of people with the disease who were not detected by the test $= \frac{\text{FN}}{\text{TP} + \text{FN}} \times 100$

Percentage specificity = percentage of people without the disease who were correctly labelled by the test as not diseased $= \frac{\text{TN}}{\text{TN}+\text{FP}} \times 100$

Percentage false positives = percentage of people without the disease who were incorrectly labelled by the test as having disease $= \frac{\text{FP}}{\text{TN} + \text{FP}} \times 100$

---

[*]Note the analogy between the selection of the screening level and of the significance (α) level in statistical decision making. The inverse relation between false positives and false negatives is comparable to the inverse relation between the risk of Type I (α) and Type II (β) errors.

Note that the determination of specificity is made with reference only to the nondiseased persons and is totally independent of the diseased group. Note also that the percentage of false negatives is the complement of sensitivity, the percentage of false positives the complement of specificity.

The following is a simple, hypothetical example which illustrates the calculation of these measures of validity:

Results of Screening Test in 990 Persons
Disease State

		Disease	No Disease
	Positive	75	50
Test Result			
	Negative	15	850
		90	900

$$\text{Sensitivity} = \frac{75}{75 + 15} = \frac{75}{90} = 83 \text{ per cent}$$

$$\text{False negative} = \frac{15}{75 + 15} = \frac{15}{90} = \frac{17 \text{ per cent}}{100 \text{ per cent}}$$

$$\text{Specificity} = \frac{850}{850 + 50} = \frac{850}{900} = 94 \text{ per cent}$$

$$\text{False positive} = \frac{50}{850 + 50} = \frac{50}{900} = \frac{6 \text{ per cent}}{100 \text{ per cent}}$$

Naturally, we want a *sensitive* test, one which will identify a high proportion of those who actually have a disease and will thus create *few false negatives*. At the same time, we would like the test to be *specific* for the disease; positive reactions should be limited largely to the group which is truly diseased and there should be *few false positives*.

Evaluation of the sensitivity and specificity of a test requires that a diagnosis of disease be established or ruled out for *every person* tested by the screening procedure, *regardless of whether he screens negative or positive*. This diagnosis must be established by techniques independent of the screening test. For example, if a urine test for diabetes is to be evaluated, the diagnosis of diabetes may be established on the basis of a blood sugar or glucose tolerance test, but not on the basis of the urine test.

It is important to be aware that the validity of a test is affected not only by characteristics of the test but also by host factors, such as stage or severity of the disease and presence of other conditions. For example, false negatives may occur early in a disease [e.g., a negative serologic test for syphilis (STS) in the first weeks after syphilitic infection is acquired] or late in disease, as in some cases of tertiary syphilis. Patients with overwhelming tuberculous infection, sarcoidosis, or Hodgkin's disease may give negative responses on tuberculin test.

Conversely, the presence of one disease may cause a positive reaction to a screening test used to identify another condition. For example, malaria, leprosy, systemic lupus erythematosus, and other collagen diseases may cause false positive results on screening tests for syphilis.

Combinations of Tests. Two or more tests can be combined to enhance sensitivity or specificity of the screening process. There are two principal forms of combination — *tests in series* and *tests in parallel*. With tests in series, the person is called positive only if he tests positive to all of a series of tests, negative if he tests negative to any. When tests are done in parallel, the person is labelled positive if he tests positive to any of the tests. The former approach (i.e., tests in series) enhances the specificity of the testing, the latter (i.e., tests in parallel) enhances sensitivity.

Combination in series is perhaps more common. It typically employs a sequence of tests of increasing specificity. A test widely employed in routine screening for syphilis is the VDRL (Venereal Disease Research Laboratories) slide test, a broadly sensitive serologic test based on the presence of reagin, a nonspecific (nontreponemal) antigen prepared from beef heart. Since many conditions can produce false positives on this test, every positive result is followed up with a more specific test, such as the fluorescent treponemal antibody-absorption test (FTA-ABS), which is positive only as a result of past or current treponemal infection. Diabetes, hyperthyroidism, and glaucoma are other diseases for which screening tests are often combined in sequence.

An example of tests combined in parallel can be found in screening for breast cancer. Since 1963 the Health Insurance Plan (HIP) of Greater New York has been carrying out a large-scale, controlled study to evaluate the usefulness of mammography as a screening device. Women in the test group are screened concurrently by physical examination and mammography. The control women receive only physical examinations. Women abnormal on either physical examination or mammography are considered "positive" and are studied further by biopsy. The results to date indicate that each of these procedures contributes independently to the diagnosis (Strax et al., 1970). That is, some women later confirmed as having breast cancer have been detected through mammography but have been negative on physical examination. For others the reverse has been true; the addition of mammography to the screening procedure has served to increase the sensitivity of the screening.

Reliability (Precision)

A reliable screening test is one which gives consistent results when the test is performed more than once on the same individual under the same conditions. Two major factors affect consistency of results: the *variation inherent in the method* and *observer variation (observer error)*. The variability of a method depends upon such factors as the stability of the reagents used and fluctuation in the substance being measured (e.g., in relation to meals, diurnal variation). Observer variation can stem from differences among observers (*interobserver variation*) and also from variation in readings by the same observer on separate occasions (*intraobserver variation*). These variations can usually be reduced by careful standardization of procedures, by an intensive training period for all observers (or interviewers), by periodic checks on their work, and by the use of two or more observers making independent observations.

Yield

The *yield* of a screening program may be defined as the amount of previously unrecognized disease which is diagnosed and brought to treatment as a result of the screening. The yield from screening is dependent on several factors.

The Sensitivity of the Test. Obviously, a screening test must detect a sufficient proportion of the cases to be useful. If the test has low sensitivity and, therefore, identifies only a fraction of the diseased individuals, the yield may be poor regardless of other factors.

Prevalence of Unrecognized Disease. The higher the prevalence of unrecognized disease in a population, the higher will be the yield from screening. In turn, the prevalence of unrecognized disease is at least partially dependent on the level of medical care which has prevailed in a community. Where little medical care has been available prior to the screening, there will be much undiagnosed and untreated disease (e.g., tuberculosis or malaria in underdeveloped tropical areas) and the yield from screening will be high.

Extent of Previous Screening. The yield from screening will also vary depending on whether an initial or a repeat screening is being done. Since an initial screening detects cases which may have developed over a period of years, the yield may be much higher than that obtained by repeat screening. Referring to Chapter 7, we can see that an initial screening reflects prevalence of disease, repeat screening an incidence value.

Health Behavior. Screening will not improve health unless people both participate in the program and act on any problems uncovered. Psychologic and social factors affecting participation in preventive care, usually referred to as "health behavior," are therefore relevant to the success of screening programs. In a classic analysis of participation in mass chest x-ray surveys, Hochbaum (1958) identified four factors which determine the likelihood of participation in screening. First, a threat of disease must be perceived; that is, the disease must be known to the individual. It must also be regarded as a serious threat to health. Further, it must be defined as relevant to the patient; he must feel vulnerable. A feeling of invulnerability will inhibit action. Lastly, there must be a firm belief that action will have meaningful consequences. Fatalism will also inhibit action. In summary, if the disease being studied is perceived as a serious, personal threat, and if action is expected to abort the threat, then participation is likely. If any of these factors is not present, the person is not likely to respond to appeals to participate in the program.

The behavioral aspects of secondary prevention extend beyond participation in screening. Follow-up of positive screening results and compliance with any treatment outlined are also essential components. All of the factors enumerated in relation to screening also help to determine whether a person will follow through on the results of screening. In addition, factors of convenience, expense, and attitudes towards physicians and medical care undoubtedly come into play.

The yield from screening should be monitored periodically so that programs are revised as needed. Recent changes in screening programs for tuberculosis in this country illustrate this point. Mass chest x-rays, for many years a mainstay of tuberculosis case-finding programs, were gradually abandoned because of the progressive decrease in yield, as well as growing concern about exposure to ionizing radiation. In 1963 a Child-Centered Program was formulated, which stressed routine tuberculin testing of children entering school; it was hoped that identification of child reactors would lead to the adult source cases. Within a few years this procedure too was abandoned because of low reactor rates (e.g., 0.2 to 0.3 per cent) in young children (Edwards, 1971). Currently, efforts are being concentrated in high-risk groups and communities.

While screening programs generally aim for a high yield, programs which yield a small number of cases may be warranted if the condition being detected, such as phenylketonuria (PKU), has serious consequences which can be averted.

A popular approach to increasing yield is *multiphasic screening*, the simultaneous use of multiple tests to detect several pathologic conditions in the same screening program. When many parameters of health are tested, the probability of finding any positive result is increased. The recent trend toward automation of laboratory procedures has favored the development of multiphasic screening efforts. Of course, since each test produces some false positives, the total expense of investigating false positives also goes up as the number of tests is increased.

Predictive Value. One important problem in screening concerns the relationship between sensitivity, specificity, and prevalence of disease. It has been pointed out (Vecchio, 1966) that when prevalence is low even a highly specific test will give a relatively large number of false positives because of the many nondiseased persons being tested. Vecchio has referred to this as the *predictive value* of a test. The concept of predictive value can actually be applied to either positive or negative test results. That is, the predictive value of a positive test is defined as the likelihood that an individual with a positive test has the disease. The predictive value of a negative test refers to the likelihood that a person with a negative test does not have the disease. Referring to Figure 11–5, we see that the predictive value of a positive test is $\frac{TP}{TP + FP}$ and that of a negative test is $\frac{TN}{TN + FN}$.

The importance of prevalence to predictive value of a positive test can be seen from the following example. Table 11–1 shows predictive values for a population of 1000 people screened with a test of 99 per cent sensitivity and 95 per cent specificity at two levels of prevalence, 1 per cent and 2 per cent.

TABLE 11–1 Predictive Values of a Positive Test with 99 Per Cent Sensitivity and 95 Per Cent Specificity at Two Levels of Prevalence

Item	1 Per Cent	2 Per Cent
a. Number in population	1000	1000
b. Diseased	10	20
c. Nondiseased	990	980
d. True positives (b × .99)	10 (9.9)	20 (19.8)
e. False positives (c × 1 − .95)	50 (49.5)	49
f. Total positives (d + e)	60	69
g. Predictive value of a positive (d/f)	$\frac{10}{60} = 17$ per cent	$\frac{20}{69} = 29$ per cent

Note that at the lower level of prevalence only one-sixth of the positives, 17 per cent, would be true positives. In other words, five out of six persons who tested positive would not have the disease. With an increment of only 1 per cent in prevalence, the predictive value of the test would be appreciably higher, 29 per cent.

Figure 11-6 shows the relation between prevalence and predictive value under an assumption of constant sensitivity (95 per cent) and specificity (95 per cent). The graph makes it clear that the

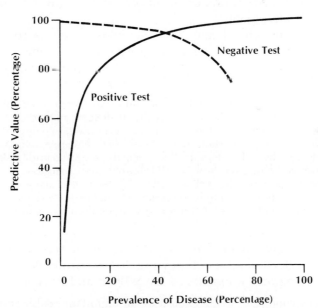

Figure 11–6 Relationship between prevalence of disease and predictive value, with sensitivity and specificity held constant at 95 per cent. (Adapted from Vecchio, T. J.: Predictive value of a single diagnostic test in unselected populations. N. Engl. J. Med., 274:1171, 1966.)

predictive value of a positive test is poor if prevalence is low. Other analyses indicate that this remains true even with tests of excellent specificity and sensitivity. Therefore, screening is generally directed toward high prevalence groups. For example, diabetes screening programs are often limited to high prevalence groups such as persons over 40, the obese, or those with a family history of diabetes.

PRINCIPLES UNDERLYING SCREENING PROGRAMS

We might turn now from the technical aspects of screening to some more general issues. We should note that screening may have one of several aims. It may be undertaken as part of an epidemiologic survey to determine the frequency or natural history of a condition (e.g., the Framingham study of coronary heart disease). Its primary purpose may also be prevention of contagion and protection of the public's health, such as the mass x-ray surveys formerly carried out to detect pulmonary tuberculosis. However, at this point we are concerned with *prescriptive screening,* i.e., the detection of disease, or precursors of disease, as a guide to the medical care of individuals.

The special ethical and practical considerations relevant to prescriptive screening of populations have been summarized well in a book of essays, *Screening in Medical Care,* published in Britain for the Nuffield Provincial Hospitals Trust (1968).

... although the requirements which should be met by a screening procedure — evidence that it is effective and that it deserves priority over competing medical measures — are not unique to screening, two considerations make them unusually important in this field. First, because investigation is initiated by or on behalf of doctors, there is a presumptive undertaking, not only that the screening method is reliable, but that treatment is possible and will be made available to those who require it. And second, the large scale on which screening should be practiced makes it essential to ensure that it will make better use of limited resources than competing medical measures.

The implications of these requirements for screening procedures are reflected in the following list of principles for mass screening programs enumerated by Wilson and Jungner in 1968:

(1) The condition sought should be an important health problem.
(2) There should be an accepted treatment for patients with recognized disease.
(3) Facilities for diagnosis and treatment should be available.
(4) There should be a recognizable latent or early symptomatic stage.

(5) There should be a suitable test or examination.

(6) The test should be acceptable to the population.

(7) The natural history of the condition, including development from latent to declared disease, should be adequately understood.

(8) There should be an agreed policy on whom to treat as patients.

(9) The cost of case-finding (including diagnosis and treatment of patients diagnosed) should be economically balanced in relation to possible expenditure on medical care as a whole.

(10) Case-finding should be a continuing process and not a "once and for all" project.

It can be seen quite readily that screening programs for many conditions, particularly some of our major chronic disease problems, do not fulfill all of the principles set forth by Wilson and Jungner.

Facilities for diagnosis and treatment should be available. Many screening programs have had little effect because planning for them did not include adequate and effective mechanisms for follow-up of positives. This has been a major weakness of school health programs in this country.

The test should be acceptable to the population. Cancer of the rectosigmoid should lend itself to early detection, but overall acceptance of proctosigmoidoscopy has been poor. Thus, while this procedure continues to be used in clinical settings, it is generally not incorporated into programs for population screening.

The natural history of the condition, including development from latent to declared disease, should be adequately understood. Consider the case for screening for lung cancer, the leading cancer in men. There is only scant evidence (Brett, 1969) which indicates that the prognosis is improved even by semiannual screening with chest x-rays. After following over 6000 middle-aged men for ten years with semiannual chest x-rays, Boucot and Weiss (1973) concluded that the cost-benefit ratio of screening for lung cancer is high, that the cost per cure in Brett's study was about $83,000, and that further research on prevention of smoking "would do far more to solve the problem of lung cancer than semi-annual screening."

There should be an agreed policy on whom to treat as patients. For mild cases of diabetes mellitus this criterion is not satisfied.

Thus, although the *concept* of screening is widely accepted, the above limitations make the place of screening in the total spectrum of health care programming somewhat controversial. Differences of opinion arise from the assessment of its benefits and costs in relation to the costs and benefits of alternative programs.

The costs of screening should not be underestimated. Any substantial screening program imposes a heavy load on the medical care system. To the costs of the screening itself must be added the expenses related to medical investigation of the "positives" and long-term follow-up of those diagnosed as having disease. The diseases for which screening is carried out (tuberculosis, diabetes, hypertension, and glaucoma) require sustained supervision. Many patients require drug therapy over a period of years. The expenses and risks secondary to these medications must also be included in the ultimate costs of screening.

One organizational setting for medical care suitable for screening on a large scale is the health maintenance organization (or HMO), which has recently been promoted by the federal government. The prototype of the HMO may be found in large prepaid group health plans, such as Kaiser Permanente, HIP in New York City, and Group Health of America in Washington, D.C.

In this type of organization screening and periodic examination can be incorporated into a comprehensive program of health care for a defined group of people. The large number of persons enrolled in each unit, as well as current technologic advances, makes it economically feasible to perform many tests for a variety of disease conditions. The existence of advanced technology permits diagnostic accuracy to be high. On the other hand, the ease with which multiple tests can be performed may lead to the purposeless ordering of a large number of tests.

The concept of screening is being applied to children as well as adults. The federal government has mandated that all children (under age 21) who are eligible for care under Medical Assistance programs be offered a program known as Early and Periodic Screening, Diagnosis, and Treatment (EPSDT). The purpose is "to require states to take aggressive steps to screen, diagnose and treat children with health problems" (Medical Services Administration).

In suitable contexts the word "screening" can have an expanded and quite different meaning from earlier usage, in which it referred to testing for a single disease, often by an agency without responsibility or resources for adequate follow-up and continuing care. Further, this newer approach to screening is designed not merely to detect disease (secondary prevention) but also to identify persons at high risk. For example, elevated blood lipids, hypertension, and cigarette smoking are known to increase the risk of coronary heart disease. A large scale controlled trial, the Multiple Risk Factor Intervention Trial, is now underway to evaluate the effectiveness of active intervention for high risk individuals. If morbidity and mortality can be reduced, then identification of high risk persons by screening could contribute to true primary prevention.

CURRENT STATUS OF SCREENING FOR SPECIFIC DISEASES

Despite the controversies alluded to in the previous section, there are several diseases for which widespread screening either is well established or appears to be imminent. These will be discussed briefly.

Carcinoma of the Cervix

Screening for this condition goes back to the demonstration by Papanicolaou (1943) that cytologic screening of the cervix by examination of exfoliated cells from a vaginal smear can provide evidence of malignancy even before invasion has occurred. The concept of mass screening for cervical cancer by "Pap smear" is based on the assumptions, which are not entirely proven, that a high proportion of cancers detected *in situ* would progress to invasive cancer over time and, conversely, that most invasive cancers remain *in situ* long enough for screening at reasonable intervals to detect a high proportion of the potential cases of invasive neoplasia.

Since 1950 or so Pap screening has been performed on a large number of women through examination by private physicians and in organized public health programs. Mortality from this disease

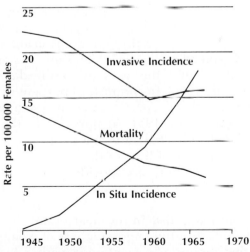

Figure 11–7 The changing status of cancer of the cervix. Cervical cancer incidence and mortality, New York State except New York City, 1945–1970. (From Christopherson, W. M.: The changing patterns of cervix cancer. CA, *21*:282, 1971.)

began to decline before screening programs could have had any impact. Since no controlled trial of the effects of mass screening on death rates was done, the extent of its contribution to the drop in mortality cannot be quantified. Nevertheless, the continuing decrease in mortality from the disease and the increase in the ratio of *in situ* to invasive cases (Figure 11–7) have encouraged continued application of this test as an effective preventive measure.

Unfortunately, the women at greatest risk of this disease tend to avail themselves of cervical cytologic screening less than others in the population. In a study of the utilization of cervical screening in Alameda County, California, Breslow and Hochstim (1964) found that utilization rates were relatively low among minority racial and ethnic groups and those low on the socioeconomic ladder.

Cancer of the Breast

As the leading cause of cancer deaths in women in this country, cancer of the breast presents a particular challenge. The mortality from this condition has varied little over the years. The essentially steady mortality rates are the net results of a slight rising trend in incidence coupled with a modest increase in survival.

Of course, primary prevention of this disease should be the ultimate goal, but until this is feasible it is desirable to detect and treat the disease early in its evolution. The main factor influencing prognosis in cancer of the breast appears to be stage at diagnosis. For those with localized disease, five-year survival is approximately 80 per cent. The survival figure drops to about 50 per cent once lymph node spread has occurred. Studies over the years have shown that less than half of the cases are localized at time of diagnosis (Mausner et al., 1969). In contrast, 70 per cent of the cases detected in women enrolled in special screening programs have been localized (Gershon-Cohen, 1961; Shapiro et al., 1971). The HIP study reported by Shapiro et al. indicates approximately a one-year lead time (i.e., shortening of time to diagnosis) as a result of their screening program. The study also provides some evidence that the ultimate prognosis of breast cancer can be improved by earlier detection.

It is therefore likely that in the near future there will be an increase in attempts to bring large numbers of women under surveillance for this disease. As mentioned earlier in the chapter, screening programs for breast cancer will probably combine tests in parallel, i.e., several modes of screening will probably be applied at the same visit. Mammography, although expensive, is well developed as a screening modality, and other approaches, such as thermography and xeroradiography, are also being explored as possible supplements to physical examination. Monthly self-examination of the breasts is an additional approach to detection of the disease.

Hypertension

Programs for detection of hypertension have been sparked by several developments. One was the identification of hypertension as a major risk factor in coronary heart disease and stroke, another the demonstration in the trials by the Veterans Administration Cooperative Study Group that treatment of hypertension could lower morbidity and mortality rates. These facts have particular significance against the background of studies which indicate that only half of the total number of persons with hypertension in technically advanced countries have been identified and that of the known hypertensives only one-quarter are receiving adequate therapy. In view of the greater prevalence of hypertension and the higher death rate from hypertensive cardiovascular disease in Blacks than in whites, control of hypertension among Blacks is a particularly urgent problem. Complicating the picture are factors relating to health behavior and inadequacies of the medical care system. These sets of factors interact to produce low levels of participation by inner city ghetto residents.

Mention has already been made (page 254) of the high costs of a public health program directed against hypertension which would include screening and treatment. Nevertheless, the effects of continued high blood pressure on the heart, brain, kidneys, and retina are so devastating that there is widespread interest in initiating such programs. Research now in progress should shed some light on the relative costs and benefits of this approach.*

Sickle Cell Disease

This disease raises interesting questions about nonmedical implications of screening programs. Sickle cell refers to red blood

---

*The discussion of hypertension refers to the usual type of hypertension, essential hypertension; as the word "essential" implies, this is a disease of unknown etiology. A small fraction of the total load of hypertension can be attributed to specific causes, such as a tumor of the adrenal gland or kidney disease. In any screening program some proportion of those found to have hypertension will need study to rule out hypertension of specific etiology.

TABLE 11-2 Conditions in Various Age Periods for Which Case-finding Is Now Done or Should Be Considered°

Prenatal and Pregnancy	Neonatal	Infancy and Preschool	Childhood
		Congenital	
Suspected hereditary disorders (amniocentesis)	Birth defects Inborn errors of metabolism (e.g., PKU, Tay-Sachs)		
		Developmental	
		Growth and development.................	
		Vision...	
		(especially strabismus)	(especially refractive errors, amblyopia)
		Speech, language, hearing	Speech and hearing
		Social and Behavioral	
		Social and mental development...........	
		Hematologic	
Rh factor		G-6-PD deficiency Hemoglobin disorders......................................	
Anemia			Anemia................
		Infectious and Parasitic	
Asymptomatic bacteriuria			Bacteriuria........... (females)
Syphilis Gonorrhea Rubella titer			
		Tuberculin sensitivity...................................... Parasitic infestation......................................	
		Metabolic and Other	
Diabetes mellitus			Diabetes..............
		Dental disease....................................	
Toxemia		Obesity	
		Lead poisoning (especially in inner city areas)	
		Neoplastic	

°Adapted from Wilson, J. M. G., and Jungner, G.: Principles and practice of screening for disease (Public Health Papers No. 34). WHO, Geneva, 1968 with the assistance of Dr. I. Renner, Maryland State Department of Health and Mental Hygiene.

TABLE 11–2 Conditions in Various Age Periods for Which Case-finding Is Now Done or Should Be Considered* (*Continued*)

Adolescence	Adulthood	Old Age
	(especially glaucoma)	(especially cataracts, macular degeneration, poor night vision)
	Hearing	
	Problem drinking	Unmet social and emotional needs
	(reproductive years only)	
Iron deficiency anemia .... (especially females)		
Syphilis		
Gonorrhea..		
.... Pulmonary	tuberculosis .... (high risk groups only)	
Hypertension		
	Hypercholesterolemia	
	Hyperlipidemia	
	Chronic respiratory disease (especially smokers)	
	Cancer (especially high risk groups)...................... skin cervix (pap smear) oral cavity (smokers) breast rectosigmoid	

cells which contain an abnormal form of hemoglobin (Hgb S). The gene is found primarily in Blacks, with a frequency of approximately 10 per cent. *Sickle cell trait* is said to exist when the Hgb S gene is inherited from only one parent. Roughly 1 per cent of marriages between Blacks occur between two carriers of the trait, and one-fourth of their offspring would have two SS genes (i.e., would be homozygous, and have *sickle cell disease*). The disadvantage of having sickle cell trait may be slight, although this needs further study. However, children with homozygous condition do very poorly. They are subject to painful crises; their growth may be impaired, their susceptibility to infection and bone infarct increased, and their life expectancy markedly shortened.

Interest in sickle cell disease in the late 1960's and subsequent passage by Congress in 1971 of a National Sickle Cell Anemia Control Act led to rapid expansion of research and the inauguration of large-scale screening programs. Widespread confusion about the difference between sickle cell disease and sickle cell trait became apparent. Identification of persons with hemoglobin S led to anxiety and a sense of stigma in Black communities. Children with sickle cell trait were kept from participating in school athletics; some adults were denied employment; some insurance companies increased premiums. It is obvious that better conceived programs of screening and counselling are needed.

Overview of Current Screening Practices

Table 11–2 summarizes, in terms of current knowledge, the major conditions for which case-finding is now done or should be considered in different age groups.

SUMMARY

In this chapter screening was presented as a form of secondary prevention. High validity, reliability, and yield, as well as feasibility and low cost, were outlined as characteristics desired in screening tests. Sensitivity and specificity were defined as aspects of validity. The particular obligations of physicians toward patients derived from the nature of prescriptive screening were stressed. Some of the major current problems associated with screening were outlined, including cost, lack of public acceptance, and inadequate follow-up of positives. These were presented as background for current controversy over the proper role of screening programs in the spectrum of health care services. The expanding potentialities for screening inherent in large, prepaid groups offering comprehensive care were also noted. Finally, the current status of screening for certain diseases was discussed briefly.

STUDY QUESTIONS

11–1 Define the following terms and give an example when appropriate:
Screening vs. diagnosis (page 239)
"Normal" values (page 240 ff.)
Validity (page 242)
Sensitivity (page 242)
Specificity (page 242)
False negative (page 244)
False positive (page 245)
Tests in series and in parallel (page 247)
Reliability (precision) (page 248)
Observer variation (page 248)
Yield (page 248)
Health behavior (page 249)
Multiphasic screening (page 250)
Predictive value (page 250)
Prescriptive screening (page 252)

11–2 A new screening test for a certain disease is being evaluated. The test was administered to 480 persons, 60 of whom are known to have the disease. This new test was found to be positive in 50 of the 60 people with the disease, as well as in 15 people who do not have the disease.

    A. Calculate the following values:
        (1) The sensitivity of the test
        (2) The specificity of the test
        (3) The percentage of false positives
        (4) The percentage of false negatives
        (5) The prevalence of disease
        (6) The predictive value of a positive test
        (7) The predictive value of a negative test
    B. Assume that sensitivity and specificity remained the same but that prevalence increased to 20 per cent. Now what would be the predictive value of a positive test?

Answer on page 355.

11-3 Two screening tests, A and B, are available for one disease. The sensitivity and specificity of each test are shown below

	Test A	Test B
Percentage Sensitivity	70	80
Percentage Specificity	95	90

    A. Which test produces the greater percentage of false negatives? Which the greater percentage of false positives?

    B. What general principle does this example illustrate?

Answer on page 356.

11-4 In the past few years, there has been interest in using ultrasound as a screening modality. Sigel et al. (1970) have compared Doppler ultrasound with clinical examination as a way of detecting venous disease of the lower extremities. Confirmation of deep vein occlusion has usually been done by venography (x-ray visualization of the veins after injection of radiopaque dye). For a few patients, confirmation is based on findings at surgery or autopsy.

    In a series of 140 patients, 248 extremities were tested both by clinical examination for tenderness and swelling and by Doppler ultrasound. The results were as follows:

	Occlusion Confirmed	Patency Confirmed
Doppler Ultrasound		
Positive	63	15
Negative	20	150
Total	83	165
Clinical Examination		
Positive	45	59
Negative	38	106
Total	83	165

    A. Calculate for both Doppler ultrasound and clinical examination: (1) sensitivity, and (2) specificity. Is either test superior to the other?

    To determine whether some combination of the two tests would increase the sensitivity of the testing procedure, we next examine the results of both tests for the 83 extremities in which occlusion was confirmed:

		Doppler Ultrasound		
		Positive	Negative	Total
Clinical	Positive	35	10	45
Examination	Negative	28	10	38
	Total	63	20	83

    B. What is the sensitivity of the testing procedure: (1) with the two tests in parallel, and (2) with the two tests in series? Which type of combination yields the greater sensitivity?

Answer on page 356.

REFERENCES

Boucot, K. R., and Weiss, W.: Is curable lung cancer detected by semiannual screening? J.A.M.A., 224:1361, 1973.

Breslow, L., and Hochstim, J. R.: Sociocultural aspects of cervical cytology in Alameda County, California. Public Health Rep., 79:107, 1964.

Brett, G. Z.: Earlier diagnosis and survival in lung cancer. Br. Med. J., 4:260, 1969.

Commission on Chronic Illness: Chronic Illness in the United States, Vol. 1. Commonwealth Fund, Harvard University Press, Cambridge, 1957, p. 45.

Edwards, P. Q., and Ogasawara, F. R.: Phasing out the child-centered TB program. National Tuberculosis and Resp. Dis. Assn. Bull., Nov., 1971, pp. 12–13.

Elveback, L. R.: How high is high? A proposed alternative to the normal range. Mayo Clin. Proc., 47:93, 1972.

Elveback, L. R., Guillier, C. L., et al.: Health, normality and the ghost of Gauss. J.A.M.A., 211:69, 1970.

Gershon-Cohen, J., Hermel, M. B., et al.: Detection of breast cancer by periodic X-ray examinations. J.A.M.A., 176:1114, 1961.

Hackett, T. P., Cassem, N. H., et al.: Patient delay in cancer. N. Engl. J. Med., 289:14, 1973.

Hochbaum, G. M.: Public participation in medical screening programs. USPHS Pub. No. 572, U.S. Govt. Printing Office, Washington, D.C., 1958.

Mausner, J. S., Shimkin, M. B., et al.: Cancer of the breast in Philadelphia hospitals, 1951–1964. Cancer, 23:260, 1969.

Medical Services Administration: Program Regulation Guide–21, Medical Assistance Manual, Part J, 70–20 Implementation. Social and Rehabilitation Service, Dept. of Health, Education, and Welfare, 1972.

Papanicolaou, G. N., and Traut, H. F.: Diagnosis of uterine cancer by the vaginal smear. The Commonwealth Fund, New York, 1943.

Screening in Medical Care: Reviewing the Evidence. A Collection of Essays. Nuffield Provincial Hospitals Trust, Oxford University Press, London, 1968.

Shapiro, S., Strax, P., et al.: Periodic breast cancer screening in reducing mortality from breast cancer. J.A.M.A., 215:1777, 1971.

Sigel, B., Popky, G. L., et al.: Evaluation of Doppler ultrasound examination. Arch. Surg., 100:535, 1970.

Strax, P., Venet, L., et al.: Breast cancer found on repetitive examination in mass screening. Arch. Environ. Health, 20:758, 1970.

Thorner, R. M., and Remein, Q. R.: Principles and procedures in the evaluation of screening for diseases. USPHS Pub. No. 846, U.S. Govt. Printing Office, Washington, D.C., 1961.

Vecchio, T. J.: Predictive value of a single diagnostic test in unselected populations. N. Engl. J. Med., 274:1171, 1966.

Wilson, J. M. G., and Jungner, F.: Principles and practice of screening for disease (Public Health Papers No. 34). WHO, Geneva, 1968.

EPIDEMIOLOGIC ASPECTS OF INFECTIOUS DISEASE

12

Despite the great scientific advances which have reduced morbidity and mortality from infectious diseases over the past decades, these conditions continue to account for a major proportion of acute illness, even in technically advanced countries. Current estimates put the toll from infectious disease in the United States at 145 million school-loss days and 130 million days lost from work, in addition to 140,000 deaths annually.

In this chapter we will expand upon some of the epidemiologic concepts related to infectious disease introduced previously (Chapter 2). We will outline host-parasite interactions, methods of transmission, and the investigation of an epidemic. We will also discuss current approaches to control of several infectious diseases of major concern in the United States today.

HOST-PARASITE RELATIONS

To prevent or control diseases in man due to an infectious agent, we must be able to answer questions about the cycle by which the organism maintains its existence in nature and the means by which it reaches man. What is the nature of the infectious agent? In what reservoirs does it normally reproduce and multiply? What are the conditions of temperature and humidity needed for its survival outside human or animal hosts? How does it spread from one host to another? What are the portals of entry and exit?

Infectious Agents

A wide variety of infectious agents, from the simplest viral particles to complex multicellular organisms, can produce disease in man. No discussion of infectious disease would be complete without specification of infectious agents as essential links in the chain of events resulting in infection in man. However, a detailed or comprehensive account of the various agents is beyond the scope of this text.

In Chapter 2 we introduced the concept of a spectrum of disease severity. We noted that infectious agents differ in their characteristic extent of severity. Two terms are frequently used to specify the gradient of severity: pathogenicity and virulence. *Pathogenicity* refers to the capacity of an agent to cause disease in an infected host. *Virulence* refers to the ability of an agent to produce serious illness; it refers to the proportion of cases which are severe. Figure 12–1 presents the diagrammatic classification of disease severity shown previously (Figure 2–1). Using this schema, we can define pathogenicity and virulence as follows:

$$\text{Pathogenicity} = \frac{\text{cases of disease}}{\text{total number infected}} = \frac{b+c+d+e}{a+b+c+d+e}$$

$$\text{Virulence} = \frac{\text{cases of severe and fatal disease}}{\text{all cases of disease}} = \frac{d+e}{b+c+d+e}$$

Referring to Figure 2–1 (page 23), we see that infections with Class A agents (e.g., tubercle bacillus, hepatitis A virus) are characterized by low pathogenicity and, usually, low virulence. Infections with Class B agents (viruses of measles and chickenpox) show high pathogenicity, but are relatively low in virulence in comparison with Class C infections (e.g., rabies), in which a fatal outcome is the general rule. Except for infections with very virulent organisms, host characteristics play a major role in determining the nature of an individual's reaction to infection.

Case fatality rate (defined on page 26) is closely related to virulence, but is a more restricted measure since it refers only to the proportion of cases of disease that are fatal, i.e., $\dfrac{e}{b+c+d+e}$.

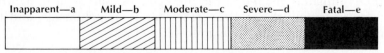

| Inapparent—a | Mild—b | Moderate—c | Severe—d | Fatal—e |

Figure 12–1   Classification of severity of infection.

TABLE 12–1 Spectrum of Pathogenetic Host-parasite Interactions*

Disease	Invasiveness	Intoxication	Hypersensitivity
Botulism	0	++++	0
Tetanus	+	++++	0
Diphtheria	++	++++	0
Staphylococcosis	+++	++	±
Pneumococcosis	++++	0	0
Streptococcosis	+++	++	++
Tuberculosis	+++	0	++++

*From Hoeprich, P. D. (ed.): Infectious Diseases: A Guide to the Understanding and Management of Infectious Processes. Harper & Row, Publishers, New York, 1972.

Several characteristics of infectious agents determine their ability to induce disease in man. These include the tendency to invade tissues, to produce toxins, and to cause damaging hypersensitive (allergic) reactions. Table 12–1 presents examples of several organisms which differ in the mechanisms by which they produce disease in man. Other aspects of organisms which also determine pathogenicity include their ability to withstand phagocytosis, to live intracellularly, and to produce endotoxin.

The ability of an agent to induce immunity in a host is known as *immunogenicity.* Organisms vary greatly in this characteristic. For example, it is possible to have repeated attacks of gonorrhea, whereas second attacks of measles are virtually unknown. More detailed discussion of the mechanisms by which specific infectious agents induce disease in man may be found in standard textbooks of microbiology.

Reservoirs

Reservoirs may be defined as the living organisms or inanimate matter (such as soil) in which an infectious agent normally lives and multiplies. Thus, the reservoirs of infection consist of human beings, animals, and environmental sources. The concept of the reservoir is central in infectious disease because the reservoir is an essential component of the cycle by which an infectious agent maintains and perpetuates itself. The specific reservoir for an agent is thus intimately related to the life cycle of that agent in nature.

In the simplest cycle the reservoir is man himself, and the cycle may be diagrammed as follows:

$$\text{Man} \longrightarrow \text{Man} \longrightarrow \text{Man}$$

This type of cycle is characteristic of most of the infectious diseases to which man is subject: most of the viral and bacterial respiratory diseases, most staphylococcal and streptococcal infections, diphtheria, venereal diseases, the childhood exanthemata, mumps, typhoid fever, amoebiasis, and many others.

In addition to the diseases which he acquires from other human beings, man is also subject to some diseases which he acquires from other species, such as bovine tuberculosis (from cows), brucellosis (from cows, pigs, and goats), anthrax (from sheep), leptospirosis (from rodents), and rabies (from dogs, bats, foxes, and other wild animals). These diseases are known as *zoonoses*, infections transmissible under natural conditions from vertebrate animals to man. In these diseases man is not an essential part (usual reservoir) of the life cycle of the agent. Thus:

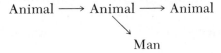

Certain other infectious diseases are characterized by more complex cycles. Features may include multiple reservoirs and different developmental stages of the agent. The cycle may involve an alternation of widely divergent host species. More complex cycles are illustrated by echinococcosis, tapeworm infestations, schistosomiasis, and malaria.

Man as Reservoir: Cases and Carriers. The section on pathogenicity and virulence was concerned primarily with characteristics of the agent. In this section the focus will be on man as a reservoir of infection.

Infection is said to have occurred if an infectious agent has entered and established itself in a host. A range of reactions to this occurrence is possible. At a minimal level, the agent may be present on the surface of the body and propagate at a rate sufficient to maintain its numbers without producing identifiable evidence of any reaction in the host. This phenomenon, which is referred to as *colonization*, is exemplified by the presence of *Staphylococcus aureus* on the nasal mucosa.*

At the next level is *inapparent infection* (covert or subclinical infection). In this type of relationship the organisms not only multiply in the host, but also cause a measurable reaction which, however, is not clinically detectable. When infection leads to clinical

---

*A related term is *contamination*. This refers to the presence on the surface of the body or on inanimate objects (fomites) of an infectious agent which can serve as a source of infection.

(overt) disease with symptoms, physical findings, or both, *infectious disease* is said to exist. Thus, infection encompasses (1) colonization, (2) inapparent infection, and (3) infectious disease. This range of interactions between host and parasite is indicated by the Venn Diagram in Figure 12–2.

All infected persons, including those with colonization only, are potential sources of infection to others. A *carrier* is an infected person who does not have apparent clinical disease, but is, nevertheless, a potential source of infection to others. The term "carrier" includes persons whose infection remains inapparent (asymptomatic) throughout, as well as those for whom the carrier state precedes or follows manifest disease (incubatory and convalescent carriers, respectively). When the carrier state persists for a long period of time, the person is referred to as a chronic carrier. Some examples of infectious agents which give rise to each of these types of carriers follow:

Type of Carrier	Examples
Inapparent throughout	Poliovirus, meningococcus, hepatitis viruses
Incubatory carrier	Viruses of chickenpox, measles, and hepatitis
Convalescent carrier	*C. diphtheriae,* hepatitis B virus, and Salmonella species
Chronic carrier	*S. typhosa,* hepatitis B virus

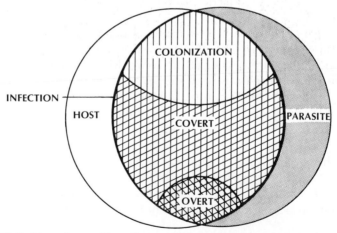

Figure 12–2 Venn diagram illustrating several types of host-parasite interaction. (Adapted from Hoeprich, P. D. (ed.): Infectious Diseases: A Guide to the Understanding and Management of Infectious Processes. Harper & Row, Publishers, New York, 1972, p. 40.)

A person with an inapparent infection is not necessarily a carrier. For example, most persons with positive tuberculin tests do not actively disseminate tubercle bacilli and, therefore, are not labelled carriers, even though they probably harbor tubercle bacilli.

MECHANISMS OF TRANSMISSION OF INFECTION

In discussing *transmission of infection*, we are concerned with the various mechanisms by which agents reach and infect the human host. This involves escape of the agent from a source or reservoir, conveyance to a susceptible host, and entry into that host. Transmission may be direct or indirect as shown in the following scheme:

Classification of the Mechanisms of Transmission

Direct transmission   Indirect transmission
                              Vehicleborne
                              Vectorborne
                              Airborne (droplet nuclei and dust)

Direct transmission consists of essentially immediate transfer of an infectious agent from an infected host or reservoir to an appropriate portal of entry. Note that this can involve not only direct contact, such as kissing and sexual intercourse, but also spray by *droplets* through sneezing and coughing onto the mucous membranes of others. Such droplet spread is classified as direct transmission because it occurs over short distances—the droplets travel only a few feet before falling to the ground. Direct transmission also includes exposure of susceptible tissues to fungal agents, bacterial spores, or other parasites (e.g., hookworm) lying in the soil or vegetation.

Indirect transmission may be vehicleborne, vectorborne, or airborne. *Vehicleborne* transmission is indirect contact through inanimate objects (fomites), such as bedding, toys, or surgical instruments, as well as contaminated food, water, and intravenously administered fluids. The agent may or may not multiply or develop in or on the vehicle before it is introduced into man.

In *vectorborne* transmission, the infectious agent is conveyed by an arthropod to a susceptible host. The arthropod may merely carry the agent mechanically, by soiling its feet or proboscis, in which case multiplication of the agent in the vector does not occur. The vector may also be truly biological if the agent multiplies in the arthropod before it is transmitted. In this case, there is an incubation period in the arthropod, known as the extrinsic incubation period, before the arthropod can become infective.

Finally, indirect transmission may be *airborne*. Two types of particles are implicated in this kind of spread—dusts and droplet nuclei. *Dusts* are particles of varying size which result from resuspension of particles which have settled on floors or bedding as well as particles blown from the soil by the wind. Coccidioidomycosis (San Joaquin Valley fever, page 64) is an example of a disease spread through airborne transmission of fungal spores.

Droplet nuclei are very tiny particles which represent the dried residue of droplets. They may be formed in several ways. One is from the evaporation of droplets which have been coughed or sneezed into the air. Droplet nuclei are also formed from aerosolization of infective materials in the course of laboratory procedures and of processes for rendering animals in slaughterhouses. Because of their small size, these droplet nuclei can remain suspended in the air for long periods of time, and are also capable of being inhaled and carried into the alveoli.

Figure 12–3 shows the relationship between particle size and retention within the alveolar spaces. Most particles over 5 microns

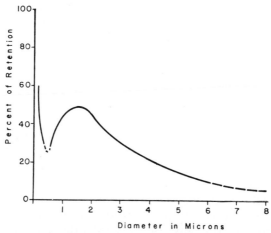

Figure 12–3 Retention of inhaled particles in the pulmonary spaces in relation to particle size. (From Langmuir, A. D.: Air-borne infection. In Sartwell, P. E. (ed.), Maxcy-Rosenau Preventive Medicine and Public Health, 9th ed. Appleton-Century-Crofts, New York, 1965, p. 422.)

in diameter do not reach the lungs because they are removed in the upper respiratory passages. As particle size decreases, more of the inhaled particles penetrate into the lungs and are retained there. When particles 1 to 2 microns in diameter are inhaled, approximately half are deposited in the lungs.

Airborne infection is important in a number of diseases. For example, coughing by a person with an open cavitary, tuberculous lesion can result in the formation of droplets which travel only a few feet and then either fall to the ground or are inhaled (direct contact). Because of their large size, these droplets, if inhaled, are promptly removed from the upper airways. However, as described above, some droplets form droplet nuclei which can be inhaled directly into the alveoli. Airborne spread from droplet nuclei is now considered to be the major mode of transmission of tuberculosis from person-to-person.

With a few exceptions, general acceptance of the importance of airborne spread has developed only recently. Interest in airborne disease has been stimulated since World War II by research on the pulmonary effects of particle size (see above), by experimental studies related to biological warfare, and by investigations of epidemics which could only be attributed to airborne transmission. Among these have been outbreaks of Q fever, histoplasmosis, and tuberculosis. For example, in one outbreak of Q fever in San Francisco Bay region, 75 cases of the disease occurred in an area approximately one-half to one mile wide and seven miles long, downwind from a rendering plant which processed sheep and goats. In addition, among laboratory personnel there have been outbreaks of Q fever, brucellosis, and psittacosis, which have clearly been airborne in origin. An important finding of these studies on airborne spread has been that with this mechanism **very small numbers of organisms** can induce infection.

The distinction between direct and indirect spread of respiratory secretions has been emphasized because of its importance to the control of disease. When disease is spread by direct transmission, control depends upon the proper handling of the source case. Reliance must be placed on treatment of the patient and on proper handling of secretions. Airborne spread of infection poses essentially an engineering problem. Measures such as adequate ventilation and proper air hygiene are needed to reduce the incidence of infection. For an historical perspective on airborne infection and on the controversies over the years between proponents of contact and airborne spread in respiratory diseases, the reader is referred to Langmuir (1965) and Riley and O'Grady (1961).

TYPES OF EPIDEMICS: COMMON SOURCE VS. PROPAGATED

We are now ready to apply the information about transmission of infectious agents to community patterns of disease occurrence. These mechanisms of spread account for the usual level of morbidity (endemic disease) as well as levels above those expected (i.e., epidemics). Two principal types of epidemics can be distinguished: (1) common source, and (2) propagated, or progressive. In general, these can be differentiated primarily be plotting the distribution of cases by time of onset (i.e., by determining the *epidemic curve.*

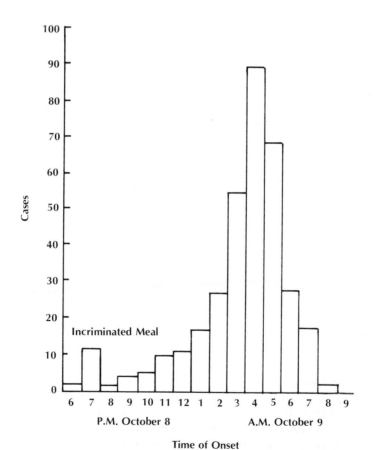

Time of Onset

Figure 12–4 Food intoxication at a military base in Texas, October 8–9, 1968. (From Morbidity and Mortality Weekly Report, CDC, USPHS, *18*:20, 1969.)

Common source epidemics are outbreaks due to exposure of a group of persons to a common, noxious influence. When the exposure is brief and essentially simultaneous (a *point or point source epidemic*), the resultant cases all develop within one incubation period of the disease. (See page 277 for further discussion of incubation period.) Figure 12–4 shows the times of onset of illness during an outbreak of food intoxication at a military base. The rapid rise and fall of the epidemic curve is compatible with a point (point source) epidemic. (This outbreak is discussed further in study question 12–5.)

Point source epidemics can also arise from common exposure to noninfectious agents, such as chemical poisons and polluted air. Figure 12–5 shows the relation between atmospheric pollution and deaths in London for the period which included the great fog of December, 1952. The figure also shows that shortly after the fog there was an epidemic of influenza, which also caused an excess number of deaths in comparison with the corresponding week of the previous year. This type of epidemic (propagated) will be discussed next.

Propagated or progressive epidemics result from transmission, either direct or indirect, of an infectious agent from one susceptible host to another. This can occur through direct person-to-person transmission or can involve more complex cycles in which the agent must pass through a vector to be transmitted from one human host to another, as in yellow fever and malaria. Figure 12–6A depicts the distribution of onsets of infectious hepatitis (hepatitis A) in an institution for the mentally retarded during an epidemic. Even though the incubation period of hepatitis A can be long, it does not generally exceed 50 days. Therefore, it is apparent that the epidemic extended over a number of incubation periods. The probable path of transmission among patient-employees, contacts, and ward groups is shown schematically in Figure 12–6B.

The upward trend at the onset of a propagated epidemic reflects an increasing number of cases in each successive time period. As a consequence, the increased probability that a susceptible will have contact with one or more cases more than offsets the decline in the number of susceptibles. However, eventually the number of susceptibles falls below a critical level and the number of cases declines.

It is clear from comparison of the point source epidemics (i.e., food intoxication and the London fog in Figures 12–4 and 12–5) with the propagated spread of influenza and hepatitis (shown in Figures 12–5 and 12–6) that the two types of epidemics show different temporal curves. Typically, the curve of onsets for a common

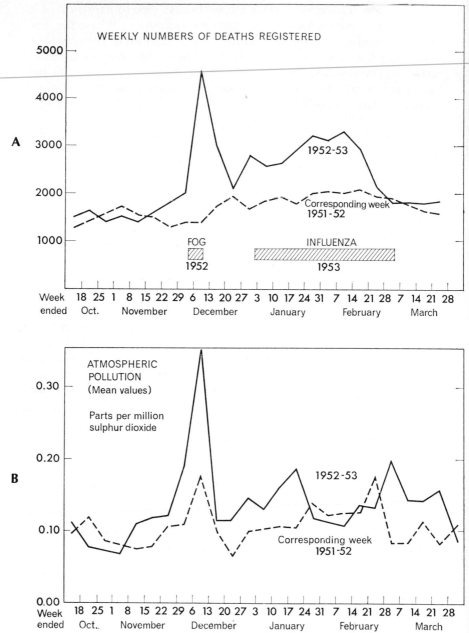

Figure 12–5 The great fog of December, 1952. Weekly numbers of deaths registered in Greater London (*A*) in relation to levels of air pollution, indicated by SO₂ (*B*). All causes of death; all ages, both sexes. Comparison of 1952 with ordinary year, 1951. Effects of the 1953 influenza epidemic are also shown. (From Morris, J. N.: Uses of epidemiology. Rep. Public Health Med. Subj. (Lond.), *95*:200, 1954; with permission of the Controller of Her Majesty's Stationery Office.)

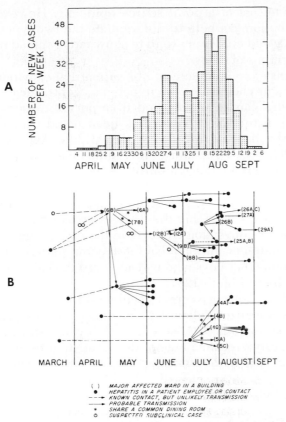

Figure 12–6 Epidemic of infectious hepatitis in an institution for the mentally retarded. A, Weekly clinical case rate. B, Schematic representation of possible hepatitis transmission. (From Matthew, E. B., Dietzman, D. E., et al.: A major epidemic of infectious hepatitis in an institution for the mentally retarded. Am. J. Epidemiol., 98:199, 1973.)

vehicle epidemic shows a rapid rise and fall within one incubation period whereas new cases in a propagated epidemic continue to develop beyond one incubation period. Sometimes it is possible to identify "generations" of cases. However, the variability in incubation periods often obscures such patterns.

It may be difficult to identify the nature of an epidemic from the shape of the epidemic curve alone. The typical point source curve may be affected by the development of secondary cases, by the continued contamination of the source, or by a long and variable incubation period. Conversely, propagated spread of a disease like influenza, which has a short incubation period and is highly infectious, can create a rapidly rising and rapidly falling epidemic curve similar to that of a point source epidemic. However, geographic distribution can help to differentiate the two types of epidemics; propagated epidemics tend to show radial spread with successive generations of cases.

The origins of an epidemic can be primarily behavioral rather than infectious or chemical. Like infectious agents, ideas and behavioral patterns can be transmitted from person to person. The communicable nature of behavior has been noted over the centuries, from the dancing manias of the Middle Ages to recent outbreaks of hysteria. Drug abuse, including cigarette smoking, is one of the most serious behavioral phenomena of our times. The development of cases is dependent not only on person-to-person transmission but also on group reinforcement. The rituals associated with the act of injecting the drug, or smoking the cigarette, are as important as physiologic effects in the early stages of initiation. The person-to-person spread of intravenous heroin use to boys in one town from other boys who had acquired the habit elsewhere is shown vividly in Figure 12–7.

The chain of events in a common vehicle epidemic is relatively simple to conceptualize. Following a common exposure, a proportion (not necessarily all) of those exposed develop an illness; the times of onset vary over the range of the incubation period for that condition. The forces determining the extent and course of a

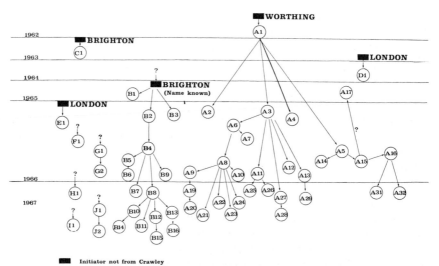

Figure 12–7 Pathways of spread of intravenous heroin use in Crawley New Town, 1967. (From de Alarcon, R.: The spread of heroin abuse in a community. Bull. Narc., 31:17, 1969.)

propagated epidemic are more complex. The rate of transmission of infection from one person to another depends upon a number of factors, especially the proportions of susceptible and immune persons in the population. A historical review of attempts to develop mathematical models of the course of propagated epidemics may be found in Serfling (1952).

SOME ASPECTS OF PERSON-TO-PERSON SPREAD OF DISEASE

We will next discuss three important aspects of person-to-person spread of disease: generation time, herd immunity, and secondary attack rates.

Generation Time

With person-to-person spread, the interval between cases is determined by the *generation time*, the period between the receipt of infection by a host and maximal communicability of that host (Sartwell and Price, 1965). In general, the generation time is roughly equivalent to the *incubation period*, the time interval between the receipt of infection and the onset of illness. However, the two terms are not identical. The time of maximal communicability may precede or follow the end of the incubation period. In mumps, for example, communicability appears to reach its height about 48 hours before the onset of swelling in the salivary glands. A further difference is that the term incubation period can only be applied to infections that result in manifest disease, whereas generation time refers to transmissions of infection, whether apparent or inapparent. Since infectious agents can be spread by persons with inapparent infection as well as clinically manifest cases, the concept of generation time is essential in studies of the dynamics of transmission of infection.

Herd Immunity

Herd immunity, the term used to express the immunity of a group or community, has been defined well by Fox (1970) as the "resistance of a group to invasion and spread of an infectious agent, based on the immunity of a high proportion of individual members of the group." We can illustrate this concept through an oversimplified diagram.

Figure 12–8 depicts two groups of people **before** and **after** an epidemic. Each group consists of Mr. Jones and two office mates, X and Y, with whom he has close contacts. Both coworkers also have close association with three other individuals. The two groups are the same except that in Figure 12–8A all individuals are susceptible to the illness, whereas in Figure 12–8B coworker X is immune. Let us assume that during the course of the epidemic Mr. Jones becomes ill, that the disease is highly contagious, and also that Mr. Jones' contacts have no other exposures.

Note that in Group A in which everyone is susceptible, all come down with the illness. In B only the contacts of Y become ill. Because of X's immunity, he does not transmit the infection from Mr. Jones to his three contacts. Thus, in Group A, Mr. Jones' illness led to eight other cases of disease. In Group B, his illness resulted in only four cases of disease even though only one of the other four

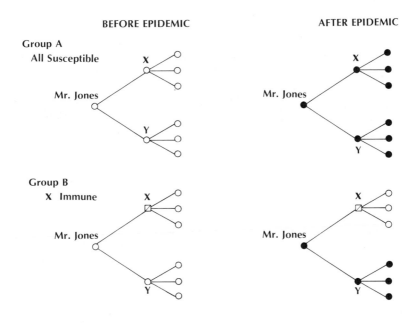

BEFORE EPIDEMIC   **AFTER EPIDEMIC**

Group A
All Susceptible

Group B
X Immune

○ Individual susceptible to the disease

☒ Individual not susceptible (previously has had the disease or has been immunized against it)

● Susceptible individual who develops the disease

Figure 12–8 Schematic illustration of herd immunity.

people was immune. By his immunity, X protected three other people against the disease.

Herd immunity is an important factor underlying the dynamics of propagated epidemics and the periodicity of diseases such as chickenpox and measles (prior to widespread use of vaccine). During the course of an epidemic a number of susceptible people come down with the disease, thus providing multiple sources of infection to others. However, since the cases develop immunity, as the epidemic progresses the proportion of nonsusceptibles in the population increases and the likelihood of effective contact between cases and remaining susceptibles declines. With the birth of additional babies or immigration of nonimmunized persons into the community, the number of susceptibles gradually increases enough to support a new wave of transmission.

This view of the dynamics of periodicity in measles was applied by Hedrich (1933). On the basis of reported cases, births, and deaths in children under age 15 he estimated the relation between number of susceptibles and monthly attack rates from measles over a 30-year period in Baltimore. A build-up in the estimated proportion of susceptibles precedes the peaks in case rates (Figure 12–9).

Another important consequence of herd immunity is that, in general, it is not necessary to achieve 100 per cent immunity in a population in order to halt an epidemic or control a disease. Just how far short of 100 per cent is safe is, of course, a crucial question. No definite answers can be given here, although it has been cus-

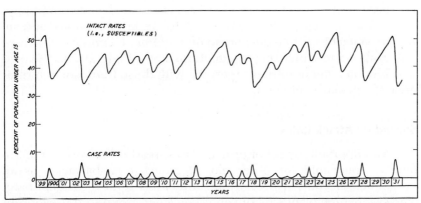

Figure 12–9 Estimated complete monthly attack rates from measles, and intact rates (proportions not previously attacked) for the population under age 15, Old Baltimore, Md., July, 1899–December, 1931. (From Hedrich, A. W.: Monthly estimates of the child population "susceptible" to measles, 1900–1931, Baltimore, Md. Am. J. Hyg. 17:626, 1933.)

tomary to cite 90 to 95 per cent for smallpox and a much lower figure (about 70 per cent) for diphtheria. However, studies of several outbreaks of diphtheria, including one which involved 196 persons in San Antonio, Texas, in 1970 (Marcuse and Grand, 1973), suggest that in densely settled areas immunization of the total population may be needed to prevent the occurrence of clinical diphtheria. Since immunized persons can harbor diphtheria organisms, they are a potential source of infection to the nonimmune portion of the population. Recent studies to evaluate the success of rubella immunization campaigns have shown that herd immunity does not operate well in prevention of rubella. Outbreaks have occurred even in populations in which 85 to 90 per cent have presumably been immune owing to natural infection or vaccination.

Another problem has been that an apparently satisfactory overall level of immunity of a population may obscure the existence of pockets of unimmunized persons. In this country, small outbreaks of poliomyelitis and diphtheria have occurred among such population subgroups. For example, in the 1970 outbreak of diphtheria in San Antonio, the 5- to 14-year olds had higher case rates than the 1- to 4-year olds, a reflection of the fact that a smaller proportion of the older children had been fully immunized.

Two situations are particularly conducive to the development of large-scale propagated epidemics. (1) A large epidemic can result from the introduction of infectious agents into populations which have never been exposed to the agent previously or from which the agent has been absent for many years (so-called virgin populations, see page 27). (2) Epidemics also occur following the introduction of a large number of susceptible persons into a closed community, such as a barracks, where crowded living arrangements and intimate contact facilitate the spread of infection. Examples of this are outbreaks of meningococcal infections and of adenovirus types 4 and 7 among young military recruits, with those from isolated rural areas particularly affected.

Secondary Attack Rates

An important aspect of propagated spread is the concept of the family, household, or other closed group (e.g., barracks) as an epidemiologic unit within which infections tend to disseminate. The case which brings a household or other group to the attention of public health personnel, is called the *index case*.* Spread within

---

*Investigation may reveal cases that antedate the index case. That is, the index case is not necessarily the first case in a family or group.

a group is measured through the *secondary attack rate.* This is defined as the number of cases of a disease developing during a stated time period among those members of a closed group who are at risk. That is:

Secondary attack rate =

$$\frac{\text{number of new cases in group minus the initial case or cases}}{\text{number of susceptible persons in the group minus the initial case or cases}} \text{ during specified time period}$$

The index case is excluded from both numerator and denominator as are *coprimaries,* cases which are related to the index case so closely in time that they are considered to belong to the same generation of cases.

Because members of a household have intimate contact with each other, much can be learned from intrahousehold spread. This value of the secondary attack rate is illustrated by study question 7–6 on tuberculosis in Bangalore which showed that the secondary at tack rate among susceptibles was higher in households with culture-positive than in those with culture-negative primary cases. Studies of intrafamilial spread also provide information on the type of family member who introduces the disease into the household. For respiratory Infections this is primarily the young school child.

OUTLINE OF THE INVESTIGATION OF AN EPIDEMIC

The investigation of an epidemic is an exciting exercise in medical detection. However, successful investigations require painstaking accumulation of information in the field ("shoeleather" epidemiology), and careful analysis of data, as well as flashes of insight. Therefore, we will present a systematic outline of the essential steps in the investigation of an outbreak even though some may seem self-evident. These steps are not necessarily accomplished in the order given and, in fact, the investigator usually sets in motion the activities needed for answering several questions simultaneously. However, *verification of the diagnosis* and *establishment of the existence of an epidemic* always deserve early attention when report of an apparent outbreak is received.

Preliminary Analysis

Verify the Diagnosis.   Do clinical and laboratory studies to confirm the diagnosis.

Always consider whether initial reports are correct. For example, an outbreak of jaundice initially diagnosed as "leptospirosis" (a spirochetal disease usually transmitted by water contaminated by the urine of infected animals) was found to be infectious hepatitis. The confirming tests indicated that one laboratory reagent was faulty. Investigation of a purported epidemic of "gonorrhea" among the girls in a grade school revealed a "phantom epidemic" based on rumors (Mausner and Gezon, 1967).

It is necessary to establish criteria for labelling persons as "cases." Depending on the type of problem being investigated, the classification will be based on symptoms, laboratory results, or both.

Verify the Existence of an Epidemic.   Attempt to compare the current incidence with past levels of the disease to determine whether an excessive number of cases have occurred.

Describe the Epidemic with Respect to Time, Place, Person.   Plot the cases by time of onset (epidemic curve).

Plot the cases by location (spot map).

Characterize persons by tabulating distribution of cases by age, sex, occupation, and other relevant attributes. The identification of "relevant" attributes may be a crucial step in the solution of the problem. For example, in the winter of 1960 to 1961 the New Jersey State Health Department became aware that an unexpectedly large proportion of the cases of hepatitis reported to them were occurring in adult males. This intelligence led eventually to identification of contaminated clams taken from Raritan Bay as the vehicle of spread for these cases (Dougherty and Altman, 1962).

Formulate and Test Hypotheses.   Identify type of epidemic—common source vs. propagated.

Using above descriptive characteristics to define the population which has been at highest risk of acquiring the disease, consider possible source or sources from which disease may have been contracted. Compare ill population (cases) with well population (controls) with regard to exposure to the postulated source. Carry out statistical tests to determine probable source. When appropriate, attempt to confirm epidemiologic findings by laboratory tests (samples of blood or feces, samples of suspect food, and so on).

Possible Further Investigation and Analysis

Search for Additional Cases.   Locate unrecognized or unreported cases by:

1. Canvass of physicians or hospitals or both in the area to determine if they have seen other patients who might have the disease under investigation.

2. Intensive investigation of asymptomatic persons or those with mild illness who may be contacts of cases. For example, in an investigation of an outbreak of hepatitis one might do liver function tests (e.g., serum transaminase levels) to search for cases of anicteric hepatitis (i.e., nonjaundiced), which ordinarily would not come to diagnosis.

Analyze the Data.   Assemble the results. Interpret findings.

Make a Decision about the Hypotheses Considered.   By the conclusion of the investigation all of the known facts should be consistent with one, and only one, hypothesis.

Report of the Investigation

At the termination of an investigation a report is usually prepared and submitted to the appropriate agency (or agencies). The report generally includes discussion of factors leading to the epidemic, evaluation of measures used for control, and recommendations for prevention of similar episodes in the future.

CENTRAL CONCEPTS UNDERLYING CONTROL OF INFECTIOUS DISEASE IN THE UNITED STATES TODAY

Many infectious diseases which are problems in other countries are of little concern in the United States. These differences are related partly to geography, but primarily to differences in levels of environmental hygiene and medical technology. A tropical climate can support parasites and vectorborne organisms not seen in more temperate areas. Enteric infections are a major problem in tropical areas, probably in great measure because of inadequate hygienic practices and sanitary protection.

In the United States the sharp decline in infectious diseases has necessitated ongoing evaluation and restructuring of control programs. (For examples, see pages 249 and 295 on control of tuberculosis and page 285 on vaccination against smallpox.) Traditional aspects of control have been supplemented by programs based on surveillance. Eradication has also been proposed as a realistic goal for several conditions. We will discuss some specific control measures first and then comment briefly on surveillance and eradication.

Specific Control Measures

These may be grouped as measures directed against the reservoir of the organism, those designed to interrupt transmission of infection, and those which reduce the susceptibility of the host.

Measures Directed Against the Reservoir.   The nature of the reservoir is of paramount importance in determining the appropriate methods of control and their likelihood of success. If the reservoir of infection is in domestic animals the problem can be approached through immunization, testing of herds, and destruction of infected animals. These procedures have been applied very successfully to brucellosis and bovine tuberculosis.

This approach is less applicable to wild animals, although experimental studies of methods of control are being conducted. Infection of wild animals with plague and rabies continues to pose a threat to domestic animals and human beings. Although for the last decade there has been an average of only one case of human rabies each year, some 20,000 persons receive postexposure prophylaxis annually.

When man is the reservoir, eradication of an infected host is not a viable option. However, in some circumstances it may be possible to remove the focus of infection (e.g., cholecystectomy in a chronic typhoid carrier). Related control measures include isolation of infected persons, treatment to render them noninfectious, and disinfection of contaminated objects.

Isolation is the separation of infected persons from those not infected for the period of communicability. While isolation is still an essential element in the control of certain diseases, there is decreasing reliance on this measure. It is futile to impose isolation if there is a large component of inapparent infection or if maximal infectivity precedes overt illness.

A control procedure closely related to isolation is quarantine. Classically, *quarantine* is the limitation of freedom of movement of apparently well persons or animals who have been exposed to a case of infectious disease. Quarantine is imposed for the duration of the usual maximal incubation period of the disease. Currently in the United States, even for the four diseases which are quarantinable by international agreement (cholera, plague, smallpox, and yellow fever), quarantine has been replaced by active *surveillance of individuals.* In such surveillance, close supervision is maintained over possible contacts of ill persons to detect infection or illness promptly; their freedom of movement is not restricted. For example, travelers from countries where there have been cases of a disease of serious concern may be required to remain in touch with their local health officer during the incubation period of the disease.

Measures Which Interrupt the Transmission of Organisms. Environmental measures to prevent transmission of disease by ingestion of contaminated vehicles include purification of water, pasteurization of milk, and inspection and other procedures designed to ensure a safe food supply. These public health measures, along with improvements in housing, nutrition, and other social conditions, are largely responsible for the great reduction in sickness and death due to infectious disease in developed countries during this century.

Attempts to reduce transmission of respiratory infection in classrooms in the 1930's by chemical disinfection of air and use of ultraviolet light gave generally disappointing results (Riley and O'Grady, 1961). Work on ventilation patterns, including unidirectional ("laminar") airflow to reduce the transmission of organisms in hospitals, is still in the process of development and evaluation (American Hospital Association, 1971).

Success in interrupting transmission of diseases whose cycle involves arthropods or alternative hosts or both has been variable. Schistosomiasis, a parasitic disease whose cycle includes snails, has no public health significance in the United States; it causes considerable debilitation and economic loss in other parts of the world. Unfortunately, in places irrigation to increase food production has also increased the prevalence of schistosomiasis. The construction of the Aswan High Dam in Egypt has provided a notable example of this particular dilemma. Other unsolved problems include the arthropod-borne viral encephalitides, such as eastern and western equine encephalitis, and various rickettsial diseases. Malaria will be discussed in conjunction with the concept of global eradication of disease.

Measures Which Reduce Host Susceptibility. Active immunization against diphtheria, tetanus, and pertussis has been a mainstay of public health practice for many decades. In the mid-1950's vaccine against poliomyelitis became available. More recently, vaccines against measles, mumps, and rubella have been added to the armamentarium. Most of these measures have been incorporated into routine pediatric practice. The immunization schedule recommended by the American Academy of Pediatrics (1974) is shown in Table 12–2. Other vaccines with more limited application include those against typhoid, typhus, and cholera for persons traveling abroad and immunizations against anthrax and rabies for persons occupationally exposed. Routine smallpox vaccination in childhood is no longer recommended in the United States, since the risk of complications from the vaccine now outweighs that of acquiring the disease (Karzon, 1972).

Annual nationwide immunization surveys provide an estimate of the overall level of immunization in the country and among subgroups of the population. Table 12–3 shows the lower levels of immunization against poliomyelitis, measles, diphtheria, tetanus,

TABLE 12–2 Recommended Schedule for Active Immunization of Normal Infants and Children[*]

2 months	DTP[1]	TOPV[2]
4 months	DTP	TOPV
6 months	DTP	TOPV
1 year	Measles[3]	Tuberculin Test[4]
	Rubella[3]	Mumps[3]
1½ years	DTP	TOPV
4–6 years	DTP	TOPV
14–16 years	Td[5] and thereafter every 10 years	

[*]Report of the Committee on Infectious Diseases, American Academy of Pediatrics, Evanston, Ill., 1974.

[1]DTP, Diptheria and tetanus toxoids combined with pertussis vaccine.

[2]TOPV, Trivalent oral poliovirus vaccine. This recommmendation is suitable for breast-fed as well as bottle-fed infants.

[3]May be given at 1 year as measles-rubella or measles-mumps-rubella combined vaccines.

[4]Frequency of repeated tuberculin tests depends on risk of exposure of the child and on the prevalence of tuberculosis in the population group. The initial test should be at the time of, or preceding, the measles immunization.

[5]Td, Combined tetanus and diphtheria toxoids (adult type) for those more than 6 years of age in contrast to diphtheria and tetanus (DT) which contains a larger amount of diphtheria antigen. *Tetanus toxoid at time of injury:* For clean, minor wounds, no booster dose is needed by a fully immunized child unless more than 10 years have elapsed since the last dose. For contaminated wounds, a booster dose should be given if more than 5 years have elapsed since the last dose.

and pertussis among preschool children from urban poverty areas than among all children of the same ages. Such differences have persisted over a number of years despite clinics where immunization is provided without cost. Laws in some states which require proof of immunization at time of school entry are helpful, but do not ensure that children will receive immunizations early enough to provide protection when it is needed most.

The prophylactic measures discussed so far are examples of *active immunization* in which either the altered organism or its product induces the host to produce antibodies. Protective antibodies produced by another host can also be introduced into a susceptible person, a procedure known as *passive immunization.* Passive immunization plays a role, albeit a somewhat lesser one than active immunization, in infectious disease control. The transfer of maternal antibodies to the fetus through the placenta is a form of passive immunization. Other examples of passive immunization include administration of immune serum globulin (ISG) for the prophylaxis of measles and infectious hepatitis (hepatitis A) and of tetanus antitoxin for unimmunized persons who receive penetrating wounds. (The latter should never be necessary as active immunization

TABLE 12-3 Percentage of Population, 1–4 Years of Age, Receiving Specified Vaccines; Total United States and Poverty Areas within Central Cities; SMSAs, with Population ≥250,000, 1971*

Vaccine	Total United States	Poverty Areas
Poliomyelitis (3+ OPV or 3+ IPV or both)	67.3	54.3
Measles	61.0	48.7
Rubella	51.2	52.0
Diphtheria-tetanus-pertussis (3+ doses)	78.7	58.4

*From United States Immunization Survey—1971 Public Health Service. U.S. Department of Health, Education, and Welfare, U.S. Govt. Printing Office, Washington, D.C., 1971.

against tetanus is far preferable.) Other substances available for passive immunization include antitoxin against *Clostridium botulinum* and antiserum against rabies following animal bites. Another prophylactic measure is the use of antibiotics for known contacts of cases—for example, in tuberculosis, gonorrhea, and syphilis.

Surveillance of Disease

Surveillance of disease is "the continuing scrutiny of all aspects of occurrence and spread of disease that are pertinent to effective control" (Benenson, 1970). The steps essential to this ongoing activity include collection, collation, and analysis of relevant data, followed by regular dissemination of reports to those responsible for disease control.

Nationwide surveillance is accomplished through cooperative arrangements between the Center for Disease Control and state health departments. Since 1952, when surveillance for malaria was initiated, an increasing number of diseases have been placed under surveillance. Techniques for surveillance vary for different diseases, ranging from routine morbidity and mortality reports to technically advanced laboratory and field investigations. Surveillance programs have provided invaluable information on the magnitude and etiologic factors of the diseases studied. This information serves as a data base for early identification of epidemics and for planning immunization campaigns and other activities necessary for the control of disease.

Eradication of Disease

The concept of *eradication of a disease*, i.e., total elimination of that disease worldwide, was considered visionary a few decades ago, but is now potentially attainable for at least two diseases. Under the leadership of the World Health Organization, major campaigns are now under way to eradicate smallpox and malaria.

The decision to make an all-out effort to eradicate smallpox was taken in the mid-1960's. Factors leading to this decision included the continual danger of importations from endemic to disease-free areas, the complications from vaccination itself, and the fact that man is the only known reservoir. Since then, substantial successes have been achieved. Figure 12–10 shows the general decline in reported incidence of smallpox between 1967 and 1971 (dark line), as contrasted with the expected values based on the average figures for the preceding five years (shaded area).

Eradication efforts have been aided by international cooperation, by the availability of lyophilized heat-stable vaccine, and by active surveillance measures; but they have been impeded by national and local conflicts and economic instability. In 1973, despite intensified case-finding, cases of smallpox were reported from only

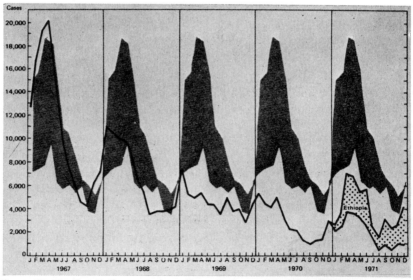

Figure 12–10 Reported cases of smallpox in the world, 1967–1971. The gray area represents the range of incidence during the five-year period 1962–1966. The cases from Ethiopia represent improved case finding and reporting. (From Karzon, D. T.: Smallpox vaccination in the United States. The end of an era. J. Pediatr., *81*:600, 1972.)

11 countries, in contrast with the 43 countries that recorded cases in 1967. Currently smallpox is considered endemic in only four countries—Bangladesh, India, Pakistan, and Ethiopia.

Malaria has now been eradicated from large areas of the world, largely owing to spraying of dwellings with insecticides. In several areas, however, advanced control efforts have met with setbacks because of the emergence of insecticide-resistant strains of Anopheles mosquitoes and of drug-resistant Plasmodium. Once importation occurs, the potential exists in the United States for the spread of malaria by indigenous vectors and by parenteral transmission through shared needles and syringes.

The prospect of eradication of diseases, such as rabies, plague, and other zoonoses, which involve an extensive reservoir among nondomestic animals, appears more remote.

CURRENT STATUS OF SPECIFIC INFECTIOUS DISEASE PROBLEMS IN THE UNITED STATES

Despite an overall decline in incidence and mortality from infectious diseases in the United States, certain infectious diseases continue to pose serious health problems. A few of the most important are discussed briefly: venereal disease, viral hepatitis, influenza, tuberculosis, foodborne disease, and nosocomial infections.

Venereal Disease

It is appropriate to discuss the venereal diseases first, since gonorrhea is currently the most frequently reported communicable disease in the nation. During 1972, more than 700,000 cases were reported. The reported cases represent only a small fraction of the actual occurrences. It is estimated that there were actually more than 2.5 million cases.

Of the several diseases transmitted sexually, the most commonly reported are syphilis and gonorrhea. The reported incidence of these two diseases has varied widely over the past three decades (Figure 12–11). From 1941 to 1947, a period which spanned the years of World War II and those immediately following, there was an increase in cases of gonorrhea and a smaller increase for syphilis. From 1948 to 1957, both diseases declined, especially early syphilis. Finally, since 1957, there has been a relentless increase in the reported incidence of gonorrhea, with a less consistent pattern for syphilis.

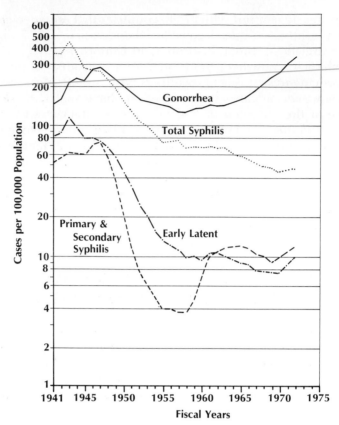

Figure 12–11 Reported cases of syphilis and gonorrhea per 100,000 population, United States, 1941–1972. (From VD Fact Sheet, 1972 (29th ed.), USPHS, U.S. Dept. of Health, Education, and Welfare Pub. No. 73-8195, U.S. Govt. Printing Office, Washington, D.C., 1973.)

The major cause of the decline in infectious syphilis between 1948 and 1957 was the introduction and widespread use of penicillin. Initially limited to military patients, the drug soon became available to civilians. Its introduction revolutionized the medical management of venereal diseases. There was a great reduction in the length of time and number of sessions required to treat syphilis.

With this newfound ability to manage patients effectively, private physicians began to treat more venereal disease patients; few of them received care in public clinics. However, although private physicians saw more patients, they reported a much smaller proportion. This, coupled with the fact that penicillin used for many other conditions masked symptoms of syphilis but did not cure it, led to a deceptive decline in reported incidence of syphilis during the 1950's.

Unfortunately, the reported decrease in cases, which was partly real but largely artifactual, led to a reduction in funding for venereal disease control programs in the misguided hope that these diseases would inevitably disappear. This was a sad error. The rates soon began to rise and have continued to soar. Gonorrhea, in particular, is now a disease completely out of control.

Societal changes during the 1960's quite likely contributed significantly to an increased incidence of venereal disease. During this period, there was a social revolution in value systems and in modes of sexual and other behavior. Unquestionably, these changes were supported by the development of effective contraceptives which removed the fear of pregnancy as a deterrent to sexual relations. The ready availability of abortion in some areas of the country has probably had a similar effect. In addition, reliance on oral contraceptives caused a decrease in the use of condoms which provide some protection against infection.

Certain features of gonorrhea make its control especially difficult. Among these are: the short incubation period, the lack of a highly sensitive and specific serologic test to detect current infection, the large proportion of infections in both women and men (Handsfield et al., 1974) which are asymptomatic, the increased resistance of the organism to penicillin, and the fact that infection does not confer immunity. While the control of syphilis is greatly aided by the existence of well-established serologic tests, certain features of this disease also pose problems for control; serology does not become positive during the incubation period and the early stage of primary infection, and the lesions in females are often unrecognized. Nevertheless, the advent of penicillin, public attention to syphilis, and systematic investigation of contacts have created some control over this disease. In particular, there has been a decrease in the number of late manifestations (Figure 12–11), including admissions to mental hospitals for general paresis and infant deaths from syphilis.

Aggressive attempts to control gonorrhea are more recent. Many institutions and physicians now screen for gonorrhea in women by taking cultures routinely in conjunction with pelvic examinations. A major advance in many states has been the passage of legislation which permits examination and treatment of minors without parental permission. Since rates of both gonorrhea and syphilis are high in teenagers, this is an important contribution to control. Intensive, continuing education programs in schools are being fostered. Research directed toward enhancing control of both diseases is proceeding on several fronts. Attempts are being made to develop a serologic test for syphilis that would be positive earlier in the course of infection. For gonorrhea, attempts are being made to develop a vaccine, to improve screening tests, and to develop methods of case finding with a high yield.

Viral Hepatitis

Like venereal disease, hepatitis is a condition whose incidence mirrors social and behavioral factors. Currently, viral hepatitis is one of our major health problems. Recent statistics show over 60,000 reported cases (1972) and over 1000 deaths from this disease (1969).

These statistics refer to two disease entities. One, known as infectious hepatitis or hepatitis A, is a usually mild disease of acute onset and relatively short incubation period (15 to 50 days), with an almost negligible case fatality rate. Serum hepatitis, or hepatitis B, has a longer incubation period (60 to 180 days or more), a more insidious onset, and a higher case fatality rate. Both hepatitis A and B can spread by a variety of mechanisms. However, hepatitis A is spread mostly by the fecal-oral route, whereas hepatitis B is spread mainly by parenteral introduction of blood or contaminated needles. Since the discovery of an antigen associated with hepatitis B, considerable advances have been made in epidemiologic knowledge about hepatitis.

Figure 12–12 shows the numbers of reported cases of hepatitis per 100,000 population from 1952 to 1972. Two years, 1954 and 1961, stand out as years of epidemic occurrence. The fact that mortality remained relatively constant during these years of fluctuating morbidity suggests that, at least until 1966, the amount of hepatitis B was relatively constant. The fluctuations in incidence of viral hepatitis were due to variations in the incidence of hepatitis A.

Since 1966 there has been a distinct change in the epidemiologic features of reported hepatitis (Garibaldi et al., 1972). This includes dampening of seasonal fluctuations, shift in age of highest incidence from 5 to 14-year olds to 15- to 24-year olds, a predominance of male cases (instead of the former 1 to 1 sex ratio), a shift from rural to urban concentration of cases, and regional trends paralleling the pattern of illicit drug use. This apparent increase in the proportion of hepatitis which is transmitted parenterally is consistent with other evidence of widespread parenteral drug use among young adults.

Clearly, a problem of this nature requires different approaches to control than those which would be appropriate for a disease

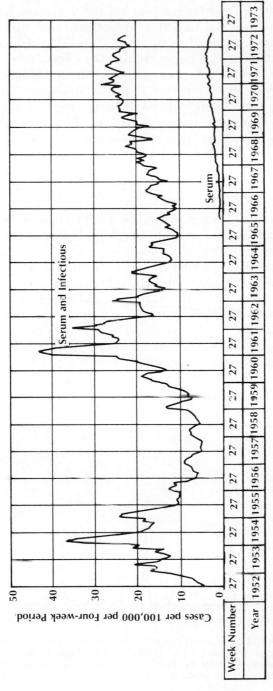

Figure 12–12 Reported cases of viral hepatitis, case rate by four-week periods since July, 1952 United States. (From Hepatitis Surveillance Report No. 36, CDC, USPHS, U.S. Govt. Printing Office, Washington, D.C., 1973.)

being spread primarily by contact or by ingestion of contaminated food or water. Of particular concern are the many anicteric cases and chronic carriers of hepatitis B antigen and the multiple methods of transmission of both viruses. Blood and blood products continue to transmit hepatitis despite efforts to detect and exclude carriers among potential donors by detailed history-taking and by laboratory screening for hepatitis B antigen. A related problem concerns occupational risks of acquiring and transmitting hepatitis virus, especially among persons working in renal dialysis units, but also among dentists, surgeons, and those performing related tasks.

Influenza

Influenza remains a serious public health problem because of the ability of influenza virus to undergo periodic antigenic shifts. Surveillance programs on local, national, and international levels monitor the activity of influenza virus and the presence of new strains. Despite the ability to predict, at least on a short-term basis, the extent of influenza activity, morbidity and mortality from influenza have continued largely unchecked. Influenza is today the one infectious disease in the United States which has a discernible impact on death rates. Fluctuations in excess mortality from pneumonia-influenza, over the 12-year period of 1957 to 1969, are shown in Figure 12–13. Each peak in mortality was associated with a

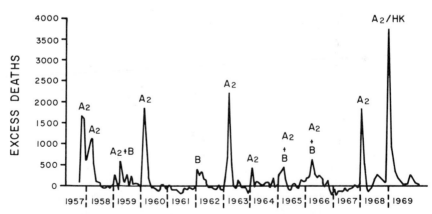

Figure 12–13 Reported excess mortality from pneumonia due to influenza, by four-week intervals, 122 cities, United States, 1957–1969. Influenza viruses known to be active at those times also are shown. (From Eickhoff, T. C.: Immunization against influenza: Rationale and recommendations. J. Infect. Dis., *123*:446, 1971.)

period of influenza activity, with the larger peaks related to influenza A outbreaks. (See also Figure 4–9).

Currently, control of influenza is based on surveillance of illness and absenteeism, on attempts to develop vaccines that will keep pace with antigenic shifts in the virus, and on immunization. The current rationale for immunization is based on studies of mortality since the first outbreak of Asian flu (influenza A_2) in 1957 (Figure 12–13). Eickhoff et al. (1961) estimated that between 1957 and 1960, 86,000 deaths above the expected number occurred in the United States in association with influenza. Analysis of these deaths, as well as deaths during subsequent outbreaks, led to identification of certain groups as being at high risk of death from influenza: elderly persons and those with chronic disease, particularly cardiovascular-renal and bronchopulmonary disease and metabolic conditions, such as diabetes mellitus. It is recommended that such persons receive annual immunization, even in years when large outbreaks are not anticipated. To date, annual immunization of the total population has not been advised because protection has been of variable effectiveness and short duration. The 1973 to 1974 epidemic of influenza B among young persons associated with a rare, highly fatal sequela (Reye's syndrome) has led to renewed efforts to develop a long-acting vaccine for general use.

Tuberculosis

Morbidity and mortality from tuberculosis have decreased remarkably over the past century. This decrease antedated any specific measures for prevention or cure of this disease. With the advent of chemotherapy, the decline accelerated, especially with regard to mortality.

Nevertheless, tuberculosis remains an important problem in the United States. The infected persons, estimated to number approximately 16 million, are a potential source of active disease and spread of infection to others with close or prolonged exposure. More than 90 per cent of all new cases apparently represent endogenous activation of dormant foci in previously infected persons. Tuberculosis rates are therefore highest in certain socioeconomic segments of the community in which the tuberculin-positive reactor rates are relatively high, such as immigrants, Blacks, American Indians, and inhabitants of slums, jails, and skid row areas.

Antimicrobial drugs are now the mainstay of tuberculosis control. The highest priority in tuberculosis control is given to prompt treatment of newly diagnosed, sputum-positive cases, as well as investigation of their contacts.

The availability of specific antimicrobial drugs has changed the nature of treatment dramatically. Because drug therapy eliminates infectivity rapidly, prolonged hospitalization in a tuberculosis sanatorium is no longer necessary. Initial treatment in a general hospital may be needed for an acutely ill patient or one with complicating medical problems. Most patients are treated entirely on an ambulatory basis in outpatient clinics or physicians' offices. The location of treatment is not important; the critical issue is that adequate treatment be given. Lapses from treatment, especially among groups such as alcoholics, create a serious problem of relapse with drug-resistant organisms. Patients who have received adequate chemotherapy can be regarded as cured and are discharged with instructions to return if they develop symptoms that could be due to tuberculosis.

Antimicrobial drugs have not only revolutionized the treatment of tuberculosis, but have also been proved effective in preventing disease in infected persons. Preventive therapy with isoniazid (INH) is now recommended for all recently infected persons (tuberculin converters) and close contacts of newly diagnosed cases, as well as certain other groups of positive reactors at high risk of developing disease: those with abnormal chest x-ray findings, persons under the age of 35, and those with specified clinical conditions (e.g., steroid treatment). INH is also recommended for persons with a previous history of tuberculosis who did not complete a full course of adequate chemotherapy.

A possible alternative to drug prophylaxis is vaccination with BCG, an attenuated strain of bovine tubercle bacillus developed by Calmette and Guérin. Such vaccination, although widely used in some countries, is not recommended in the United States except in specified circumstances. Because the risk of infection has become so low, the conversion of the tuberculin reaction following BCG vaccination is an important disadvantage, since it interferes with the ability of the test to give evidence of virulent (natural) infection.

Foodborne Disease

Foodborne disease is generally defined as illness caused by ingestion of food contaminated by a pathogenic organism or noxious agent, such as a toxin or chemical. A foodborne outbreak is such an illness occurring in two or more persons; however, single cases of botulism, trichinosis, or chemical poisoning are also handled as epidemics.

Over the past three decades reported outbreaks of waterborne and milkborne disease have declined in number. In contrast, reported morbidity from foodborne disease has remained at a relatively high and constant level (Figure 12–14). In 1971, 320 foodborne disease outbreaks affecting 13,000 individuals were reported in the United States. Intensive surveillance in one state (Barker et al., 1974) suggests that the true number of outbreaks is at least ten times as great.

The relative contributions of various etiologic agents to these

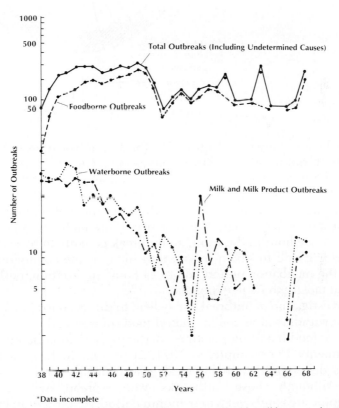

*Data incomplete

Figure 12–14 Foodborne disease outbreaks, compared with milkborne and waterborne disease outbreaks, United States, 1938–1968. (From Bryan, F. L.: Guide for Investigating Foodborne Disease Outbreaks and Analyzing Surveillance Data, Center for Disease Control Training Program. U.S. Dept. of Health, Education, and Welfare, Atlanta, 1973, p. 63.)

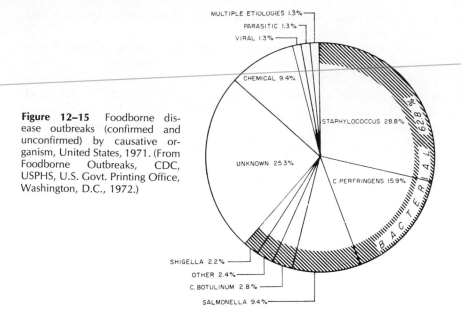

Figure 12–15 Foodborne disease outbreaks (confirmed and unconfirmed) by causative organism, United States, 1971. (From Foodborne Outbreaks, CDC, USPHS, U.S. Govt. Printing Office, Washington, D.C., 1972.)

outbreaks are shown in Figure 12–15. The majority of outbreaks were bacterial in origin, with staphylococci, *Clostridium perfringens,* and Salmonella species the most frequently identified organisms. One-quarter of the outbreaks were never traced to a specific etiologic agent. However, the length of the incubation period can provide a clue to etiology. For instance, if the incubation period is less than one hour in duration, an outbreak is likely to be chemical in origin; if one to seven hours, it is likely to be staphylococcal. When the incubation period is 8 to 14 hours in duration, outbreaks are due mostly to *C. perfringens.*

Investigation of outbreaks may lead to direct control measures, such as withdrawal of contaminated food sources and correction of improper food-handling practices, particularly in food-handling establishments. For example, in 1971, 21 persons in 12 separate incidents developed staphylococcal gastroenteritis after eating salami. Although these outbreaks were spread over a wide geographic area and over a four-month period, investigation incriminated a salami distributed nationally by two companies. When products from both companies were found to contain staphylococcal enterotoxin, they were recalled. Production was stopped until recommended changes were instituted.

Epidemiologic investigations, including environmental surveys, may also contribute to knowledge of disease etiology. When it was learned that a great deal of foodborne disease in Japan was due to *Vibrio parahemolyticus,* this organism was sought as an etiologic agent elsewhere. It has since been recovered from virtually all coastal waters in the United States. In addition, since 1971, several outbreaks due to seafood contaminated by this organism have been reported. Increased surveillance has established that *V. parahemolyticus* infection is indeed a problem in the United States. This, in turn, has led to further knowledge about reservoirs, sources, transmission patterns, and pathogenicity of this organism (Barker, 1974).

Hospital-acquired (Nosocomial) Infections

The final problem to be discussed, that of hospital-acquired or *nosocomial* infections, has come to the fore just recently. It has become apparent that the hospital constitutes an ecologic unit different from the general community, with a number of factors contributing to a high risk of infection. It has been estimated that as many as 5 to 10 per cent of patients admitted to general hospitals acquire infections while in the hospital (Cluff and Johnson, 1972).

Host, as well as environmental, factors play an important role in nosocomial infection. Patients with conditions such as lymphoma, multiple myeloma, diabetic ketoacidosis, uremia, and ascites or extensive burns have diminished resistance to infection. Immunosuppressive therapy contributes to the risk of bacteremia.

Because of impaired host resistance, many nosocomial infections are caused by organisms which are not usually pathogenic. Systemic fungi, cytomegalic inclusion virus, and *Pneumocystis carinii* are among the so-called *opportunistic* organisms, i.e., organisms which are generally saprophytic or commensal, but which can be pathogenic.

In the hospital, sick persons are exposed to a great many reservoirs of infection. Nearby patients may shed pathogenic bacteria from draining wounds or desquamating skin lesions. Staff members may be carriers. In addition, the widespread use of antibiotics favors the development of resistant organisms. The acquisition of transfer factor (R factor) by gram-negative bacteria is a particularly serious problem (Damato et al., 1974).

Invasive procedures, such as intravenous therapy, tracheostomy, and extensive surgery, also favor the development of infections. These activities bring tissues into direct contact with supposedly sterile fluids, catheters, and other devices. These may be maintained in place for days at a time, with increasing risk of infection. At times these materials have been contaminated even before use. Several deaths have been traced to contaminated intravenous fluids.

There are several mechanisms by which infectious organisms are transmitted to hospitalized patients. One important mode of transmission is transfer by the hands of personnel. This has been implicated in staphylococcal outbreaks in newborn nurseries and enteric infections occurring in institutions for the chronically ill and aged. In-service educational programs on the necessity for observance of handwashing and other precautions have been started in many institutions.

Another route of spread is provided by respiratory equipment. Reservoirs of water in humidifiers can support the presence of organisms such as Pseudomonas and Serratia, necessitating careful surveillance and frequent sterilization of equipment. Airborne transmission of disease is also of concern. Attempts at control include the substitution of single and double rooms for large wards and improvement in ventilation systems.

Urinary tract infections, by-products of indwelling catheters, instrumentation, and surgery account for a large proportion of nosocomial disease. Although the closed drainage systems now used represent an advance over open drainage, they still permit the development of infection.

Still another risk to hospitalized patients is hepatitis. Despite improved methods for detecting the antigen of hepatitis B virus, the use of blood from commercial sources and the prevalence of anicteric carriers in the general population contribute to a substantial risk of post-transfusion hepatitis.

An active infections committee and a capable nurse-epidemiologist are essential to the control of nosocomial infection. For excellent discussions of this general topic, the reader is referred to the American Hospital Association (1971) and to Alexander (1973).

SUMMARY

This chapter focussed on the epidemiology and control of infectious disease. Several dimensions of host-parasite interactions were examined, including characteristics of the infectious agent (i.e., pathogenicity, virulence, and immunogenicity) and the range of reactions to infection (i.e., colonization, inapparent infection, and overt disease). Any of these reactions can create an infected host capable of acting as a source of infection to others.

Mechanisms of spread of infection were classified as direct or indirect. Direct spread occurs through direct contact and respiratory droplets. Mechanisms of indirect transmission include fomites and other vehicles, arthropod vectors, and airborne spread through dusts and droplet nuclei. The importance of airborne droplet nuclei in the spread of tuberculosis and certain other diseases has received increasing acceptance in recent years.

The difference between spread by a common vehicle (common source) and propagated spread (person-to-person) was discussed. Generation time, herd immunity, and infection of members of a closed group by an index case (secondary attack) are features of propagated spread.

A formal outline for the investigation of an epidemic was presented. Verification that an epidemic exists, confirmation of diagnosis, and orientation as to time, place, and person were emphasized.

Specific control measures were classified as those designed to eliminate the organism, those which interrupt the transmission of infection, and those which reduce susceptibility of the host. The newer concepts of surveillance of disease and eradication were discussed in relation to current levels of infectious disease in the United States and to conditions affecting control of disease worldwide.

Finally, we reviewed several diseases of major public health importance in the United States today. These were venereal disease, viral hepatitis, influenza, tuberculosis, foodborne disease, and nosocomial infections.

STUDY QUESTIONS

12–1 Define the following terms and give an example when appropriate:

Pathogenicity (page 265)	Colonization (page 267)
Virulence (page 265)	Inapparent infection (page 267)
Immunogenicity (page 266)	Infectious disease (page 268)
Reservoir (page 266)	Carrier (page 268)
Zoonosis (page 267)	Transmission of infection—
Infection (page 267)	direct, indirect (page 269)

Droplets (page 269)
Vchicleborne transmission (page 269)
Vectorborne transmission (page 269)
Airborne transmission (page 270)
Dusts (page 270)
Droplet nuclei (page 270)
Epidemic curve (page 272)
Common source epidemic (page 273)
Point source epidemic (page 273)
Propagated (progressive) epidemic
   (page 273)
Generation time (page 277)
Incubation period (page 277)
Herd immunity (page 277)

Index case (page 280)
Secondary attack rate (page 281)
Coprimary case (page 281)
Isolation (page 284)
Quarantine (page 284)
Surveillance of individuals
   (page 284)
Active immunization (page 286)
Passive immunization (page 286)
Surveillance of disease (page 287)
Eradication of disease (page 288)
Foodborne outbreak (page 296)
Nosocomial infection (page 299)
Opportunistic organisms (page 299)

12–2 An outbreak of measles occurred in an elementary school with an enrollment of 300 pupils. During October and November, 72 of the pupils in this school were absent with measles.

  A. Compute the attack rate for October and November.

  The 72 pupils with measles had a total of 92 brothers and sisters living at home. Of these siblings, 20 subsequently developed measles during the period, October through December.

  B. Compute the secondary attack rate among the siblings.

  During the first week of November (November 1 to 5) 15 new cases developed in the school. Eight of these cases developed on Monday, November 1. During October, there had been 25 cases, of which 12 were still active on November 1.

  C. Bearing in mind that persons with known histories of measles are no longer at risk of the disease, calculate the following rates per 100: (1) incidence rate for the period November 1 to 5, (2) period prevalence rate for the period November 1 to 5, and (3) point prevalence on November 1.

  There were 35 pupils in the sixth grade of the school. Ten of these pupils were absent with measles during the October and November measles outbreak. These cases all had their onsets in October as follows: first week, four cases; second week, four cases; third week, one case; and fourth week, one case.

  D. Calculate the attack rates for the sixth grade for each of the four weeks of October. What could explain the low attack rate in the last two weeks of October and the absence of cases in November?

E. Could such an outbreak occur today?

Answer on page 357.

12–3   A city health department receives reports of three cases of typhoid fever from one health district over a ten-day period. List the steps you would take to determine whether there has been a common source outbreak of the disease.

12–4   In the fall of 1959, over 150 persons on the staff of the Veterans Administration Hospital in Denver, Colorado, became ill about 12 to 13 hours after eating a turkey dinner. The most common symptoms were diarrhea and cramps; a minority of those who became ill also had nausea, vomiting, and prostration. Information was collected about the specific foods consumed by 159 of the estimated 340 to 350 persons who ate that meal. Based on that information, the attack rates were calculated (Table 12–4).

TABLE 12–4   Food-history Attack Rate Table *

Food	Number of Persons Who Ate Specified Food				Number of Persons Who Did NOT Eat Specified Food			
	Ill	Not Ill	Total	Percentage Ill	Ill	Not Ill	Total	Percentage Ill
Turkey	97	36	133	72.9	2	23	25	8.0
Dressing	88	33	121	72.7	11	26	37	29.7
Potatoes and gravy	92	35	127	72.4	7	24	31	22.6
Peas	77	28	105	73.3	22	31	53	41.5
Rolls	50	16	66	75.8	49	43	92	53.3
Oleomargarine	50	16	66	75.8	49	43	92	53.3
Salads	1	3	4	25.0	98	56	154	63.6
Dessert	22	14	36	61.1	77	45	122	63.1
Sandwich	1	10	11	9.1	98	49	147	66.7
Coffee	59	39	98	60.2	40	20	60	66.7
Milk	12	6	18	66.7	87	53	140	62.1

*Adapted from Tong, J. L., Engle, H. M., et al., 1962.

A. What features in such a table would incriminate a particular food as being responsible for the epidemic?
B. Does the table suggest that one food must be responsible? More than one food? If the latter, what further information may be helpful in incriminating a specific food?

Answer on page 358.

12–5 In the outbreak illustrated in Figure 12–4, review of the food histories indicated that one food, mushroom gravy, was probably responsible for the outbreak. Ninety-one per cent of the people who ate mushroom gravy, but only 40 per cent of those who did not, became ill (Table 12–5).

Table 12–5 Summary of Food History Data Obtained from Personnel at a Military Base in Texas, October, 1968 *

Food or Beverage	Persons Who Ate Specified Foods				Persons Who Did Not Eat Specified Foods			
	Ill	Not Ill	Total	Attack Rate Per cent	Ill	Not Ill	Total	Attack Rate Per cent
Salisbury steak	207	115	322	64	145	13	158	92
Mushroom gravy	288	30	318	91	64	98	162	40
Rissole potatoes	275	113	388	71	77	15	92	84
Whole grain corn	236	92	328	72	116	36	152	76
Butter	182	71	253	72	170	57	227	75
Ice cream	230	97	327	70	122	31	153	80
Strawberry topping	171	77	248	69	181	51	232	78
Milk	262	61	323	81	91	67	158	58

*From Morbidity and Mortality Weekly Report, CDC, USPHS, 18:20, 1969.

A. Assume that the mushroom gravy was responsible for the outbreak. Indicate two reasons why 91 per cent rather than 100 per cent of those who ingested the gravy became ill.
B. Give three reasons which could account for an attack rate of 40 per cent among people who did not consume gravy.
C. Study the epidemic curve in Figure 12–4 and note the variability in incubation period. Why did the onsets of illness occur over so many hours? (The mean incubation period was ten and one-half hours, the range 5 to 14 hours.)

D. Judging from the incubation period, could this outbreak have been due to ingestion of food containing enterotoxin produced by *Staphylococcus aureus*? Defend your answer.

Answer on page 358.

12-6 Figure 12-16 shows the intervals between the index case and subsequent cases of infectious hepatitis (hepatitis A) in 37 families during an outbreak. The incubation period of hepatitis A is usually given as 15 to 50 days, with a median of 30 days.

A. What type of epidemic (i.e. common source or propagated) is suggested by this curve? Why?
B. Note that 11 cases developed within two weeks of the onset in the index case. Give three possible reasons for the short interval between the index case and subsequent cases.

Answer on page 359.

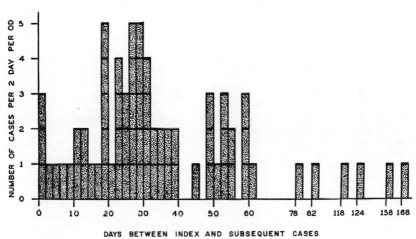

DAYS BETWEEN INDEX AND SUBSEQUENT CASES

Figure 12-16 Intervals (in days) between index and subsequent cases of infectious hepatitis in 37 families, Cooper County, Missouri, 1951. (From Knight, V., et al. Relationship of intervals between index cases and subsequent occurrence of disease in family contacts. Am. J. Hyg., 59:1, 1954.)

REFERENCES

Alexander, J. W.: Nosocomial Infections. Current Problems in Surgery. Yearbook Medical Publishers, Inc., Chicago, 1973.

American Hospital Association: Proceedings of the International Conference on Nosocomial Infections, 1970, Center for Disease Control. Waverly Press, Inc., Baltimore, 1971.

Barker, W. H., Jr.: Vibrio parahaemolyticus outbreaks in the United States. Lancet, 1:551, 1974.

Barker, W. H., Jr., Sagerser, J. C., et al.: Foodborne disease surveillance, Washington State, 1969. Am. J. Public Health, in press, 1974.

Benenson, A. S. (ed.): Control of Communicable Diseases in Man, 11th ed. Amer. Public Health Assn., New York, 1970.

Cluff, L., and Johnson, J.: Clinical Concepts in Infectious Disease. The Williams & Wilkins Company, Baltimore, 1972.

Damato, J. J., Eitzman, D. V., et al.: Persistence and dissemination in the community of R-factors of nosocomial origin. J. Infect. Dis., 129:205, 1974.

Dougherty, W. J., and Altman, R.: Viral hepatitis in New Jersey. Am. J. Med., 32: 704, 1962.

Eickhoff, T. C.: Immunization against influenza: Rationale and recommendations. J. Infect. Dis., 123:446, 1971.

Eickhoff, T. C., Sherman, I. L., et al.: Observations on excess mortality associated with epidemic influenza. J.A.M.A., 176:776, 1961.

Fox, J. P., Hall, C. E., et al.: Epidemiology: Man and Disease. Macmillan Publishing Co., Inc., New York, 1970.

Garibaldi, R. A., Hanson, B., et al.: Impact of illicit drug-associated hepatitis on viral hepatitis morbidity reports in the United States. J. Infect. Dis., 126:288, 1972.

Handsfield, H. H., Lipman, T. O., et al.: Asymptomatic gonorrhea in men: Diagnosis, natural course and prevalence. N. Engl. J. Med., 290:117, 1974.

Hedrich, A. W.: Monthly estimates of the child population "susceptible" to measles, 1900–1931, Baltimore, Md. Am. J. Hygiene, 17:626, 1933.

Hoeprich, P. D. (ed.): Infectious Diseases: A Guide to the Understanding and Management of Infectious Processes. Harper & Row, Publishers, New York, 1972.

Karzon, D. T.: Smallpox vaccination in the United States: The end of an era. J. Pediatr., 81:600, 1972.

Langmuir, A. D.: Air-borne infection. In Sartwell, P. E. (ed.): Maxcy-Rosenau Preventive Medicine and Public Health, 9th ed. Appleton-Century-Crofts, New York, 1965.

Marcuse, E. K., and Grand, M. G.: Epidemiology of diphtheria in San Antonio, Texas, 1970. J.A.M.A., 224:305, 1973.

Mausner, J. S., and Gezon, H. M.: Report on a phantom epidemic of gonorrhea. Am. J. Epidemiol., 85:320, 1967.

Riley, R. L., and O'Grady, F.: Airborne Infection: Transmission and Control. Macmillan Publishing Co., Inc., New York, 1961.

Sartwell, P. E., and Price, W.: General epidemiology of infections. In Sartwell, P. E. (ed.): Maxcy-Rosenau Preventive Medicine and Public Health, 9th ed. Appleton-Century-Crofts, New York, 1965.

Serfling, R. E.: Historical review of epidemic theory. Hum. Biol., 24:145, 1952.

Tong, J. L., Engle, H. M., et al.: Investigation of an outbreak of food poisoning traced to turkey meat. Am. J. Public Health, 52:976, 1962.

METHODS
FOR THE
STUDY
OF
CHRONIC
DISEASE
13

EMERGING IMPORTANCE OF THE CHRONIC DISEASES

Largely as a result of the decline in infectious diseases in infancy and childhood, the average length of life has increased. This improved longevity, coupled with a decrease in birth rates over the past decades, has led to an increase in the proportion of elderly persons in the population.

A result of these demographic changes has been a marked increase in long-term, or chronic, illness. A National Commission on Chronic Illness, which functioned from 1949 through 1956, defined *chronic disease* as follows:

Chronic disease comprises all impairments or deviations from normal which have one or more of the following characteristics: are permanent; leave residual disability; are caused by nonreversible pathological alteration; require special training of the patient for rehabilitation; may be expected to require a long period of supervision, observation, or care (Commission on Chronic Illness, 1957).

Our relative inability to control the diseases which afflict older persons in particular, such as cardiovascular disease, cancer, and arthritis, has resulted in a striking change in the patterns of morbidity and mortality. Since the beginning of the century infectious diseases—influenza and pneumonia, tuberculosis, and gastroenteritis—have been replaced by chronic conditions—heart disease, cancer, and stroke—as the three leading causes of death (Figure 13–1).

307

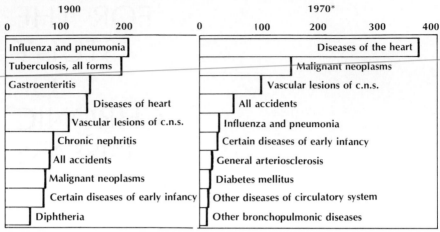

Figure 13–1 Death rates for the ten leading causes of death per 100,000 population, United States, 1900 and 1970. (From Linder, F. E., and Grove, R. D.: Vital Statistics Rates in the United States, 1900–1940. U.S. Govt. Printing Office, Washington, D.C., 1943 [data for 1900]; National Center for Health Statistics: Annual Summary for the United States, 1970. Monthly Vital Statistics Report, Vol. 19. U.S. Dept. of Health, Education, and Welfare, USPHS, U.S. Govt. Printing Office, Washington, D.C., 1971 [data for 1970].)

---

*Based on 10 per cent sample of death certificates.

It is the chronic diseases which are the major obstacles to extending the life span. As noted in Chapter 9, there has been little improvement in life expectancy among those of middle age, especially men, over the past two decades (Table 13–1).

We have used the terms "chronic disease" and "infectious disease" as if they were polar, or opposite. Actually each refers to a separate dimension of disease classification. One dimension is the temporal aspect of disease (acute vs. chronic), the other the underly-

TABLE 13–1 Expectation of Life of White Persons Aged 40, United States*

| | Years Remaining | |
Period	Men	Women
1949–1951	31.2	35.6
1959–1961	31.7	37.1
1965	31.7	37.5
1969	31.8	37.8
Gain 1950 to 1969	0.6	2.2

*Adapted from Keys, A.: Cardiology. The essentiality of prevention. Minn. Med., 52:1191, 1969.

ing etiologic mechanism (infectious vs. noninfectious). Table 13–2 shows this two-way classification of disease. Although there are four possible cells in the table, most diseases fall into two categories, acute-infectious and chronic-noninfectious.

While diseases such as measles and tuberculosis fit readily into one of the four categories, others defy such simplistic classification. Many chronic diseases have acute exacerbations (coronary heart disease, gout). Conversely, acute diseases sometimes give rise to protracted sequelae, such as post-necrotic cirrhosis after viral hepatitis, or subacute sclerosing panencephalitis following measles. Furthermore, infection may play a role in the development of certain chronic diseases previously considered noninfectious in origin, such as Hodgkin's disease and leukemia. In addition, certain chronic conditions (e.g., rheumatic heart disease) are the result of immune responses to streptococcal infection. Nevertheless, in common usage a number of conditions with an infectious component or a course characterized by remissions and acute exacerbations are grouped under the rubric "chronic disease."

Although all infectious disease problems have not been conquered, chronic diseases provide our major health challenges today. Many patients with these diseases present themselves at a stage where cure is not possible and symptomatic treatment (tertiary prevention) over a protracted period of time is all that can be offered. Attempts to intervene earlier in the natural history of a chronic disease include not only screening for early detection (secondary prevention) but also a focus on primary prevention. The necessity for primary prevention makes it imperative that we identify the etiologic factors underlying these conditions. Thus, we need to consider the methods available for unravelling the antecedents of the so-called chronic diseases.

TABLE 13–2 Classification of Diseases by Duration and Etiology, with Examples

	Acute	Chronic*
Infectious	Common cold, pneumonia, measles, mumps, pertussis, typhoid fever, cholera	Tuberculosis, rheumatic fever following streptococcal infection
Noninfectious	Poisoning (e.g., carbon monoxide, heavy metals), trauma (e.g., automotive crashes)	Diabetes, coronary heart disease, osteoarthritis, cirrhosis due to alcoholism

*The National Health Survey uses a minimum period of three months to delineate certain conditions as "chronic" on the basis of their duration.

PROBLEMS IN ETIOLOGIC INVESTIGATION OF CHRONIC DISEASES

Several aspects of the origin and natural history of chronic diseases create special problems for investigation of causality.

Absence of a Known Agent

The absence of a known agent is a troublesome feature of many chronic diseases because it makes diagnosis difficult. In most infectious diseases, one is able to confirm or rule out the presence of disease by identification of the organism, by skin test, or by serologic reaction. Similarly, in acute intoxications, such as lead poisoning, one can demonstrate the agent in body tissues. Since there is no diagnostic test of comparable specificity for many chronic diseases, the distinction between diseased and nondiseased persons may be more difficult to establish.

Multifactorial Nature of Etiology

Although infectious diseases involve host resistance and other factors in addition to the infectious agent, the operation of multiple factors is particularly important in chronic diseases. The pertinent factors may be both environmental and constitutional (e.g., ABO blood type and oral contraceptives as risk factors for thromboembolism). The interaction of factors may be purely additive or it may be synergistic (i.e., multiplicative). For example, smoking and occupational exposure were found to have an additive effect as risk factors for bladder cancer (data of Cole, cited in MacMahon, 1972). The risk for persons with a history of both exposures is similar to that which would be predicted by summing the individual effects of each factor. In contrast, smoking appears to act synergistically with occupational exposures to asbestos (Berry et al., 1972; Selikoff et al., 1968) and uranium ore (Lundin et al., 1969). The lung cancer risk in the presence of smoking and either of these occupational exposures far exceeds that predicted from the sum of the risks.

Such interactions must be taken into account in the design of etiologic studies. They also have implications for the control of disease. For example, knowledge of a synergistic interaction makes it particularly urgent for asbestos and uranium workers to abstain from smoking.

Long Latent Period

Many chronic diseases have a long latent period during which host and environmental factors interact before the disease becomes manifest. The latent period is the equivalent of the incubation period in infectious disease, except that it is generally much longer. The long duration of the latent period makes it difficult to link antecedent events with outcomes. It is easy to identify the common exposure to staphylococcal enterotoxin of a group of students or military personnel who develop gastrointestinal illnesses within a few hours. It is much more difficult to investigate a possible relation between patterns of food consumption in youth (i.e., diet high or low in saturated fats) and the occurrence of coronary heart disease in middle age, or between suspected aspects of parent-child relationships and various mental disorders in adult life.

Indefinite Onset

Many chronic conditions are characterized by an indefinite onset. Examples are the arthritides and mental illnesses. In other chronic diseases an apparently sudden onset may be merely a dramatic episode in a long-standing process, such as, acute occlusion in coronary vessels which have been undergoing atherosclerotic change for many years. Problems in pinpointing the time of onset make incidence data difficult to collect.

Differential Effect of Factors on Incidence and Course of Disease

Finally, another difficulty is that a factor may be related differently to the initial development of disease than to its later course. For example, cancer of the breast develops more frequently in women of upper than of lower socioeconomic class. However, studies from the California Tumor Registry (Linden, 1969) have shown that, within stage, survival of patients with breast cancer was better for more advantaged women (i.e., those treated in private rather than county hospitals). Thus, social class gradient seems to favor lower class women with lower incidence, but upper class women with better prognosis. This emphasizes that etiologic studies based on prevalence or mortality rates may be difficult to interpret.

Another example can be given to show how factors may act differently at various stages of disease. The Framingham study (cited in Chapter 1) has shown that the association between smoking

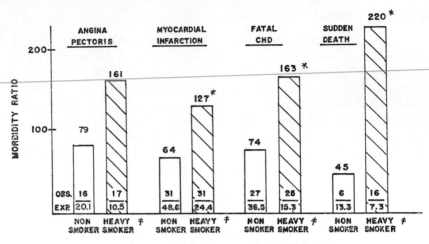

Figure 13–2 Morbidity ratio* for different manifestations of coronary heart disease (12 years) according to cigarette smoking status, men aged 30–59 years at entry, Framingham heart study. (From Kannel, W. B., Castelli, W. P., et al.: Cigarette smoking and risk of coronary heart disease. Epidemiologic clues to pathogenesis. The Framingham study. Natl. Cancer Inst. Monogr., *28*:9, 1968.)

*Morbidity ratio $= \dfrac{\text{observed number}}{\text{expected number}} \times 100$ (page 137).

and coronary heart disease varies with manifestations of the disease (Figure 13–2). That is, smoking is more strongly associated with sudden death from coronary heart disease than with less fatal forms of the disease. It follows from this that discrepant results may arise if studies do not differentiate among different stages or categories of a disease.

ANALYTIC APPROACHES TO THE ETIOLOGY OF CHRONIC DISEASE

Since chronic diseases develop over a long period of time, etiologic study of these conditions requires the analysis of events which occur over time. As mentioned in Chapter 5, two major methods are available for observational studies of etiology—one retrospective, the other prospective.

Retrospective Study. In a *retrospective study* people diagnosed as having a disease (cases) are compared with persons who do not have the disease (controls). The purpose is to determine if the two groups differ in proportion of persons who had been exposed to a specific factor or factors (Figure 13–3). Such a study is retrospective because it compares cases and controls with regard to the presence of some element in their past experience. The term "case-control method" can also be applied to this kind of study to indicate the way in which the study group is assembled.

Prospective Study.   In contrast, a *prospective study* starts with a group of people (a cohort) all considered to be free of a given disease, but who vary in exposure to a supposed noxious factor (Figure 13–3). The cohort is followed over time in order to determine differences in the rate at which disease develops in relation to exposure to the factor.

The difference between retrospective and prospective studies can be further illustrated by a diagram (Figure 13–4) in which each person is classified simply as "exposed" or "not exposed" and as "diseased" or "not diseased." The classification of each person according to both variables yields a fourfold table.

Figure 13–4 emphasizes that the essential difference between the two types of studies lies not in the time sequence but rather in the way the study groups are assembled. In retrospective studies diseased and nondiseased groups (cases and controls) are selected and compared for presence or absence of an antecedent factor. In prospective studies we begin with individuals who are free of the disease under consideration. They are classified by exposure or lack of exposure to a factor and followed for the development of disease.

With either method of study, if there is a positive association between the factor and the disease, those exposed will tend to develop the disease (group a), while those not exposed will tend not

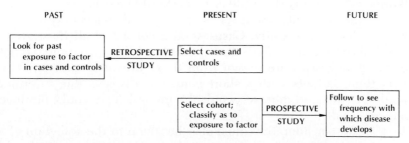

Figure 13–3 Schematic diagram of time factor in epidemiologic studies.

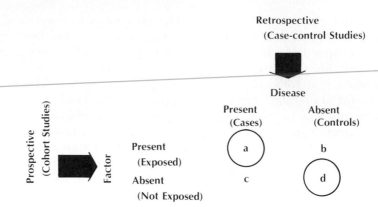

Figure 13–4 Fourfold (2 × 2) table showing retrospective and prospective study designs.

to develop it (group d). Thus, there will be a disproportionate aggregation of study subjects in groups a and d vs. b and c.

We should note that the model presented in Figure 13–4 is the simplest possible. It is often desirable to analyze a factor in terms of level of exposure (e.g., number of cigarettes smoked, estimated person-years of contact with an industrial hazard, and so on). It may also be desirable to divide a disease into several categories, e.g., coronary heart disease may be subdivided according to its different manifestations (Figure 13–2). Therefore, analysis may yield a more complicated matrix than the fourfold table shown for illustrative purposes.

RETROSPECTIVE STUDIES

Selection of Cases and Controls

In a retrospective study the nature of the study group must be delineated precisely. Definite criteria should be established so that there is no ambiguity about types of cases and stages of disease to be included in the study. Cases should consist of all those diagnosed during a specified time period. If this principle is not followed and cases are drawn from those prevalent at a point in time, then patients with a short course of disease, due to either rapid cure or rapid demise, would be missed. This could produce biassed results.

Careful consideration must also be given to the selection of a control group; the important principle is that the controls should resemble the cases closely except for the presence of the disease under study. Thus, if the cases are derived from a defined geographic area, the population of that area should be used as the source of the controls. If, as is more usual, the cases are derived from institutional rosters, then the controls should be selected to duplicate the selective factors (e.g., financial standing, area of residence, and ethnicity) which bring people to these hospitals or clinics. This is usually accomplished by selecting from among other patients who have attended the same facilities. It is generally advisable to include a wide range of diagnostic entities in the control group. However, because of the likelihood of bias with hospitalized patients as controls, some studies have selected controls from relatives, neighbors, classmates, or other associates of the cases. Of course, cases and controls should be concurrent. Once the source of the control group has been determined, the controls selected may be the entire pool of eligible subjects, a sample of the group, or, more commonly, individuals paired to specific cases.

It is apparent that there are many factors (e.g., age, sex, and color) which may confound the relationship between the factor under study and the outcome. Therefore, a retrospective study usually entails some matching, either on a group or individual basis (person-to-person matching). *Matching* is the process of selecting controls so that they are similar to the cases in specific characteristics. Age, sex, color, race, and socioeconomic status are the most commonly used matching variables. Once the controls have been selected, by whatever matching procedures the study uses, information is then obtained and recorded for variables which may be of etiologic significance.

It should be emphasized that when a variable is used for matching, its etiologic role cannot be investigated in that study because cases and controls are then automatically alike with respect to that characteristic. For example, suppose that we did not know that breast cancer rates are higher among single than among married women. A study to identify risk factors in breast cancer which used matching on marital status could not detect any difference between cases and controls with respect to that factor. However, once the role of a factor has been established, an investigator might then choose to match cases and controls on that factor while investigating other variables.

Some issues related to the pros and cons of matching in epidemiologic studies have been reviewed recently (Miettinen, 1970). When controls are matched to cases, the pairing should be maintained in analysis of the data (Pike and Morrow, 1970). Sartwell (1971) has demonstrated that if the analysis ignores the fact that matching has been done, an underestimate of relative risk (see below) can be obtained.

Analysis of Results

Analytic studies are designed to determine if an association exists between a factor and a disease and, if so, the strength of the association. Ideally, one would like to estimate the incidence rate of the disease under study among those with and without the factor. However, incidence rates usually cannot be derived from a retrospective study because there are no appropriate denominators (populations at risk). Because of the way the study group is assembled in retrospective studies, groups (a + b) and (c + d) in such studies (see Figure 13–4) do not represent the total populations exposed and not exposed to the factor.

Nevertheless, even though the magnitude of the two rates (incidence) cannot be determined from a retrospective study, the ratio of these rates (e.g., is one rate five times the other?) can often be estimated. This ratio is known as the relative risk. *Relative risk* is defined as the ratio of the incidence rate of those exposed to a factor to the incidence rate of those not exposed:

$$\text{Relative risk} = \frac{\text{incidence rate among exposed}}{\text{incidence rate among nonexposed}}$$

The relative risk can be estimated from a retrospective (case-control) study if the assumptions can be made that: (1) the controls are representative of the general population; (2) the assembled cases are representative of all cases; and (3) the frequency of the disease in the population is small. If these assumptions are satisfied, a term known as the *odds ratio* or *risk ratio* can be used as an estimate of the relative risk. An abbreviated derivation follows. (See Cornfield and Haenszel, 1960, for a fuller explanation.)

A total population may be divided by proportions as follows:

	Disease Present	Absent	Total
Exposed to Factor	P_1	P_2	$P_1 + P_2$
Not Exposed to Factor	P_3	P_4	$P_3 + P_4$
Total	$P_1 + P_3$	$P_2 + P_4$	

The ratio of incidence rates (relative risk) would be:

$$\frac{P_1}{P_1 + P_2} \div \frac{P_3}{P_3 + P_4}$$

If, as is often true, the proportion of diseased persons is small, then P_1 is small in relation to P_2, and P_3 is small in relation to P_4. The denominators then reduce to P_2 and P_4 yielding

$$\frac{P_1}{P_2} \div \frac{P_3}{P_4}, \text{ or } \frac{P_1 P_4}{P_2 P_3},$$

as an approximation of the relative risk.

The expression $\frac{P_1}{P_2} \div \frac{P_3}{P_4}$ is called the odds ratio because the quantities can be considered as the odds in favor of having the disease with the factor present and with the factor absent, respectively.

The above analysis of relative risk is applicable to prospective studies. However, under the assumptions mentioned previously, in a retrospective (case-control) study the formula $\frac{ad}{bc}$ (using the symbols for frequencies in Figure 13–4) can be substituted for $\frac{P_1 P_4}{P_2 P_3}$, yielding a reasonable approximation of relative risk. The odds ratio can thus be obtained easily by multiplying diagonally in the four-fold table (cross-products).

For an example of the calculation of estimated relative risk, consider the data from a study to determine whether tonsillectomy is associated with subsequent development of Hodgkin's disease (Vianna et al., 1971). The 109 patients and 109 controls were found to have the following histories of tonsillectomy:

		Cases	Controls
	Yes	67(a)	43(b)
Prior Tonsillectomy	No	34(c)	64(d)
	Unknown	8	2
		109	109

Ignoring the unknowns, the estimated relative risk from the formula $\frac{ad}{bc} = \frac{(67)(64)}{(43)(34)} = 2.9$. This study thus yielded an estimate that the relative risk of developing Hodgkin's disease was about three times greater for those with a prior tonsillectomy than for persons with intact tonsils.

Advantages

Retrospective studies are rather inexpensive to carry out, at least compared with prospective studies. The number of subjects can be small since the study is initiated by the identification of cases, which are often compared with a like number of controls. Even when two or three controls are selected for each case, the number of persons studied is small in comparison with the numbers needed for prospective studies. This is particularly important for etiologic study of rare diseases. Retrospective studies may provide the only practical approach to studies of the causes of such conditions. In addition, the results of a retrospective study can be obtained relatively quickly, whereas results from a prospective study are not available until the disease develops, which may require months or years.

All these advantages of the retrospective method are illustrated by a recent demonstration of transplacental carcinogenesis (Herbst et al., 1971). Between 1966 and 1969 seven cases of adenocarcinoma of the vagina were seen in young women (aged 15 to 22 years) in one Boston hospital. This was a most unexpected occur-

TABLE 13–3 Comparison of Cases of Adenocarcinoma of the Vagina and Controls for Specified Variables

Case No.	Maternal Age (years) Case	Maternal Age (years) Mean of 4 Controls	Maternal Smoking Case	Maternal Smoking Control	Bleeding in This Pregnancy Case	Bleeding in This Pregnancy Control	Any Prior Pregnancy Loss Case	Any Prior Pregnancy Loss Control	Estrogen Given in This Pregnancy Case	Estrogen Given in This Pregnancy Control
1	25	32	Yes	2/4	No	0/4	Yes	1/4	Yes	0/4
2	30	30	Yes	3/4	No	0/4	Yes	1/4	Yes	0/4
3	22	31	Yes	1/4	Yes	0/4	No	1/4	Yes	0/4
4	33	30	Yes	3/4	Yes	0/4	Yes	0/4	Yes	0/4
5	22	27	Yes	3/4	No	1/4	No	1/4	No	0/4
6	21	29	Yes	3/4	Yes	0/4	Yes	0/4	Yes	0/4
7	30	27	No	3/4	No	0/4	Yes	1/4	Yes	0/4
8	26	28	Yes	3/4	No	0/4	Yes	0/4	Yes	0/4
Total			7/8	21/32	3/8	1/32	6/8	5/32	7/8	0/32
Mean	26.1	29.3								
χ^2 (1 df)[**]				0.53		4.52		7.16		23.22
p value	(N.S.)[†]			0.50 (N.S.)		<0.05		<0.01		<0.00001

[*]Adapted from Herbst, A. L., Ulfelder, H., et al.: Association of maternal stilbestrol therapy with tumor appearance in young women. N. Engl. J. Med., 284:878, 1971.

[**]Matched control χ^2 test as described by Pike and Morrow.

[†]Standard error of difference 1.7 years (paired t-test); NS, not statistically significant.

rence. Not only is carcinoma of the vagina a rare disease, but also the usual victim is past 50 years of age and the histologic type is generally different (i.e., epidermoid).

The cause of this puzzling occurrence was investigated by a retrospective study which drew on four controls for each of the eight cases of adenocarcinoma of the vagina (the seven cases mentioned above plus one other treated at another hospital). The controls were matched to the cases by sex, date of birth, hospital of birth, and type of hospital service (private vs. ward). As shown in Table 13–3 the cases differed dramatically from the controls in past history. All but one of the cases, and none of the controls, had been exposed to an estrogenic substance, diethylstilbestrol (DES) in fetal life. This drug had been given to the mother because of bleeding, or prior pregnancy loss, or both. Since this study additional cases have been reported; these have confirmed the association with DES.

In addition to illustrating the usefulness of the retrospective study method for investigating a rare disease, this particular outbreak has profound significance because it provided the first example of transplacental carcinogenesis. It serves to remind us that ill effects from therapeutic procedures may not become manifest until years after exposure has occurred.

Disadvantages

The first problem with a retrospective study is that needed information about past events may not be available from routine records or may be inaccurately recorded. If information is sought by an interview or questionnaire, the informant (patient, relative, or physician) may have inadequate information about, or recall of, events in the distant past.

Further, information supplied by an informant may be biassed. At the time of the study, the disease has already been diagnosed in the cases. As a result, informants about cases may have a different recall of past events than informants for controls. People may be more likely to search for explanations for the disease in the cases and, therefore, may assign more significance to past events. The more severe the disease (e.g., leukemia, cancer, or severe congenital defect), the greater may be the likelihood of such bias.

At times it may be possible to test for the presence of bias. For example, in one of the early retrospective studies of cigarette smoking and lung cancer (Doll and Hill, 1950), after the cases and controls had been interviewed it was discovered that some patients had erroneously been thought at time of interview to have lung cancer. The fact that the smoking histories of these patients were subsequently found to resemble those of controls rather than cases was reassuring evidence that the difference between cases and controls in smoking could not be attributed to interviewer bias.

However, the most serious problems associated with the use of the retrospective method are perhaps those related to the selection of an appropriate control group, the "Achilles' heel" of any retrospective study (Kannel and Dawber, 1973). The selection of controls from hospital or clinic rosters can readily introduce serious bias. If the disease among the controls is affected (either positively or negatively) by the factor being investigated, a true association may be partially masked or a spurious association found. For example, in a retrospective study (Jick et al., 1973) an association between coffee drinking and coronary heart disease was found which had not emerged from prospective studies. One possible explanation is that the hospitalized control group might contain individuals who had been advised against coffee drinking for medical reasons, such as peptic ulcer. As a result, consumption of the coffee in the control group might be unrepresentative of the patterns of consumption in the general population.

The opposite effect, that of minimizing a positive association, occurred in some early retrospective studies of the role of cigarette smoking in lung cancer (Wynder, 1950). Because the association of smoking with chronic pulmonary disease was not appreciated at that time, patients with such disease were included among the controls for the lung cancer patients.

For these reasons it is often advisable to select more than one control series, including a general population control, as in the Oleinick study discussed earlier. If several control series resemble each other and if all show a much lower frequency of exposure to the factor than do the cases, then this is good evidence for the validity of the association of the factor with the disease under study. Alternatively, if other types of patients are to serve as the control group, it may be possible to elicit items of information (e.g., marital status, distribution of occupations, and smoking habits) for which general population values are known. Comparison of the population and the control group for these variables would then provide some measure of the extent to which the controls were representative of the population.

A final disadvantage of the retrospective method has been discussed under Analysis of Results. Although a relative risk can sometimes be estimated from retrospective studies, it is usually not possible to calculate the incidence rates in persons exposed and not exposed to a given factor. This fact has not always been considered. The first indication that rubella in pregnant women is associated with congenital defects in their offspring was Gregg's report (1941) of a series of babies with congenital cataract. This Australian ophthalmologist noted that almost 90 per cent of the mothers of these infants gave a history of German measles during the pregnancy. Other retrospective studies gave similarly high estimates. This was taken by some to mean that if a pregnant woman has German measles the risk of cataracts in the offspring is 90 per cent. This, of course, does not necessarily follow; the babies who did not develop cataracts following rubella in their mothers were not brought to the ophthalmologist's attention. Indeed, subsequent prospective studies have indicated that the risk of congenital defect is much lower.

Further discussions of issues related to retrospective studies may be found in Mantel and Haenszel (1959) and Cornfield and Haenszel (1960).

PROSPECTIVE STUDIES

Selection of the Study Group, or Cohort

In prospective studies several approaches to selection of a cohort are possible. A particular group may be chosen for study because it is accessible (e.g., volunteers), or because its medical records are readily available (e.g., armed forces), or because the group is known to have experienced some particular exposure, such as that arising during the course of work.

The cohort may thus be heterogeneous with respect to some previous exposure or may be restricted to a group of either high or low exposure. Examples of heterogeneous cohorts can be found in the studies of lung cancer described in Chapter 5, in which each study population included both smokers and nonsmokers.

When the study group is essentially homogeneous in exposure, comparison can be made with another cohort differing in previous exposure or with rates derived from vital statistics. The latter type of comparison was utilized by Selikoff and his colleagues (1968) in studies of the frequency of cancer among asbestos workers. By setting up comparisons with general population values, they were able to demonstrate a marked excess of deaths among the asbestos workers from cancer of the lung, stomach, and colon, as well as several deaths from a rare tumor, mesothelioma of the pleura and peritoneum.*

---

*This is actually an example of an historical prospective study to be described later. The principles in selection of cohorts for study is the same in both types of investigations.

Analysis of Results: Measures of Excess Risk

Prospective studies permit determination of the magnitude of risk of disease for the populations exposed and not exposed. Therefore, the excess risk due to exposure to a given factor can be calculated directly. There are two major ways of expressing this excess: relative risk and attributable risk. Relative risk was discussed on page 316, where it was defined as the ratio of the incidence rate of those exposed to a factor to the incidence rate of those not exposed. Attributable risk can be defined in several ways, depending upon the question being asked. One might ask about the extent to which incidence of disease in a group of exposed persons can be attributed to their exposure. One might also ask about the proportion of all cases of the disease in the *total* population that can be attributed to the exposure. We will consider these in turn.

According to the first question, *attributable risk* can be defined as the arithmetic or absolute difference in incidence rates between an exposed group and a nonexposed group. We will illustrate this concept with data on the mortality experience of British physicians (Doll and Hill, 1956). Table 13–4 shows annual death rates from lung cancer and from coronary heart disease for heavy smokers and nonsmokers, along with the two measures of excess risk (relative risk and attributable risk).

In this example, the very high relative risk for heavy smokers as compared to nonsmokers (about 24) is evidence of a strong association between heavy smoking and lung cancer. The relative

TABLE 13–4 Comparison of Relative Risk and Attributable Risk in Mortality from Lung Cancer and from Coronary Heart Disease for Heavy Smokers and Nonsmokers[*]

	Annual Death Rates per 100,000 Persons	
Exposure Category	Lung Cancer	Coronary Heart Disease
Heavy smokers	166	599
Nonsmokers	7	422
Measure of Excess Risk		
Relative risk:	$\frac{166}{7} = 23.7$	$\frac{599}{422} = 1.4$
Attributable risk:	$166 - 7 = 159$	$599 - 422 = 177$

[*]Doll, R., and Hill, A. B.: Lung cancer and other causes of death in relation to smoking. A second report on the mortality of British doctors. Br. Med. J., 2:1071, 1956.

risk of coronary heart disease for heavy smokers is much smaller, only 1.4. This suggests that prevention of coronary heart disease would require alteration of other factors in addition to smoking. Nevertheless, because death from coronary heart disease is so common among the nonexposed (annual death rate of 422 per 100,000 persons), even a fairly small relative increase in this rate attributable to smoking can create an absolute increase in death rate that is as large as that for lung cancer (177 per 100,000 for coronary heart disease vs. 159 for lung cancer).

The second measure of attributable risk indicates the proportion of all cases in a total defined population which can be ascribed to a factor. This measure, which has been called the *population attributable risk proportion,* is a compound measure which reflects both relative risk and frequency of the factor in the population. This measure would show, for example, that a large proportion of the deaths from lung cancer in the total population are due to smoking, not only because of the high relative risk associated with smoking, but also because of the large proportion of the population that smoke. Thus, it has been estimated that 80 to 85 per cent of lung cancer deaths in the United States can be attributed to smoking. If a smaller proportion of the population smoked, there would be fewer lung cancer deaths attributable to smoking even if the relative risk due to smoking remained constant.

In summary, then, relative risk is the critical measure for assessing the etiologic role of a factor in disease. Both measures of attributable risk have utility from a public health standpoint. Lilienfeld (1973) has suggested that population attributable risk deserves more attention from epidemiologists than it has received heretofore. The various definitions and formulas for attributable risk given by several authors have been summarized by Leviton (1973).

Advantages

Although some merits and limitations of the prospective approach have already been implied, it may be helpful to state them explicitly. A major advantage of prospective studies is that the cohort is classified in relation to exposure to the factor **before** the disease develops. Therefore, this classification cannot be influenced by knowledge that disease exists, as may be true of retrospective studies. Of course, knowledge of exposure to the factor could introduce bias into the ascertainment of disease, but this is less likely to be a serious problem.

Prospective studies also permit calculation of incidence rates among those exposed and those not exposed. Therefore, the absolute difference in incidence rates between groups (attributable risk) and also the true relative risk can be measured.

Further, prospective studies permit observation of many outcomes. For example, although prospective studies of smokers and nonsmokers were originally designed to detect association of smoking with lung cancer, they also showed that smoking is associated with the development of a host of additional ailments: emphysema, coronary heart disease, peptic ulcer, and cancers of the larynx, oral cavity, esophagus, and urinary bladder (page 106).

Disadvantages

The main disadvantage of such a study is that it is usually a long, expensive, and large-scale undertaking. A large cohort must be followed, particularly if the disease has a low incidence. For example, in seven major prospective studies of smoking and lung

TABLE 13–5   Retrospective and Prospective Studies: Summary of Advantages and Disadvantages

	Advantages	**Disadvantages**
Retrospective Study	Relatively inexpensive	Incomplete information
	Smaller number of subjects	Biassed recall
	Relatively quick results	Problems of selecting control group and
	Suitable for rare diseases	matching variables
		Yields only relative risk
Prospective Study	Lack of bias in factor	Possible bias in ascertainment of disease
	Yields incidence rates as well as relative risk	Large numbers of subjects required
	Can yield associations with additional disease as by-product	Long follow-up period
		Problem of attrition
		Changes over time in criteria and methods
		Very costly

cancer, the 1833 deaths from lung cancer in cigarette smokers came from follow-up data for more than one million persons. The larger the number of factors or variables to be studied (race, area of residence, and so on), the larger the cohort must be.

In addition, the need to follow a cohort over a long period of time (longitudinal study) results in special obstacles. Perhaps the outstanding problem is attrition, the loss of patients from follow-up due to lack of interest, migration, or death from other causes. Other difficulties arise from change in the status of subjects with respect to variables of interest (e.g., the subject may change area of residence, occupation, or smoking habits) leading to error in classification of exposure. There may also be changes in diagnostic criteria and methods over time affecting the classification of individuals as diseased or not diseased. Administrative problems include loss of staff, loss of funding, and the high costs of the extensive record-keeping required. For all these reasons, prospective studies even more than retrospective should not be undertaken without careful planning.

The advantages and disadvantages of retrospective and prospective study methods are summarized in Table 13–5.

HISTORICAL PROSPECTIVE STUDIES

One additional type of study deserves mention because it combines the advantages of both the retrospective and the prospective study designs. This type of study, which may be called *historical prospective*, consists of the identification of a group at some point in the past and analysis of their subsequent morbidity or mortality experience (Figure 13–5).

To conduct such a study it must be possible to identify from records the membership of some previously existing group, such as all the employees of a given industry or all the students in a certain school at a specific date in the past. Secondly, it is necessary that the factors of interest had been recorded adequately at that time, or can be reconstructed from other sources. Thirdly, it must be possible to obtain the needed information about outcome (i.e., disease or death) for almost all the cohort. This may be accomplished through routine records maintained by the organization itself, or it may be possible to obtain the necessary follow-up information through death certificates, hospital records, disability pensions, and so on. Figure 13–5 illustrates the time sequence of this kind of study in relation to the two study designs presented earlier, the purely retrospective and prospective studies.

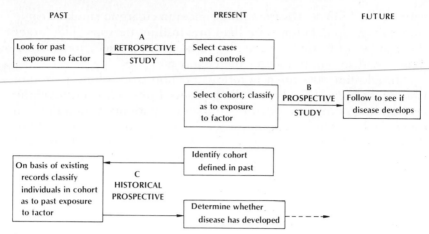

Figure 13–5 Comparison of three different study designs: *A,* retrospective, *B,* prospective, and *C,* historical prospective.

Conceptually, despite the fact that it utilizes previously assembled data, the historical prospective study is essentially longitudinal. It is more akin to a cohort (prospective) study than to a case-control (retrospective) approach. Unlike the purely prospective cohort study, the longitudinal information covers a time interval extending from past to present rather than present to future. However, it is also possible to set up a cohort study retrospectively and then continue it forward prospectively (dotted lines in Figure 13–5), adding contemporaneous data to that assembled retrospectively.

Several studies have taken advantage of previously assembled data on cohorts to study the biological effects of radiation. Court-Brown and Doll (1957) examined the deaths over 20 years (1934 to 1954) among some 13,000 patients who had received large doses of radiation for treatment of rheumatoid arthritis of the spine (ankylosing spondylitis). They found that the death rate from aplastic anemia and leukemia in this cohort was substantially higher than that of the general population. The investigation by Seltser and Sartwell of the mortality of groups of physicians in relation to their probable exposure to radiation (page 55) is another example. We have also mentioned the study by Selikoff (page 54) in which the hazards associated with occupational exposure to asbestos were estimated in a retrospectively identified cohort of asbestos workers.

More recently Paffenbarger (1966 a, b; 1967) has applied this approach to the identification of precursor factors for coronary heart disease, suicide, stroke, and other conditions in former students at the University of Pennsylvania (1931 to 1940) and Harvard (1916 to 1950). His studies have utilized the detailed personal and health histories recorded for college students and the routine follow-up information gathered by the alumni offices of the two institutions.

It is likely that an increasing number of studies will be based on already assembled cohorts as large numbers of people come under medical care in organizations, such as Kaiser Permanente and the Health Insurance Plan of Greater New York, which utilize uniform and mechanized methods for recording, storing, and retrieving data about health. When institutions, such as the universities in Paffenbarger's studies, have an independent need to maintain current information on the status and location of their members, this eases the burden and expense of follow-up.

CHOICE OF STUDY METHODS

It should be apparent that each type of study can make a distinctive contribution to elucidating etiologic factors in disease. Any one of the available study methods may be the most appropriate strategy, depending on such factors as the state of existing knowledge about a disease, its incidence, the interval between exposure and development of disease, and the nature of the factors to be studied for possible etiologic significance.

In general, when there is relatively little information about etiologic factors, the first step is a retrospective study to search for possible factors, a so-called "fishing expedition." If a factor has proved to be important in one or two retrospective studies, replication with another group of patients might seem the procedure of choice. However, once there is fairly clear evidence of the etiologic role of a factor from retrospective studies, the limitations of the retrospective method have often led to prospective investigation for confirmation of the original findings. On the whole, prospective studies have tended to confirm associations uncovered by the retrospective method.

The incidence of the disease is a crucial factor in determining the choice of study methods. If the disease is rare, a very large number of persons would have to be observed prospectively to yield an adequate number of affected individuals. Thus, a high proportion of the efforts and resources would be devoted to the study of persons who do not develop the disease. Fortunately, it is precisely in rare diseases that relative risk can be estimated through retrospective study. Conversely, the more common a disease, the more feasible is a prospective study, since fewer individuals need be followed.

In addition, the shorter the time-span between exposure to the suspected factor and a discernible outcome, the more practical is a prospective study. Thus, it would be easier to study prospectively the relation between events during pregnancy and an outcome observable at birth than to determine possible carcinogenic hazards manifest only after a twenty-year latent period.

Another factor in choice of method is the nature and availability of the desired information. If the information is both objective and uniformly available for most or all study subjects, a retrospective study can be satisfactorily and economically carried out. For example, if one wished to study the relationship between prematurity and subsequent scholastic performance, it would be quite feasible to obtain birth weights for most, if not all, potential subjects since this information is routinely recorded at time of birth.

The need to design a special questionnaire or form for recording past information of interest does not rule out a retrospective investigation. However, in such circumstances, if there are likely to be problems with memory or bias about crucial information without the possibility of checking its validity, a prospective study may be preferable. The historical prospective approach combines the advantages of both methods and should be used if possible.

As a concluding note, we would emphasize that in all types of studies, retrospective and prospective, it is necessary to evaluate carefully the comparability of the groups being surveyed with respect to any other variables (e.g., age, socio-economic status) which could affect the findings. If such differences between groups are found, they should be eliminated in the analyses through statistical techniques, such as age-adjustment, analysis by subgroups, or analysis of covariance.

SURVIVORSHIP (PROGNOSIS) IN CHRONIC DISEASE

An important epidemiologic aspect of any disease is its outcome or prognosis. Different criteria of outcome may be used — survival vs. death, survival with or without recurrence, and so on. Certainly the quality as well as duration of life is of concern to health workers. However, for simplicity we will consider only two outcomes, survival or death.

For acute diseases, the case fatality rate is a useful measure of survival. However, it is not satisfactory for the study of chronic diseases in which the course is characteristically long and variable. In chronic diseases a *cohort life table* is used to calculate the probability of surviving or dying within specified time periods after diagnosis. For example, the mortality experience of one cohort of persons (e.g., patients diagnosed as having cancer of the colon in 1970) is followed at successive periods of time after diagnosis. The cohort life-table is therefore based on successive death rates over a long period of time for the same cohort. It thus differs from the demographic life table (Chapter 0) which is based on cross-sectional data, i.e., age-specific death rates for many cohorts for one calendar year.

To prevent bias in studies of survivorship, it is important to include in the cohort all patients who meet the diagnostic and other criteria for entry. All persons should be enrolled at time of diagnosis, not at the time treatment is begun. No patient should be excluded because he dies shortly after diagnosis, remains untreated, or represents an operative death. Moore (1963) in an article entitled "How to achieve surgical results by really trying" has shown that misleading "improvement" in survivorship may be achieved by careful selection of patients for analysis.

The problem of defining a total cohort is particularly crucial in arteriosclerotic heart disease. A number of studies indicate that many patients with myocardial infarction die suddenly, before they can be hospitalized (Kuller, 1969). Studies of prognosis based only on hospitalized patients thus present the survival experience of only a portion of the total number of persons who suffer a myocardial infarction.

Five-year survival is a commonly used end-point, particularly for evaluating survival following treatment for cancer, but it should be remembered that other end-points, e.g., one, two, or ten years, can be used. Moreover, five-year survival is not necessarily synonymous with cure, as may be seen from long-term studies of survival in breast cancer. Figure 13–6A shows the observed survival rates for women with breast cancer as recorded in the Connecticut Cancer Registry, as well as rates for women of the same age and color in the general population (i.e., expected rates). Figure 13–6B presents the same data in the form of relative survival rates, or the ratio of observed to expected survival.* It is apparent that the women with breast cancer continue to be at considerably greater risk of death

---

*A person with one disease is still at risk of dying from other diseases. Since women with breast cancer tend to be of middle or older age, the risk of dying from other causes may be substantial. The relative survival rate provides an adjustment for competing causes of death.

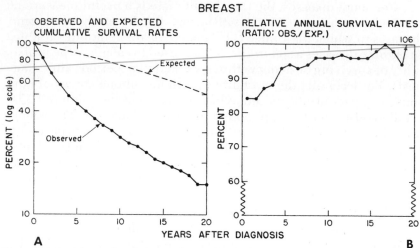

Figure 13–6 Observed and expected survival rates for 20 years of follow-up for patients with cancer of the breast diagnosed, Connecticut, 1935–1944. (From Cutler, S. J., Ederer, F., et al.: Survival of patients with breast cancer. J. Nat. Cancer Inst., 23:1146, 1959.)

than the general population of females for at least 15 years after initial diagnosis. (After 15 years the number of survivors is so small that the rates are unstable.)

The life table is a versatile tool. Life-table methodology has been applied not only to data on survival from chronic disease but also to such diverse processes as the success or failure of contraceptive practices and the probability of release from, or readmission to, a hospital for mental illness (Kramer et al., 1956; Bahn and Bodian, 1964).

When people are followed for unequal time periods because of loss of follow-up, migration, or late entry into the study, a technique known as the *modified cohort life table* is particularly useful. In this method each person is counted for the period during which he is actually observed and then dropped from subsequent computations. If only cases followed for the entire duration of the study were included, the sample size would be smaller and the standard error larger (Cutler and Ederer, 1958). Appendix 13–1 presents further details of the method and some illustrations.

SUMMARY

The aging of the population, largely owing to reduction in mortality from infectious disease, has increased the incidence and prevalence of chronic conditions. The absence of a known agent, multifactorial nature of etiology, long latent period, indefinite onset, and differential effect of factors at different stages of disease were noted to contribute to the difficulty of studying the etiology of chronic disease.

The two principal approaches for observational study, i.e., retrospective and prospective, were discussed from the standpoint of selection of study groups and analysis of results. The terms "relative risk" and "odds ratio" were introduced. The advantages and disadvantages of the two types of studies were compared. The method of historical prospective study was also presented. This method incorporates the advantages of both types of studies.

The final section of the chapter presented the methods of analyzing survivorship (prognosis) in chronic disease by use of the cohort life table.

COHORT LIFE TABLES (SURVIVORSHIP STUDIES)

The cohort life table is a method for studying outcomes of cases followed for long periods of time. It provides the probability that an event, such as death, will occur in successive intervals of time after diagnosis and, conversely, the probability of surviving each interval. The multiplication of these probabilities of survival for each time interval for those alive at the beginning of that interval yields a cumulative probability of surviving for the total period of study.

The *modified* form of the cohort life table is used for studies in which all subjects are not followed for equal lengths of time. The individuals who are followed for shorter periods may include persons lost to follow-up because of lack of cooperation or migration from the area, as well as those who entered the study after it was initiated. In the modified life table such individuals are included in the analysis during the period when they are observed and then dropped from subsequent calculations of interval probabilities.

This method, which makes maximum utilization of the available data, is unbiassed if (1) there is no change over calendar time in survival rates so that those who enter the study after it has begun experience the same survivorship as those who enter initially, and (2) those lost to follow-up actually experience the same subsequent survivorship as those who are followed. Because assumption (2) is often not true or cannot be tested, the ability to utilize life-table methods depends on high rates of follow-up.*

We will illustrate the modified life table first with a study of breast cancer in Philadelphia hospitals (Mausner et al., 1969). Table 13–6 is based on a 10 per cent random sample of the patients enrolled in a centralized register over a 12-year period. Each patient was classified by the number of years of follow-up since diagnosis and by most recently determined status. The life-table calculations are shown for the first five years after diagnosis. Columns 2 through 5, taken directly from the data, show the number alive at

---

*If a substantial proportion of the cohort is lost to follow-up, the method cannot be applied. Minimum and maximum estimates of survival, based on the assumptions that those lost to follow-up all die or all live, can help an investigator to make a judgment about the usefulness of the data.

TABLE 13-6 Life Table Showing Survival of 840 Patients with Initial Diagnosis of Breast Cancer, Philadelphia Hospitals, 1951–1964

(1) Year of Last Observation	(2) Alive at Beginning of Year	(3) Died During Year	(4) Lost to Follow-up	(5) Last Seen Alive During Year[*]	(6) Effective No. Exposed to Risk of Dying (Col. 2) − ½ (Cols. 4 + 5)	Of Those Alive at Beginning of Year:		
						(7) Proportion Dying During Year (Col. 3) ÷ (Col. 6)	(8) Proportion Surviving Year 1 − (Col. 7)	(9) Proportion Surviving from Diagnosis to End of Year ($p_1 \times p_2 \ldots$)
x	l_x	d_x	u_x	w_x	l'_x	q_x	p_x	P_x
0–1	840	93	2	2	838.0	0.111	0.889	0.889
1–2	743	93	—	63	711.5	0.131	0.869	0.773
2–3	587	55	—	67	554.5	0.099	0.901	0.696
3–4	465	55	—	42	445.0	0.124	0.876	0.610
4–5	368	25	—	32	353.0	0.071	0.929	0.567

[*]These patients entered the study late in its course and were therefore followed for less than five years.

the beginning of each year, (column 2), the number who died during each year, (column 3), the number lost to follow-up (column 4), and the number last seen alive during a follow-up year (i.e., follow-up incomplete because of late entry into the study) (column 5).

From this basic information several calculations were performed. It was assumed that each person seen for the last time during any year because of loss to follow-up or late entry, (columns 4 and 5), had been followed for exactly half a year. Thus, the effective number at risk of dying in the first year (column 6) equals the initial number, 840, minus one-half of the number lost or last seen that year, or $840 - (\frac{1}{2})(2 + 2) = 838$. The proportion dying in a year (column 7) is then calculated by dividing the number who died during that year of follow-up (column 3) by the effective number at risk (column 6). The proportion surviving during each year, (column 8) is obtained by subtracting the proportion dying during the year

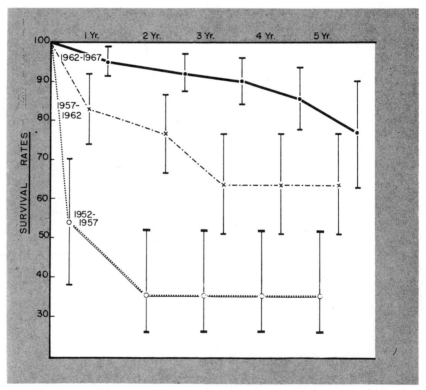

Figure 13–7 Cumulative survival rates and 95 per cent confidence limits (vertical lines) of patients with cystic fibrosis followed from first observation through intervals of one to five years during period of 1952–1957, 1957–1962, and 1962–1967. (From Huang, N. N., Macri, C. N., et al.: Survival of patients with cystic fibrosis. Am. J. Dis. Child., *120*:289, 1970.)

(column 7) from 1. The figures in column 8, therefore, represent the conditional probability of surviving until the next year for those who have already survived to the beginning of that year. The probability that the initial cohort will survive to a given year (column 9) (i.e., cumulative survival probability) is obtained by multiplying the successive annual probabilities in column 8. For example, the probability of surviving from time of diagnosis through year 2 is $0.889 \times 0.869 = 0.773$; the probability of survival from time of diagnosis through year 3 is $0.773 \times 0.901 = 0.696$, and so on.

The application of the modified life table to secular changes in survival can be seen in Figure 13–7. This figure shows cumulative survival rates for patients with cystic fibrosis in three successive five-year periods. The improvement in survival for the successive cohorts is impressive.

For a simple explanation of how the lifetable method can be applied to the study of survival of relatively small series of patients, the reader is referred to Axtell (1963).

STUDY QUESTIONS

13–1 Define the following terms and give an example when appropriate:

Chronic disease (page 307)
Retrospective (case-control) study (page 312)
Prospective (cohort) study (page 313)
Matching (page 315)
Relative risk (page 316)
Odds ratio (page 316)
Attributable risk (page 322)
Historical prospective study (page 325)
Cohort life table (page 329)
Modified cohort life table (page 330)

13–2 Retrospective and prospective study designs each have particular advantages and disadvantages. Contrast these two kinds of studies with respect to the following factors.

A. Cost
B. Time required for completion of the study
C. Size of study population
D. Usefulness for studying rare diseases
E. Problems in design
F. Problems in obtaining required information
G. Problems of bias
H. Nature of results

Answer on page 359.

13-3 On January 14, 1960, a one-day census of mental hospitals was carried out in 12 Caribbean islands. The report of this census noted:

When we examine the first admissions by length of stay, we find that 18 per cent . . . have been hospitalized under one year; 19 per cent between one and five years, and 63 per cent have been in hospital five years or longer. That is, the majority of first admissions are long-stay patients (Report on the Census of Mental Hospitals in the Caribbean, 1960).

    A. What kind of study was this — retrospective, prospective, or cross-sectional?

    B. Is the inference valid? If not, why not?

    C. What type of study would be necessary to answer questions about duration of stay in long-term hospitals?

Answer on page 360.

13-4 Classify each of the following studies as (1) prospective (cohort), (2) retrospective (case-control), (3) historical prospective, or (4) study of survivorship. Discuss the basis for each decision.

    A. Morbidity reports received by a county health department indicated that a number of young women who developed viral hepatitis after no known exposure to the disease had had their ears pierced during the preceding months. For comparison, a group of young women of similar age who attended a family planning clinic were also queried about recent ear piercing. It was found that 7 of the 48 women with hepatitis, but only 1 of the 100 women attending the family planning clinic, had had their ears pierced within the preceding seven months (Johnson et al., 1973).

    B. The records of over 8000 premenopausal women (55 years or younger) who had been admitted to two Boston hospitals between 1920 and 1940 for various types of pelvic surgery or cholecystectomy were studied in 1960 for evidence that breast cancer had developed in the interim. It was found that women who had undergone an artificial menopause (hysterectomy and bilateral oophorectomy) before age 40 had a lower risk of developing breast cancer in later life than women who had had a natural menopause (Feinleib, 1968).

    C. The authors report the course of 99 cases of systemic lupus erythematosus diagnosed at the Johns Hopkins University during the years 1949 through 1953. Life-table analysis was used to indicate status at specified years after diagnosis (Merrell and Shulman, 1955).

    D. Antenatal interviews with pregnant women during 1965 to 1968 included information on smoking history. Information on hospital admissions of the infants of these mothers was obtained from a record-linked file opened for each child at birth. The infants of mothers who smoked were found to have significantly more admissions for bronchitis and pneumonia than the infants of nonsmokers (Harlap and Davies, 1974).

Answer on page 360.

13–5 Evidence of an increased risk of lung cancer associated with cigarette smoking was sought by Doll and Hill in a series of studies.

1. In one study, 649 lung cancer cases were matched by age and sex to 649 controls; 647 of the cases and 622 of the controls had a history of smoking cigarettes (Doll and Hill, 1950).

2. In another study, the smoking habits of 34,445 male physicians were obtained by mailed questionnaries (Doll and Hill, 1964). Deaths among these physicians over the subsequent years were identified through contact with the office of the Registrar General. The death rates from lung cancer of these physicians classified by smoking habits were:

	Standardized Death Rates per 1000 Persons Aged 35 or More per Year
Nonsmokers	0.07
Cigarette Smokers (Current and Ex-smokers)	0.96

A. Name the type of study represented by (1) and (2).
B. Calculate the estimated relative risk or relative risk for smokers as compared with nonsmokers in each study.

Answer on page 360.

13–6 Figure 13–8 depicts the survival experience of a hypothetic cohort of newly diagnosed cancer cases.

A. Derive the median survival time from the graph.
B. If an individual survives the first year, what is the probability that he will survive for at least five years?
C. Compute the death rates for the initial cohort: (1) during the first year, (2) during the second year, and (3) during the first five years.
D. Compute the death rate during the second year for those who are still alive at the end of the first year.
E. Why is the death rate larger in D than in C(2)?

Answer on page 361.

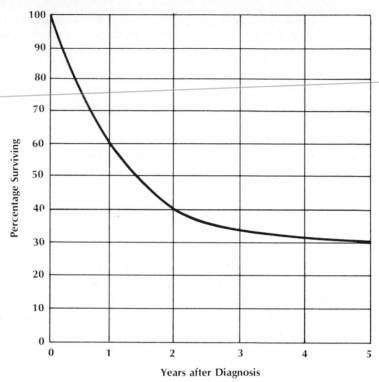

Figure 13–8 Survival experience of a hypothetic cohort of newly diagnosed cancer cases.

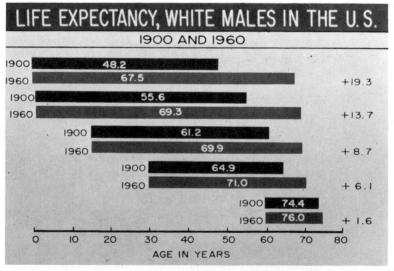

Figure 13–9 The change in life expectancy between 1900 and 1960 for white males. (Graph obtained through courtesy of Center for Disease Control, Atlanta, Ga.)

13–7 The change in life expectancy between 1900 and 1960 for white males is illustrated in Figure 13–9.

   A. What does the length of each bar represent?
   B. What does the number in each bar represent?
   C. Compare the change in life expectancy over the 60-year period at different ages.

Answer on page 362.

REFERENCES

Axtell, L. M.: Computing survival rates for chronic disease patients. A simple procedure. J.A.M.A., *186*:1125, 1963.

Bahn, A. K. and Bodian, C.: A life table method for studying recurrent episodes of illness or care. J. Chronic Dis., *17*:1019, 1964.

Berry, G., Newhouse, M. L., et al.: Combined effect of asbestos exposure and smoking on mortality from lung cancer in factory workers. Lancet, *2*:476, 1972.

Data of Cole, P. cited in MacMahon, B.: Chapter 1, Introduction: Concepts of multiple factors In Lee, D. H. K., and Kotin, P. (eds.), Multiple Factors in the Causation of Environmentally Induced Disease, Fogarty International Center Proceedings No. 12. Academic Press, New York and London, 1972.

Commission on Chronic Illness: Chronic illness in the United States, Vol. I. Harvard University Press, Cambridge, Mass., 1957.

Cornfield, J., and Haenszel, W.: Some aspects of retrospective studies. J. Chronic Dis., *11*:523, 1960.

Court-Brown, W. M., and Doll, R.: Mortality from cancer and other causes after radiotherapy for ankylosing spondylitis. Br. Med. J., *2*:1327, 1965.

Cutler, S. J., and Ederer, F.: Maximum utilization of the life table method in analyzing survival. J. Chronic Dis., *8*:659, 1958.

Doll, R., and Hill, A. B.: Smoking and carcinoma of the lung. Preliminary report. Br. Med. J., *2*:739, 1950.

Doll, R., and Hill, A. B.: Study of aetiology of carcinoma of lung. Br. Med. J., *2*:1271, 1952.

Doll, R., and Hill, A. B.: Lung cancer and other causes of death in relation to smoking. A second report on the mortality of British doctors. Br. Med. J., *2*:1071, 1956.

Doll, R., and Hill, A. B.: Mortality in relation to smoking. Ten years' observations of British doctors. Br. Med. J., *1*:1399, 1964.

Feinleib, M.: Breast cancer and artificial menopause: A cohort study. J. Natl. Cancer Inst., *41*:315, 1968.

Gregg, N. M.: Congenital cataract following German measles in the mother. Trans. Aust. Coll. Ophthalmol., *3*:35, 1941.

Harlap, S., and Davies, A. M.: Infant admissions to hospital and maternal smoking. Lancet, *1*:529, 1974.

Herbst, A. L., Ulfedler, H., et al.: Association of maternal stilbestrol therapy with tumor appearance in young women. N. Engl. J. Med., *284*:878, 1971.

Jick, H., Miettinen, O. S., et al.: Coffee and myocardial infarction. N. Engl. J. Med., *289*:63, 1973.

Johnson, C. J., Anderson, A., et al.: Paper presented to the Epidemiological Section at the Annual Meeting of the American Public Health Association, 1973.

Kannel, W. B., and Dawber, T. R.: Coffee and coronary disease (editorial). N. Engl. J. Med., *289*:100, 1973.

Kramer, M., Goldstein, H., et al.: Applications of life table methodology to the study of mental hospital populations. Psychiatric Research Reports No. 5. Am. Psych. Association, Washington, D.C., 1956.

Kuller, L.: Sudden death in arteriosclerotic heart disease; The case for preventive medicine. Am. J. Cardiol., 24:617, 1969.

Leviton, A.: Definitions of attributable risk. Am. J. Epidemiol., 98:231, 1973.

Lilienfeld, A. M.: Epidemiology of infectious and non-infectious disease: Some comparisons. Am. J. Epidemiol., 97:135, 1973.

Linden, G.: The influence of social class in the survival of cancer patients. Am. J. Public Health, 59:267, 1969.

Lundin, F. E., Lloyd, J. W., et al.: Mortality of uranium miners in relation to radiation exposure, hard-rock mining and cigarette smoking—1950 through September 1967. Health Phys., 16:571, 1969.

Mantel, N., and Haenszel, W.: Statistical aspects of the analysis of data from retrospective studies of disease. J. Natl. Cancer Inst., 22:719, 1959.

Mausner, J. S., Shimkin, M. B., et al.: Cancer of the breast in Philadelphia hospitals 1951–1964. Cancer, 12:260, 1969.

Merrell, M., and Shulman, L. E.: Determination of prognosis in chronic disease, illustrated by systemic lupus erythematosus. J. Chronic Dis., 1:12, 1955.

Miettinen, O. S.: Matching and design efficiency in retrospective studies. Am. J. Epidemiol., 91:111, 1970.

Moore, G. E.: How to achieve surgical results by really trying. Surg. Gynecol. Obstet., 116:497, 1963.

Paffenbarger, R. S., Jr., and Asnes, D. P.: Chronic disease in former college students. III. Precursors of suicide in early and middle life. Am. J. Public Health, 56:962, 1966a.

Paffenbarger, R. S., Jr., Notkin, J., et al.: Chronic disease in former college students. II. Methods of study and observations on mortality from coronary heart disease. Am. J. Public Health, 56:962, 1966b.

Paffenbarger, R. S., Jr., and Williams, J. L.: Chronic disease in former college students. V. Early precursors of fatal stroke. Am. J. Public Health, 57:1290, 1967.

Pike, M. C., and Morrow, R. H.: Statistical analysis of patient control studies in epidemiology. Factor under investigation an all-or-none variable. Br. J. Prev. Soc. Med., 24:42, 1970.

Report on the Census of Mental Hospitals in the Caribbean. Research Institute for the Study of Man, New York, 1960.

Sartwell, P. E.: Oral contraceptives and thromboembolism: A further report. Am. J. Epidemiol., 94:192, 1971.

Vianna, N. J., Greenwald, P., et al.: Tonsillectomy and Hodgkin's disease: The lymphoid tissue barrier. Lancet, 1:431, 1971.

Wynder, E. L., and Graham, E. A.: Tobacco smoking as a possible etiologic factor in bronchiogenic carcinoma. A study of six hundred and eighty-four proved cases. J.A.M.A., 143:329, 1950.

ANSWERS TO STUDY QUESTIONS

Answer to 1–2

The error in analysis here is an example of a common mistake. Raw frequency has been used instead of rate. To determine the relation of age to the probability of having an accident, one must relate the cases to the population at risk. In this problem the appropriate denominator, or population at risk, would be the number of patient-days in each age category. Therefore, one would calculate the following rate for each age group:

$$\frac{\text{Number of accidents among persons in a given age group}}{\text{Number of patient-days among persons in that age group}} \text{ per unit time}$$

Answer to 1–3

	Clinical Approach	Epidemiologic Approach
Prevention	Genetic counselling of parents	Studies to identify causes of mental retardation
	Use of immune globulin in Rh-negative women	Programs to provide care for women with high-risk pregnancies
	Testing of infants for PKU	Elimination of lead, other toxins, and infectious agents from the environment
	Amniocentesis	
		Screening of children for lead poisoning

Identification (Diagnosis)	Family history	Case-finding in schools
	History of pregnancy	Epidemiologic studies— to assess magnitude of problem (descriptive) and to search for causal factors (analytic)
	History of delivery	
	Physical examination of child, including developmental screening	
	Laboratory studies, including chromosomal analysis	
Management	Diet, e.g., for PKU	Planning of programs for care: day care centers schools sheltered workshops
	Decision about placement—home vs. institutional care	
		Establishment of facilities
		Development of training programs for personnel
		Setting standards for training and facilities
		Evaluation of programs and facilities

Answer to 1–4

    A. Primary
    B. Secondary
    C. Primary
    D. Primary
    E. Secondary
    F. Tertiary

Answer to 1–5

PRIMARY PREVENTION—Applicable to the total population.

1. Education of the general public regarding the hazards of smoking and need for prompt treatment of respiratory infection. Pulmonary infections render the individual more susceptible to permanent damage of lung tissues.

2. Environmental control programs to reduce urban air pollution and industrial exposures to dust and fumes.

SECONDARY PREVENTION—applicable to those at high risk (detection) and those known to have emphysema (prompt treatment and avoidance of further insults).

1. Screening of high-risk population groups (e.g., urban, adult males who are cigarette smokers or exposed to fumes in certain industries) by symptoms, chest x-rays, and pulmonary function tests.

2. Cessation of cigarette smoking; avoidance of exposure to excessively hot or cold air, to airborne allergens, and to urban air pollution whenever possible. Change from occupations which involve the inhalation of dust and fumes. Encouragement of yearly immunization against influenza.

3. Treatment with appropriate antibiotics, expectorants, drugs which aid in dilatation of bronchioles, breathing exercises, and so on.

TERTIARY PREVENTION—applicable to patients with advanced obstructive pulmonary disease.

Specialized treatment at pulmonary rehabilitation centers and use of assistive, mechanical breathing devices.

For a further reference see Witorsch, P.: Chronic obstructive lung disease. Am. Fam. Physician, 7:87, 1973.

Answer to 2-2

No. The greater number of reported cases of measles (almost 100-fold difference) can be attributed largely to the difference in the spectrums of these two organisms. Most infections with measles virus lead to readily diagnosable cases, whereas most infections with poliovirus are inapparent. Serologic surveys have shown that people with no prior history of poliomyelitis can have protective antibodies and, therefore, must have been infected in the past.

Answer to 2-3

A. The following outline is based on the model of the wheel (page 35).

HOST FACTORS

Age and driving experience: crash rates are high for young, new drivers.

Sex: crash rates are much higher for males than females.

Drinking habits: half of the approximately 60,000 annual highway fatalities are related to excessive alcohol use, especially problem drinking.

Senility and medical conditions which might impair ability to drive.

Personality factors such as risk-taking tendencies and antisocial behavior.

SOCIAL ENVIRONMENT (SOCIOCULTURAL-POLITICAL FACTORS)

Cultural attitudes toward products such as motorcycles, often reinforced by advertising.

State and local policies controlling such matters as licensing and reexamination of drivers, speed limits, and sanctions against violators of traffic ordinances.*

Federal regulations governing safety features in vehicles.

Organization of emergency services.

Mandatory inspection of vehicles.

Programs for driver education.

PHYSICAL ENVIRONMENT†

Vehicle factors that influence the likelihood of crashes (i.e., pre-crash): speed potential, brake and steering failure, limitations of the driver's visual field.

Vehicle factors that determine the probability and severity of injury in a crash: speed potential, door latches, restraint systems, padded dashboards, energy-absorbing steering wheels and bumpers.

Vehicle factors that affect postcrash rescue: likelihood of fire, tendency of doors to jam.

Highway design: adequate visibility, surfaces that reduce skidding, separation of streams of traffic; guardrails with buried ends, breakaway signposts.

Weather, especially fog, rain, and ice.

BIOLOGICAL ENVIRONMENT

Animals on the road.

Pets and insects in the car.

Actions of other drivers and pedestrians (may also be classified under social environment).

B. From the above listing, it is clear that intervention may be directed at either host or environment. Until recently, emphasis has been on the host, with attempts (largely unsuccessful) to prevent crashes by modifying driving behavior, for instance, through driver education and sanctions relating to alcohol usage.

However, failure to achieve a major impact on injury and death rates by educational and regulatory approaches has led to a focus on modification of the physical environment. Improvements in vehicle and road design reduce the burden for the driver, who would otherwise have to compensate for any inadequacies in vehicles, highways, or other drivers. Protective devices (e.g., airbags) that reduce the contribution individuals must make to their own safety are the most likely to be effective.

For a summary of current thinking about injury control, Baker‡ may be consulted. In addition, papers by Haddon§ are particularly helpful.

---

*Klein, D., and Waller, J. A.: Causation, Culpability and Deterrence in Highway Crashes, U.S. Dept. of Transportation, U.S. Govt. Printing Office, Washington, D.C., 1970.

†The etiologic agent of injury in motor vehicle crashes is mechanical energy. Recognition of the agent is essential to understanding the importance of the physical environment.

‡Baker, S. P.: Injury control. In Sartwell, P. E., Preventive Medicine and Public Health, 10th ed, Maxcy, K. F., and Rosenau, M. J. (eds.). Appleton-Century-Crofts, 1973.

§Haddon, W., Jr.: The changing approach to the epidemiology, prevention and amelioration of trauma: The transition to approaches etiologically rather than descriptively based. Am. J. Public Health, 58:1431, 1968; Haddon, W., Jr.: Energy damage and the ten countermeasure strategies. J. Trauma, *13*:321, 1973.

Answer to 3–2

A. The high suicide rate among elderly white males is striking. It is important for physicians and other health workers to be aware that this is a high risk group for completed suicide. Males make fewer suicidal gestures than females, or it may be that their threats are more subtle.

B. Relevant factors other than age, sex, and color include marital and family conditions, socioeconomic status, area of residence, and psychiatric history.

High suicide rates have been reported for young widowers and widows, especially the former, and for older divorcees.* Persons who suffer a major bereavement (death of spouse or other close relative, marital separation) are at particular risk for a period of some months after the event. Mental health programs such as crisis intervention provide an approach to this problem.

Gardner et al.† found that many elderly, white male suicides had been socially isolated persons living in low socioeconomic areas of a city. A high proportion had been alcoholic; many had recently been treated for depression or other psychiatric disorder. Appreciation of these risk factors can help to identify suicide-prone patients.

Answer to 4–2‡

A. Males: 1930 – stomach, 1968 – lung. Females: 1930 – uterus; 1968 – breast.

B. (1) decreasing, (2) stationary, (3) decreasing, (4) increasing, (5) stationary.

Answer to 4–3

A. The graph portrays a **secular** trend. The mortality rates from rheumatic fever and chorea were relatively steady in the 1920's. Starting about 1930, there was a downward trend whose slope became even steeper after 1950.

B. A decline in mortality rates may reflect a decrease in the rate of occurrence of a disease, an improvement in survival, or both. In the current problem, both could contribute to the drop in death rates. The downward trend in mortality from rheumatic fever and chorea parallels a decrease in incidence and severity of other manifestations of streptococcal infection as well. Since the decline antedates the introduction of sulfonamides and antibiotics, other factors must be responsible. Improvement in environmental factors such as improved nutrition and lessened overcrowding

---

*Kramer, M., Pollack, E. S., et al.: Mental Disorders/Suicide. Harvard University Press, Cambridge, Mass., 1972.

†Gardner, E. A., Bahn, A. K., et al.: Suicide and psychiatric care in the aging. Arch. Gen. Psychiatry, 10:547, 1964.

‡Answers are based on the data displayed in Figures 4–7 and 4–8.

could have contributed to the decline. After 1950, the use of sulfonamides and later of antibiotics probably accounts for the more rapid drop in rates.

C. (1) A logarithmic scale shows a trend in terms of relative or percentage change over time. A straight line on this scale therefore indicates a constant percentage decrease from one time period to another. (In Figure 4–11, note the almost straight downward slope from 1930 to the early 1950's and the still steeper linear decline thereafter.) In contrast, a straight line on an arithmetic scale indicates a constant (absolute) amount of change.

(2) A logarithmic scale can depict in one graph a marked change in magnitude of rates. The 100-fold decline in death rate from rheumatic fever between 1921 and 1966, from about 10 to 0.1 per 100,000, would be difficult to show on an arithmetic scale.

Answer to 4–4

A. This question can be answered by inspection of the graph, since the slope of the line on a semi-logarithmic scale reflects percentage (relative) change. However, calculation of percentage change helps to confirm the visual impression. Percentage change is defined as the amount of change during a time period divided by the initial value $\times 100$. For example, for males during T_1 the percentage change in lung cancer mortality rate was $\dfrac{23.4 - 13.0}{13.0} = \dfrac{10.4}{13} = 80$ per cent.

	T_1	T_2
Males	$\dfrac{10.4}{13} = 80$ per cent	$\dfrac{7.4}{33.7} = 22$ per cent
Females	$\dfrac{1}{3.5} = 29$ per cent	$\dfrac{1.7}{4.7} = 36.2$ per cent

There is a difference in trend for the two sexes. The percentage increase was higher for males than females during T_1; but higher for females during T_2, even though their actual mortality rate from lung cancer was still lower at the end of T_2.

B. No, the change in the size of the population is not responsible. Rates refer not to number of deaths but rather to number of deaths *per unit population*. In addition, change in rates cannot be ascribed to differences in the age composition over time since the rates are age-adjusted.

C. (1) A change in diagnostic criteria or diagnostic accuracy;

(2) A true increase in incidence of lung cancer or case fatality rate or both.

Answer to 5–2

The rates as given do not prove a causal relation between climate and bronchopulmonary disease. Several factors might produce regional differences in death rates from such conditions:

1. Differences among states in demographic composition. It would be

necessary to adjust for differences in age, and possibly also color, to permit valid comparisons.

2. There may well be differences in diagnostic practices.

3. Persons with chronic respiratory disease may be attracted to hot, dry areas of the country. In fact, selective migration of persons with chronic respiratory disease into these areas is a likely explanation of the high death rates in the Southwest.

Answer to 5–3

The higher death rate from lung cancer among recent ex-smokers (one pack or more per day) than among current smokers can probably be explained by selection. Many of those who had recently given up smoking probably did so because of symptoms. This illustrates the dangers of comparing groups of persons, such as current vs. ex-smokers, without knowing whether the groups are comparable in other respects (e.g., health status).

It is noteworthy that, for heavy smokers as well as for light smokers, death rates from lung cancer decrease with increasing duration of abstinence from smoking.

Answer to 6–2

A. Only the placebo control study conforms to commonly accepted standards for a scientific trial. Volunteers were randomized between vaccine and placebo groups, and double-blind procedures were used. In contrast, the observed control study, which did not use blind techniques, was subject to bias. Everyone—physicians, school personnel, parents—knew which children had received vaccine. This is not a crucial problem if one is studying only severe manifestations of disease, such as paralysis or death, but is important when a high proportion of infections are mild.

Both trials showed a high degree of efficacy of the vaccine, with about three times as many cases among those given placebo as among those given vaccine. Thus, the two study plans led to similar results. However, with a less effective vaccine, a poor research design might lead to incorrect conclusions.

B. Counterbalancing the weaknesses indicated above is the fact that the observed control study was much simpler to administer since it did not entail randomization, use of code numbers, or administration of placebo. Its simplicity was probably the reason for its adoption by the National Foundation.

Answer to 7–2

A. $\dfrac{4 \text{ (cases 1, 2, 3, 6)}}{300}$

B. $\dfrac{2 \text{ (cases 4 and 5)}}{296}$

Recurrent cases such as three are excluded from the numerator; denominator excludes cases one, two, three, and six since those persons are not at risk of acquiring new disease.

C. $\dfrac{6 \text{ (all cases)}}{300}$

Case three which had two episodes during the year is counted only once in the numerator and once in the denominator.

Answer to 7–3

A. The fact that the population of the United States is larger than that of Guyana cannot explain a difference in rates since the death rate refers to number of deaths **per 1000 persons.**

B. (1) Age-specific death rates are lower in Guyana than in the United States.

(2) Age-specific death rates are the same or higher in Guyana, but the population in Guyana is younger. High age-specific death rates in the first decades of life, typical of developing countries, can lead to a relatively young population. Thus, paradoxically, the crude death rate in developing countries can be low, despite high age-specific death rates, because of the small proportion of elderly persons.

C. The high crude birth and infant mortality rates in Guyana are compatible with the second explanation above, i.e., that there is a relatively high proportion of young people in Guyana. The rates are typical of those found in developing countries.

Answer to 7–4

Age-adjusted rates.

Crude death rates reflect not only age-specific death rates but also the age composition of the population. Since Chile, like Guyana (study question 7–3), has a younger population than the United States, age-adjusted (standardized) rates are needed for comparing the risk of death from heart disease in the two countries. When the differences in age composition are "removed" by standardization, the death rate from heart disease in the United States is only 2.3 times that of Chile, rather than 4.7.

Answer to 7–5

A. Yes. Because the incidence rate indicates the rate at which individuals who are at risk develop a disease during a specified time period, it is necessary to determine (1) the number of new cases that occur during the period, and (2) the number of persons who did not have the disease at the beginning of the period and therefore were at risk of developing it. Prevalence survey one permitted identification of the persons initially free of active tuberculosis, i.e., the denominator of the incidence rate. Prevalence surveys two and three indicated which of these persons became new cases, i.e., formed the numerator for the incidence rate.

B. The rates are expressed in person-years because all of the "nega tives" at survey one were not examined at uniform intervals thereafter. Some were examined in survey two, some in survey three, others in both two and three. Since the period of observation was not the same for all, the incidence rates are based on the number of years of observation for each person, summed for all the persons in the study.

Answer to 7–6

Table 7–11 shows that the incidence rate was ten times higher among persons whose household included a culture-positive case than in either culture-negative or no-case households. This indicates where case-finding efforts should be focussed (i.e., among contacts of sputum-positive active cases). Since health dollars are limited in India and other countries, it is particularly important to allocate resources efficiently.

Answer to 7–7

A. Incidence and prevalence are related through duration of disease ($P \sim I \times d$). Duration is affected by cure or death. One cannot tell from the data given which of these two factors is more important. However, the sex difference in prevalence is certainly affected by relative case fatality.

The case fatality rate was very high (overall it was more than 100 per 1000 per year). Further, case fatality rates were markedly higher for females than for males at most ages, with the disparity greatest at ages 15 to 24. Therefore, the disease ran a more protracted course in males who thus had a higher prevalence despite the greater incidence in females.

The very high incidence and case fatality rates for young women sug gest that childbearing or child rearing or both in this population were as sociated with increased risks of both acquiring the disease and experienc ing a fatal outcome.

B. It is apparent from Figure 7–5 that prevalence rates can give a mis leading impression of the relative risk of acquiring a disease for various subgroups of the population. Incidence rates are needed for this purpose.

Answer to 7–8

A. The population of 1940 must have been used as the standard, since crude and adjusted rates were the same for that year. When the age-specific rates for any year are applied to the population of that same year, the resultant age-adjusted death rate is identical to the crude rate.

B. (1) Age-adjusted death rate; (2) crude death rate.

Since 1900, there has been a decline in age-specific death rates, especially in the early years of life. This, coupled with a decline in birth rates, has led to a gradual "aging" of the population. Since the population of 1940 is older than that of 1900, the crude rate (which is based on the 1900 age distribution) is lower than the age-adjusted rate (which is based on the 1940 age distribution).

C. In the past few decades, the increasing proportion of elderly persons in the population has counterbalanced the continued fall in age-specific death rates. The crude death rate has, therefore, remained stationary. In contrast, since secular changes in age-adjusted rates reflect only age-specific rates (and not age composition of the population), the age-adjusted death rate has continued to fall. Thus, just as age-adjustment is necessary for comparing the force of mortality in different countries at a point in time, it is also necessary for comparing mortality in the same country over a period of years because of changes in age composition.

Answer to 8–2

A. Death certificates. Since cancer of the pancreas is a rapidly fatal disease, death certificates provide an adequate reflection of incidence.

B. Household surveys. Since most cases do not require hospitalization or continuous outpatient treatment, household surveys, such as the home interviews carried out as part of the National Health Survey, can provide some information on the prevalence of arthritis. For better delineation of specific types of arthritis, interview data must be supplemented by physical examination and laboratory studies.

C. Reports from pathology laboratories (in hospital and elsewhere). Since the case fatality rate for most forms of skin cancer is very low, death certificates would be a poor source of information on incidence. So would hospital records, since diagnosis and treatment of skin cancer are usually done on an outpatient basis. Therefore, the single best source of routinely recorded information would be the files of pathologists. A certain number of cases would be missed, however, since treatment may be carried out without pathologic confirmation of the diagnosis.

D. Death certificates (and records from cancer registers). Acute leukemia is primarily a disease of children. Since all cases would probably be hospitalized at some time during the course of illness, hospital records would provide the most complete count of cases. However, unless the area were covered by a population-based cancer register, death certificates would be the most readily available source of information. These should provide an adequate measure of incidence since survival rates remain low despite recent improvement due to multiple drug therapy.

E. Pathology reports. Unlike acute leukemia, chronic lymphocytic leukemia is principally a disease of older persons. It tends to run an indolent course and is often diagnosed when the patient presents to the physician with some unrelated complaint. Diagnosis is made from pathologic specimens.

F. Morbidity reports to the health department. Meningococcal meningitis forms one end of a spectrum of infection from the meningococcus, which ranges from inapparent infection to severe disease. Diagnosis of meningitis is made by microscopic examination and culture of the cerebrospinal fluid. Most cases probably are reported to the health department by the physician or hospital or both.

G. Tumor registers. Registers of cancers diagnosed and treated are maintained in each accredited hospital. However, many registers are of limited value because of selective factors influencing admission or inadequate follow-up of all cases. Nationwide information on survival for various types of cancer is available from the End Results Group, described on page 177.

H. The local health department. Each local health department is responsible for maintaining a register of all newly diagnosed cases of active tuberculosis reported to it. The department also maintains a follow-up system on those cases it supervises, but not those under the supervision of private physicians. Although the local health department provides reports to the state health department, the local agency would have more detailed information on the current status of its patients.

I. The answer to this question depends upon the severity of mental retardation of the children. If severe, the child would be in an institution for the mentally retarded. Some children with moderate retardation may be living at home. Those with mild retardation may not be diagnosed until school years; school records, including records from schools for exceptional children, would be the best source of information about such cases. Those with physical as well as mental handicaps may also be located on a crippled children's register in the state health department.

Answer 9–2

A. $\dfrac{\text{Live births}}{\text{Population}} \times 1000 = \dfrac{2000}{80,000} \times 1000 = 25.0 \text{ per } 1000$

B. $\dfrac{\text{Total deaths}}{\text{Midyear population}} \times 100,000 = \dfrac{648}{80,000} \times 1000 = 8.1 \text{ per } 1000$

C. $\dfrac{\text{Deaths under 1 year}}{\text{Live births}} \times 1000 = \dfrac{42}{2000} \times 1000 = 21.0 \text{ per } 1000$

D. $\dfrac{\text{Fetal deaths}}{\text{Live births}} \times 1000 = \dfrac{32}{2000} \times 1000 = 16.0 \text{ per } 1000$

E. $\dfrac{\text{Maternal deaths}}{\text{Live births}} \times 100,000 = \dfrac{1}{2000} \times 100,000 = 50.0 \text{ per } 100,000$

F. $\dfrac{\text{Deaths 45 and over}}{\text{Population 45 and over}} \times 1000 = \dfrac{300}{20,000} \times 1000 = 15.0 \text{ per } 1000$

G. (1) $\dfrac{\text{Deaths from heart disease}}{\text{Population 45 and over}} \times 100,000$

$= \dfrac{98}{20,000} \times 100,000 = 490.0 \text{ per } 100,000$

(2) $\dfrac{\text{Deaths from cancer}}{\text{Population 45 and over}} \times 100,000$

$= \dfrac{60}{20,000} \times 100,000 = 300.0 \text{ per } 100,000$

H. (1) $\dfrac{\text{Deaths from cancer}}{\text{All deaths}} \times 100 = \dfrac{60}{300} \times 100 = 20 \text{ per cent}$

(2) $\dfrac{\text{Deaths from stroke}}{\text{All deaths}} \times 100 = \dfrac{48}{300} \times 100 = 16 \text{ per cent}$

Answer to 9–3

No, one cannot conclude from these data that the risk of death from cancer is greater in the older age group. These figures refer only to the contribution cancer makes to total deaths in each of the two age groups. Proportionate mortality ratios can be misleading. One would have to examine the cause (cancer) specific death rate for the two groups to determine the relative risk.

Answer to 9–4

An infant death rate based on a census count would tend to overstate greatly the probability of an infant death. Because of the relatively high force of mortality early in the first year of life, the population of infants (age 0 to 12 months) at a point in time is appreciably lower than the true population at risk (i.e., the cohort of live births). In addition, infants are grossly underenumerated in the census.

Answer to 9–5

The increase in legal abortions has been followed by declines in all of the indices of health listed, except for the crude death rate. This measure has remained stable because most deaths occur among the elderly. It is difficult to determine the exact contribution of legal abortion to the changes in the other health indices, since other factors (i.e., widespread use of effective contraception, improved prenatal and neonatal care, and reduction in the number of illegal abortions) also play a role. Nevertheless, several recent trends are probably related, at least in part, to the increased availability of legal abortion.

The decline in infant mortality rate has been most pronounced for the neonatal period, and reflects a marked reduction in the proportion of low-birth-weight babies. The fall in maternal mortality has also been substantial. The improvement may be ascribed in part to the large proportion of legal abortions performed on young girls, a group at high risk of maternal death (Figure 9–5). Another group which has benefited from the opportunity for legal abortion has been women of high parity.

It should be noted that the current figures understate the decline in maternal mortality. Because of the way maternal mortality is defined, any deaths related to abortion are counted in the numerator of the rate, but the abortions do not contribute to the denominator, which consists only of live births. If abortions contributed to both numerator and denominator, as they should, then the current figures for maternal mortality would be even lower.

For further information on the effects of liberalized abortion laws, see Pakter, J., O'Hare, D., et al.: Two years experience in New York City with the liberalized abortion law — Progress and problems. Am. J. Public Health, 63:524, 1973.

Answers to 9–6

For all the countries shown in the table (except India), females have a higher life expectancy than males. In the United States, there has been a trend toward an increasing gap in life expectancy between the males and females, from approximately three years in 1900 to more than seven years now. Death rates are higher for males than females for many common causes of death, as shown in Table 3–1.

Answer to 9–7

Life expectancy is higher at one year of age than at birth because the infant mortality rate is greater than the death rate in subsequent childhood years. Therefore, a child's chances of survival to adulthood are appreciably greater after the first year of life than at birth.

Answer to 10–2

The four successive pyramids for Germany over a 40-year period demonstrate usefulness of population pyramids for following birth cohorts, or groups of people born in the same year. At successive points in time, each cohort appears at an older age.

The 1910 pyramid is a fairly regular triangle, typical of a population with steady high birth and death rates over a long period of time.

The striking features of the pyramid 15 years later (1925) are: (1) a marked constriction around the age of approximately ten years, and (2) a relative deficit at approximately 25 to 40 years of age. Both findings can be attributed to World War 1. The relative lack of ten year olds is due to the small number of births during the war, the paucity of adult males to loss of fighting men.

In the pyramid of 1939, both features noted above persist. However, each of them appears at a later age. That is, the waist-like constriction has moved from age 10 to a little past age 20, and the relative paucity of men has moved upwards from ages 25 to 40 toward 40 to 55. In addition, there is a small constriction opposite ages five and six representing fewer births and, possibly, increased mortality among infants and young children, during the economic depression of the early 1930's. The decrease in births is probably due to low birth rates as well as to the paucity of young adults of reproductive age.

The final pyramid (1950) continues to show all of the previous trends, but at successively later ages. Additional irregularities below age ten suggest marked fluctuations in the birth rates during the years immediately preceding the date of the pyramid. The large proportion of ten year olds may reflect pronatalist Nazi policies in the early years of World War II. The smaller percentage of children at about five years of age is due to the lowered birth rates consequent upon the continued prosecution of the war and the collapse of the Third Reich. Note also that by 1950 the shape of the pyramid is approaching the rectangular configuration characteristic of a developed country.

Answer to 10–3

A. The first step in answering this question is to determine the percentages of the white and nonwhite populations in each of the three age groups:

Whites	Male	Female	Both Sexes
0–19	16.2	16.0	32.2
20–64	27.8	30.7	58.5
65 and over	3.5	5.8	9.3
			100.0

Nonwhites	Male	Female	Both Sexes
0–19	20.5	20.3	40.8
20–64	26.1	30.5	56.6
65 and over	1.0	1.5	2.5
			99.9

Dependency Ratios	White	Nonwhite
Youth	$\frac{32.2}{58.5} \times 100 = 55.0$ per cent	$\frac{40.8}{56.6} \times 100 = 72.1$ per cent
Old Age	$\frac{9.3}{58.5} \times 100 = 15.9$ per cent	$\frac{2.5}{56.6} \times 100 = 4.4$ per cent
Total	$\frac{41.5}{58.5} \times 100 = 70.9$ per cent	$\frac{43.3}{56.6} \times 100 = 76.5$ per cent

The youth dependency ratio is considerably higher for nonwhites than for whites, while that for elderly dependent persons is higher among whites. In this particular example, these two components of the dependency ratio tend to cancel each other out. That is, the overall dependency ratio is only slightly higher for nonwhites (76.5 per cent) than for whites (70.9 per cent).

B. It is obvious that the needs of the nonwhite population center heavily on services for young children and their parents (i.e., day care, well-baby, youth, and family planning services). In contrast, services for the white population should focus to a greater extent on geriatric needs (i.e., convalescent and rehabilitative facilities, meals on wheels, home-nursing care, and home-health aides) and on programs for detection and prevention of chronic illness. Examples would be cancer screening, monitoring of blood pressure, ready availability of primary care, and so on.

C. Additional types of information valuable for planning health and related services include: household composition, family size and structure, ethnic membership, condition of housing, poverty level, community instability, and style of life.

These indices, their derivation from the census, and the general uses of a demographic profile for estimating health needs of an area are well presented in Rosen, B. M.: A model for estimating mental health needs using 1970 census socioeconomic data, NIMH Mental Health Statistics, Methodology Reports, Series C9. Dept of Health, Education, and Welfare Pub. No. 74–63, U.S. Govt. Printing Office, Washington, D.C., 1974.

Answer to 10–4

A. (5)
B. (3)

Answer to 11–2

A. The first step is to set up a fourfold table and, from the information given, calculate the figures for the missing cells and marginal totals.

		Disease State		
		Present	Absent	Total
	Positive	50	15	65
Test Result	Negative	10	405	415
	Total	60	420	480

It is then relatively easy to calculate the needed values:

(1) $\qquad \frac{50}{60} \times 100 = 83.3$ per cent

(2) $\qquad \frac{405}{420} \times 100 = 96.4$ per cent

(3) $\qquad \frac{15}{420} \times 100 = 3.6$ per cent

(4) $\qquad \frac{10}{60} \times 100 = 16.7$ per cent

(5) $\qquad \frac{60}{480} \times 100 = 12.5$ per cent

(6) $\qquad \frac{50}{65} \times 100 = 76.9$ per cent

(7) $\qquad \frac{405}{415} \times 100 = 97.6$ per cent

B. With the higher prevalence rate the number of diseased persons in the population increases to 20 per cent × 480 = 96. Applying the same sensitivity and specificity values given above, the remainder of the fourfold table can be derived. For example, true positives = 83.3 per cent × 96 = 80, and so on.

		Disease State		
		Present	Absent	Total
	Positive	80	14	94
Test Result	Negative	16	370	386
	Total	96	384	480

The predictive value of a positive test is now higher, 80/94 or 85 per cent, as compared with 77 per cent at the lower prevalence rate.

Answer to 11–3

A. To answer this question calculate the complement of the sensitivity and specificity values:

	Test A	Test B
Percentage False Negatives	30	20
Percentage False Positives	5	10

It is apparent that Test A produces a higher percentage of false negatives, and Test B a higher percentage of false positives.

B. This example illustrates that sensitivity and specificity are usually inversely related and, therefore, that one may be increased only at the expense of the other.

Answer to 11–4

A. DOPPLER ULTRASOUND

$$\text{Sensitivity: } \frac{63}{83} = 75.9 \text{ per cent}$$

$$\text{Specificity: } \frac{150}{165} = 90.9 \text{ per cent}$$

CLINICAL EXAMINATION

$$\text{Sensitivity: } \frac{45}{83} = 54.2 \text{ per cent}$$

$$\text{Specificity: } \frac{106}{165} = 64.2 \text{ per cent}$$

It is thus apparent that Doppler examination is both more sensitive and more specific than clinical examination.

B. SENSITIVITY

Combination in parallel:

$$\frac{\text{Number positive on either test}}{\text{Number diseased}} = \frac{35 + 10 + 28}{83} = \frac{73}{83} = 88.0 \text{ per cent}$$

Combination in series:

$$\frac{\text{Number positive on both tests}}{\text{Number diseased}} = \frac{35}{83} = 42.2 \text{ per cent}$$

Thus, combination in parallel increases sensitivity (88.0 per cent vs. 75.9 per cent for Doppler ultrasound alone) while combination in series decreases sensitivity (42.2 per cent). For further information on this study, see Sigel, B., Popky, G. L., et al.: Evaluation of Doppler ultrasound examination. Arch. Surg., *100*:535, 1970.

Answer to 12–2

A. $\frac{72}{300} \times 100 = 24.0$ per cent

B. $\frac{20}{92} \times 100 = 21.7$ per cent

C. (1) $\frac{15}{(300 - 25)} \times 100 = \frac{15}{275} \times 100 = 5.4$ per cent

(2) $\frac{(12 + 15)}{300} \times 100 = \frac{27}{300} \times 100 = 9.0$ per cent

(3) $\frac{(12 + 8)}{300} \times 100 = \frac{20}{300} \times 100 = 6.7$ per cent

D. First week: $\frac{4}{35} \times 100 = 11.4$ per cent

Second week: $\frac{4}{(35 - 4)} \times 100 = \frac{4}{31} \times 100 = 12.9$ per cent

Third week: $\frac{1}{(31 - 4)} \times 100 = \frac{1}{27} \times 100 = 3.7$ per cent

Fourth week: $\frac{1}{(27 - 1)} \times 100 = \frac{1}{26} \times 100 = 3.8$ per cent

Note that the persons known to have had the disease are excluded from the denominator subsequent to their illness.

The downward trend in the sixth grade attack rate during October probably reflects the fact that few of the remaining sixth graders were susceptible, either because they had had measles in the past or had been immunized against it.

E. Yes, with low immunization rates, outbreaks of measles still occur.

Answer to 12–4

A. In order to incriminate a specific food as the cause of the illness, there should be a high attack rate for persons who ate the food and a low attack rate for those who did not eat the food. That is, there should be a large and statistically significant difference in attack rates between those who ate and those who did not eat the particular food.*

B. Table 12–4 suggests that turkey is most likely the vehicle of transmission. However, for several other foods (i.e., dressing, potatoes and gravy), there was also a large difference in attack rates between those who ate and those who did not eat the particular food, probably because people usually eat turkey with dressing and gravy. It would therefore be helpful to see tables arranged to show attack rates for those who ate, for example, both turkey and dressing, only one of these two foods, or neither of them. An analysis by this type of grouping is shown in Table 12–5.

TABLE 12–5   Food Cross-Reference Table Comparing Attack Rates for Those Eating and Not Eating Turkey and Dressing

		Ate Dressing	Did Not Eat Dressing	Totals
Ate turkey	Ill	88	9	97
	Well	33	3	36
	Total	121	12	133
	Percentage ill	72.7	75.0	72.9
Did not eat turkey	Ill	0	2	2
	Well	0	23	23
	Total	0	25	25
	Percentage ill	0	8.0	8.0

It is apparent from this table that the attack rate was high when turkey was eaten, regardless of whether or not dressing was also eaten; the reverse is not true. Similar results were obtained from analysis of the other suspect foods; i.e., turkey vs. potatoes and gravy, and turkey vs. peas. Therefore, it seems quite certain that the turkey, and not the other foods, served as the vehicle of transmission.

Answer to 12–5

A. (1) Not everyone who reported eating gravy may, in fact, have actually eaten it (confusion, misunderstanding of the question, faulty memory, and so on).

---

*The χ^2 test is commonly used to test for association between illness and the ingestion of a specific food. If the numbers are small, Fisher's exact test is used instead.

(2) Even if everyone **did** eat the gravy, it would not be surprising if some people were to remain symptom free because (a) they may have eaten only a small quantity of food; (b) contamination may not have involved the entire lot of food, but perhaps just one dish or serving tray; or (c) there may be differences in individual susceptibility.

B. (1) Failure to recall consumption of gravy.

(2) An increased tendency to report minor symptoms during investigation of an outbreak.

(3) Reporting of symptoms due to other enteric infections difficult to differentiate from the disease under investigation.

(4) Contaminated ingredients used to prepare gravy may have been used in other foods.

C. Even when a group is exposed almost simultaneously to one agent of disease (point source epidemic) there is variation in the time of onset of symptoms due to biological variability (host differences) and differences in dose of agent received.

D. Contamination of food with staphylococcal enterotoxin leads to a much shorter incubation period (one to seven hours). In the investigation of this outbreak, two serotypes of *Clostridium perfringens* were recovered from food and feces of patients. *C. perfringens,* a common contaminant of meat and meat products, is associated with an incubation period of about 8 to 14 hours.

Answer to 12–6

A. The epidemic curve is typical of a propagated rather than a common source epidemic. Note that there are two peaks of incidence, each about 30 days apart. This interval coincides with the median incubation period for the disease.

B. The short intervals between the index case and subsequent cases may reflect:

(1) Exposure to incubatory carriers. The index cases may have been infectious before they developed symptoms.

(2) Exposure to inapparent infections in the family. There may have been persons who did not develop signs and symptoms of disease and yet were infective to others.

(3) Exposures outside the family. There may have been contact with infected persons outside the family.

Answer to 13–2

Retrospective Studies	Prospective Studies
A. Relatively inexpensive	Relatively expensive
B. Relatively quick results	Long follow-up period often needed
C. Smaller number of subjects	Large number of subjects required

D. Can be used in study of rare diseases	Inappropriate for study of rare diseases owing to very large number of subjects required
E. Problems in selecting control group and in matching controls to cases	There may be problems in selecting comparison cohort
F. Past information may be incomplete	Losses due to attrition
G. Bias in recall of factor	Changes over time in criteria and methods
H. Generally yields only estimated relative risk	Possible bias in ascertainment of disease Yields incidence rates (attributable as well as relative risks)
Cannot yield information about diseases other than that selected for study	Can yield information about more than one disease outcome

Answer to 13–3

A. Cross-sectional. This kind of study yields point prevalence data.

B. The inference is not valid. A census count reflects the "residue" of persons admitted over a period of time. Therefore, long-stay patients are overrepresented and short-term patients underrepresented. From such a count, it is not possible to make valid inferences about the probability of length of stay.

C. To study duration of stay one must follow a defined cohort of admissions over time. This is the life-table approach discussed at the end of the chapter.

Answer to 13–4

A. (2)
B. (3)
C. (4)
D. (1)

Answer to 13–5

A. (1) Retrospective (case-control)
(2) Prospective (cohort)

B. (1) To obtain the estimated relative risk in the retrospective study, we first set up a fourfold table:

	Lung Cancer	Controls
Smokers	647	622
Nonsmokers	2	27
Total	649	649

The estimated relative risk obtained from the cross-products (odds ratio) is:

$$\frac{ad}{bc} = \frac{(647)\,(27)}{(622)\,(2)} = 14.0$$

(2) The relative risk from the prospective study is:

$$\frac{\text{Mortality rate in exposed}}{\text{Mortality rate in nonexposed}} = \frac{0.96}{0.07} = 13.7$$

It is interesting that the two estimates agree very closely even though they are based on different methods of study and different populations.

Answer to 13–6

A. The median survival time (i.e., time by which half of the cohort have died) is one and one-half years (Fig. 13–10). Note that the mean (average) survival time cannot be computed until all persons in the cohort have died.)

B. $\dfrac{\text{Probability of surviving five years}}{\text{Probability of surviving one year}} = \dfrac{0.30}{0.60} = 0.50$, or 50 per cent

This is referred to as a conditional probability because only those who have survived the first year can be followed for the next four years.

C. Note: Death rate is 1−survival rate. Death rates for initial cohort are:

(1) $1 - 0.60 = 0.40$, or 40 per cent
(2) $0.60 - 0.40 = 0.20$, or 20 per cent
(3) $1 - 0.30 = 0.70$, or 70 per cent

D. $\dfrac{\text{Probability of member of initial cohort dying in second year}}{\text{Probability of member of initial cohort being alive at end of first year}}$

$$= \frac{0.60 - 0.40}{0.60} = 0.33, \text{ or 33 per cent}$$

Thus, the conditional probability of dying during the second year for those alive at the beginning of that year is 33 per cent.

E. The numerator is the same in both questions. However the denominator in C(2) consists of the entire initial cohort, whereas in D it consists only of those still alive at the beginning of the second year. Therefore, in D the number at risk is smaller and the resultant fraction is larger.

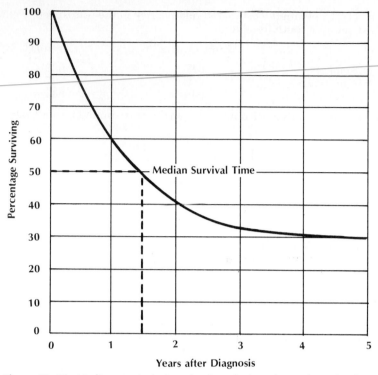

Figure 13-10 Median survival time for hypothetic cohort of newly diagnosed cancer cases.

Answer to 13–7

A. The length of the bars indicates the average remaining years of life at a given age (i.e., the age corresponding to the beginning point of the bar).

B. The number in each bar represents the average expected age at death, i.e., the number of years already lived plus the average remaining years of life.

C. The striking feature of the graph is the difference in extent to which life expectancy has changed between 1900 and 1960 for different age groups. There was a gain of over 19 years for newborns and of almost 14 years for one year olds. In contrast, at age 15, the increase was less than 9 years, and at age 60, there was an increment of only one and one-half years between 1900 and 1960. The relevant factors have been discussed in Chapters 9 and 13.

AUTHOR INDEX

363

INDEX

Note: Page numbers in *italics* refer to illustrations. Page numbers followed by the letter "t" refer to tables.